Implantology

Fixed Teeth in a Day

- **50 Cases**
- **271 Implants**
- **1104 Images on Immediate Restoration**

F. Schrader

Dentist, Implantology Specialist
Zerbst, Germany

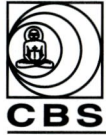

CBS

CBS Publishers & Distributors Pvt Ltd

New Delhi • Bengaluru • Chennai • Kochi • Kolkata • Mumbai
Hyderabad • Nagpur • Patna • Pune • Vijayawada

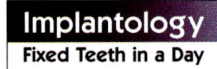

ISBN: 978-93-85915-91-8

Copyright © 2014 by mediaSign-Verlags-GbR, Jütrichau, Germany

Translation: Melanie Schneider, Nörten-Hardenberg, Germany
Edited by Dr. Daniel McEowen, USA

CBS Edition: 2017

Published in India by CBS Publishers & Distributors Pvt Ltd as an English translation under special arrangement with the original publishers mediaSign-Verlags-GbR, Jütrichau, Germany

Published by Satish Kumar Jain and produced by Varun Jain for

CBS Publishers & Distributors Pvt Ltd

4819/XI Prahlad Street, 24 Ansari Road, Daryaganj, New Delhi 110 002, India.
Ph: 23289259, 23266861, 23266867
Fax: 011-23243014
Website: www.cbspd.com
e-mail: delhi@cbspd.com; cbspubs@airtelmail.in.
Corporate Office: 204 FIE, Industrial Area, Patparganj, Delhi 110 092
Ph: 4934 4934   Fax: 4934 4935   e-mail: publishing@cbspd.com; publicity@cbspd.com

Branches

- **Bengaluru:** Seema House 2975, 17th Cross, K.R. Road,
  Banasankari 2nd Stage, Bengaluru 560 070, Karnataka
  Ph: +91-80-26771678/79   Fax: +91-80-26771680   e-mail: bangalore@cbspd.com

- **Chennai:** 7, Subbaraya Street, Shenoy Nagar, Chennai 600 030, Tamil Nadu
  Ph: +91-44-26680620, 26681266   Fax: +91-44-42032115   e-mail: chennai@cbspd.com

- **Kochi:** Ashana House, No. 39/1904, AM Thomas Road, Valanjambalam,
  Ernakulam 682 016, Kochi, Kerala
  Ph: +91-484-4059061-62-64-65   Fax: +91-484-4059065   e-mail: kochi@cbspd.com

- **Kolkata:** 6/B, Ground Floor, Rameswar Shaw Road, Kolkata-700 014, West Bengal
  Ph: +91-33-22891126, 22891127, 22891128   e-mail: kolkata@cbspd.com

- **Mumbai:** 83-C, Dr E Moses Road, Worli, Mumbai-400018, Maharashtra
  Ph: +91-22-24902340/41   Fax: +91-22-24902342   e-mail: mumbai@cbspd.com

Representatives

- **Hyderabad** 0-9885175004   • **Nagpur** 0-9021734563   • **Patna** 0-9334159340
- **Pune** 0-9623451994   • **Vijayawada** 0-9000660880

Printed at Rashtriya Printers, Delhi 110095, India

Content

Preface

Frank Schrader is a gifted dentist, a great colleague, who really deserves it to be called "colleague". Furthermore, he is my friend too! When he asked me to write this preface for the book, at first I wasn't entirely sure what I should actually write, after all it is my first preface for a book! Should I write that the Champions systems has gained an immense popularity in our online forum also thanks to his articles? Should I write that we have managed to stand up to the "big ones" in an effective manner? Should I write that in the meantime the other systems and their self-appointed "experts" use the same operating protocols and prosthetics strategies which we have used for almost 16 years now? Should I write that we as Champions users are able to offer our patients in our dental offices much more and finally can also implement it thanks to our excellent cost-effectiveness, since "affordability" with optimum quality often enough determines our patients' choice of dental prosthesis?

No, Frank has literally absorbed the entire Champions philosophy, further developed it and wonderfully implemented it in the patients' interest in his everyday practice. Not only is Frank an extraordinarily good surgeon, but also an equally excellent prosthodontist. This is surely just as important! Certainly, in Germany someone who is successful will not only win friends but also attract some envy. For that reason, also a strong human character is required.

Frank is someone, you can trust a 100% as colleague, friend and patient! I for one would be one of his patients, if I ever needed a "Champion". To my mind, Frank Schrader has been a real "champion" for a long time! He doesn't even need the title of professor to make himself understood by his patients -also in "their language"- and to put his enormous expertise into practice working with them- often enough in the field of immediate restoration/loading.

Anyhow, I wish the reader great pleasure studying his first book...

Sincerely yours, Dr. Armin Nedjat

October 2011, Flonheim

Dentist
Implantology Specialist
ICOI Diplomate
CEO Champions- Implants GmbH

Foreword

Around 60 years ago the US American Leonhard I. LINKOW invented his "leaf implant". What was celebrated as a pioneering work in the field of oral implantology at that time, today can only be found under the section "physical injury" in the forensic part of legal magazines.

Definitely, Linkow was a pioneer in his commitment to "fixed teeth" and thus, his place in the upper echelons of implantology is justified and deserved.

Developments do not stand still. The once hailed design rapidly became less important. Today, the focus in research is on the anatomical shape of the dental root. Scientists and practitioners generally agree on the design.

Other topics are being discussed instead: immediate restoration of implants, implant placement directly after extraction, immediate loading, one-piece, two-piece implants and so on.

Topics that are and should be of burning interest to dentists, implantologists and oral surgeons, after all it is about the practical use in patients. Patients who demand the best value for their money have highest demands for the money and are no (longer) willing to endure hours-long painful treatment sessions and intervals for years on end.

It was only a question of time for the "CHAMPIONS®" of Armin NEDJAT from Flonheim to cause a stir in the implantology scene in Germany. However, *one* brilliant mind is not enough. Equally important are, many brilliant practitioners who are able to understand these ideas and concepts, take them up and implement the stirring visions for the patients as well as for the colleagues in the everyday practice.

Today, one of these brilliant practitioners and currently one of the most prominent users of CHAMPIONS® implants in Germany is the dentist and implantologist Frank SCHRADER from Zerbst in Germany.

In his own implant education centre, he places more than 700 implants per year. In this centre, he provides surgical and prosthetic training to dentists. To colleagues who have recognised the tide is turning. He shares his knowledge enthusiastically and vividly- without any reservations of getting in contact with the universitites' state of the art.

Frank Schrader particularly focuses his activities on fields such as "immediate restoration" and "immediate implant placement- immediate loading".

The amount of his national and international publications is constantly growing.

Therefore, it is only a logical consequence to summarise the large number of interesting and ambitious documents of his treatments in book form. For the colleagues who know Frank the book will be a reliable guide in the everyday practice. That's why I am happy that he decided to publish his complex wealth of experience and to share it with us in this form.

For colleagues, who hesitate to deal with this matter, it represents an invitation to a discussion.

Only through critical discussion creativity can arise!

I wish Frank's book a lot of success- it will find its audience".

Dr. Ulrich Brause
December, 2011, Pottenstein, Germany

Introduction

When I started working in the field of dental implantology in 1999, the world was still intact in Germany. All pulled together. The goal was the improvement of the overall performance in the field of implantology.

The implantologists and the prosthodontist created techniques in order to improve the osseointegration and the "red-white-aesthetic". Apart from innovative mesio-structures the industry also designed new implant structures and improved implant surfaces. The laboratories integrated new materials and methods in dental work.

And that was a good thing.

Although the big secrets in the field of implantology had been lifted within the following years, the industry developed and still develops new implant types, abutments, connection elements, prosthetic elements and a vast set of equipment. Therefore, those who work in the field of implantology can no longer find in many catalogues what they really need without experts or a helpline.
The industry wants us to believe that a new implant set every year is indispensable including all instruments, DVT or dental GPS systems.
For that reason in the 2nd half of the last decade implantologists - unnoticed by many- divided into two groups.
The first group believes in all new "inventions" and positions itself between their own beliefs and the available budget.
I belong to the second group. To those, who challenge the benefit of every measure with scientific facts for implant success. The point is not to reject new things in general. It is necessary to find out if these actions are reasonable.
We try to reduce the vast amount of available information to the essentials and make use of them. For example which aspects are important for a successful osseointegration? There are primarily two factors:

1. Primary stability of the inserted titanium implant
2. to prevent movement of the implant during the healing period

The supporters of the first group are going to argue now:
But what is with all the many other factors such as immediate implant placement, immediate restoration or loading, inflammations, peri-implantitis, hygienic potential, general diseases and the like?
Based on the 2 quoted "strong" factors for the osseointegration I have looked for years to find possibilities to prevent these problems.
The biggest difficulty was to question the traditional implantology method (KIV).

I still remember it exactly. When I read his first studies, articles and images about minimally invasive implantology methods 4-5 years ago, it made my hair stand on end to think about inserting "blind" into the bone. And the notion to restore these one-piece implants *immediately* was a case of extreme madness to my mind.

I did not think it could be possible that I had laid flaps with difficulty, performed internal and external sinus lifts, bone block graftings and operated distraction osteogenesis, while these MIMI®-tologists simply inserted the implant through the finished hole after some minimally invasive pre-drillings.

I thought about these concepts for several months, and then I did it!

I pursued these "mad assumptions". For Christmas I bought myself a starter set of Champions® implants with a drill and tried it. I tested the concept using chipboard to simulate the maxilla and a harder solid pine board for the mandible. The method is similar to working with wood screws, a small pilot hole in the wood followed by an expanding wood screw. Taken to the mouth, a small pilot hole, expanders/condensors in the bone and screwing in the implant.

It was similar to working with wood screws. So I asked myself why this technique should not also work in bones? The mechanical procedures are similar.

And the success was astounding. Everything was great.

Following my intial success with the concept and the system, I began to think I could place as much as 50% of all my implants using these techniques. To my surprise, I was able to increase the percentage even higher as daily use of the system helped me overcome the challenges of the method and overcome the conventional methods I knew before.

This method is predominately minimally invasive and 95% of the cases we do are one piece implants without grafting or augmentation. The remaining cases can be done with the two piece implants and some form of augmentation or grafting.

What this means for the patient is: *always* immediate loading and immediate restoration.

The most important advantages of the minimally invasive method of the (MIMI) implantation are:

1. almost painless and almost without swelling
2. no suction-pump effect (at the implant-abutment transition)
3. as a result no bone loss
4. significantly faster restoration
5. cost effective

At present, many deride, ignore or condemn this method. In my opinion, the future will show the following: An implantologist, who does not throw light on these methods is guilty of an offence just like a dentist who does not throw light on implants. Regardless of whether he applies this method or not.

This book is not a schoolbook with complete theoretical explanations.

I am a practitioner. No statistician. Neither am I representing the university. It is in my interest to reveal the fantastic opportunities of this method. This book should guide all curious and interested people to reflect and perhaps rethink or even make changes.

Nearly all of the images were taken with our intraoral cameras. This camera can photograph both x-ray and intra oral images. It is designed for sharp intraoral views which you will see in this book. Even though there are some quality limitations, I have for the "integral experience" deliberately included some blurred images in the documentation of some cases. I hope you will understand.

It would be a pleasure for me if you can send me your opinions, suggestions, proposals for improvement to my email address: *f.schrader@feste-zähne-an-1-tag.de*

Frank Schrader

Comments

1. Abbreviations

KISS	Keep It Safe & Simple
MIMI	Minimally Invasive Method of Implantology
PC	Prep-Cap
PT	Periotest

2. Implants

all implants are the German CHAMPIONS® - IMPLANTS - GMBH

3. Treatment periods

the period between the placement of the implant and the fabrication of the dental prosthesis and are well-elaborated

4. Cementation

a) all temporaries and fixed definitive dental prostheses are cemented with Havard.
b) all Pre-Caps are cemented with commercially available Glass Ionomer Base cement.

5. Impressions

a) Impregum impression material was used for all prepared and unprepared Champions® implants
b) for impressions of natural teeth and Champions® implants with restored prepcaps, we used the sandwich technique with a PVS material
c) Impregum impression material was used for combination cases

6. Prep-Caps

Pre-Caps are available in different materials (titanium, zirconium, WIN), shapes and angles. They will be cemented and have the following functions:

- Widening of the clinical crown
- Simplify the cast creation
- Aesthetic improvement of implants
- Compensation of abutment and insertion divergences
- Exact transfer of implant preparation from mouth to laboratory
- Improvement of the peri-implant soft-tissue situation after implant placement

7. Periotest® (PT)

This measuring device is used for the assessment of the osseointegration of dental implants. It shows the damping characteristics and by doing so indirectly the implant stability from -8 up to +50.

PT < 0   negative values are generally considered as good
PT 0 up to +9   clinical tests are required;
                   e.g. PT values in the lower jaw are principally lower
                   than those in the upper jaw
PT above 10   suspect and alarming

8. Intraoral camera- I.C. Lercher

The intra oral cameras we generally use to record implant placement are tried, tested and used for these reasons:

a) forensic security
b) detailed monitoring in normal and macro function
c) manual operation without foot switch

9. Matrices

MMT (metal matrices for tulip head implants)

a) available in 3 different pull-off forces (blue, red, black rubber rings)
b) due to the rubber they have a very good buffered locking
c) due to their location below the ball a compensation for divergences is not possible

Preci-Clix

a) available in 3 different pull-off forces (white, yellow, red plastic caps)
     b)   thanks to this plastic the retention is stronger
c) due to their location on the ball a compensation for divergences is possible
d) in a case of limited space the plastic caps can also be cured into the denture resin without metal sleeves

Matrix integration

a) it is preferential to integrate the matrices directly into the existing prosthesis on the day of surgery and implant placement
b) if the case is to be done with a new prosthetic device, our laboratory integrates the matrices into the prosthetics before final delivery

10. The 3rd level

All cross-sectional images are taken by a non-linear spiral computed tomography

11. Up to date

My discontent concerning old, obsolete presentations in conventional books has prompted me to present mainly relevant cases.
However, I also added some older cases in order to present the practicability of our proceeding. By this means, the X-ray images allow a documentation of a long-term success of these cases.

12. Additional implant placements

"Fixed teeth in one day" mean that you only have to place the implant "once"!

If possible, we always try to ensure that additional implants are not required at a later date. For this reason we insert 1 or more extra implants at the first visit. Because we cannot control osseointegration factors such as chewing behaviour, poor oral hygiene or patient behaviour we cannot as implantologist provide any guarantee against the loss of the dental implants. By placing extra implants, the loss of a single implant will not affect the overall success of the case.

For example: In the upper jaw with a removable dental prosthesis. We would place **8 + 2** extra implants.

The patient receives a total of 10 ball head implants. 2 of the 10 are charged only for the material costs. If 1 or 2 of the implants fail to integrate, a palatal free dental prosthesis can still be placed without the need for additional implants.

13. Implant diameter, implant minimum thickness and number of implants

In jaws with adequate and mature bone we use implants with a diameter of 3.5 mm in approximately 90% of the cases. In addition, we aim for a reproduction of the natural root arrangement. "Mother Earth" has a long preliminary phase of 100,000 years and there is a reason some teeth have more than one root. We mimic this natural anatomy by restoring molar teeth with 2 implants. This provides security for the static forces and guarantees anti-rotation protection.

14. Bone cavity control (BCC)

In the case of minimally invasive implant placements (flapless technique) there is no view of the bone. In order to guarantee that the implant is fixed in the bone, we *always* perform a bone cavity control. For this control we always use a WHO probe or - in case of deeper implant cavities - an endo plugger. In doing so, we examine all implant cavity walls (mesial, distal, vestibular, oral and apical) for wall integrity.

Further procedure:

1. If all bone walls are present and adapted for the implant placement, continue on with Minimally Invasive Implant Placement
2. Occasionally, there is insufficiant bone in the vestibular area. If this occurs, the Minimally Invasive pilot hole requires a change in the axial direction. It is at this point you must decide if option 1 above or option 3 below is the best approach for implant success
3. Flap reflection and implant insertion into the open bone

Note:
The Minimally Invasive technique is always the 1st choice. Even in marginal bone cases we use this technique first. Only when Minimally Invasive techniques fail do we reflect a flap for implant placement.

15. Definition with reference to our procedure

Classification of the implant protocol for one-piece implants

Immediate implant placement	immediate implant placement after extraction
Early implant placement	implant placement within 2 weeks after extraction
Late implant placement	implant placement in the healed jaw
Immediate loading	immediate functional loading after implant placement, at latest after 48 hours
Immediate restoration	immediate non-functional restoration with fixed temporaries
Early loading	prosthetic restoration with final dental prosthesis within 2 weeks
Late loading	prosthetic restoration 8 weeks after implant placement

What are we doing differently?

Progress happens today so fast that while someone declares something not to be realizable at all, someone who has already realized it, interrupts him.

(Albert Einstein)

Based on actual knowledge, we have set "the clock at 0".

Back to the roots

The **KISS rule** is valid: **k**eep **it s**afe & **s**imple

The successful osseointegration of an implant requires two prerequisites:

1. Primary stability (40 – 70 Ncm)
2. No movement during the healing period (in the first 8 weeks)

How can we implement that in practice?

Rule 1- Primary stability (40 – 70 Ncm)

Implant cavity is prepared in an undersized manner. In the upper jaw in the most cases 1.8 mm pilot holes for a 3.5 mm implant are sufficient.

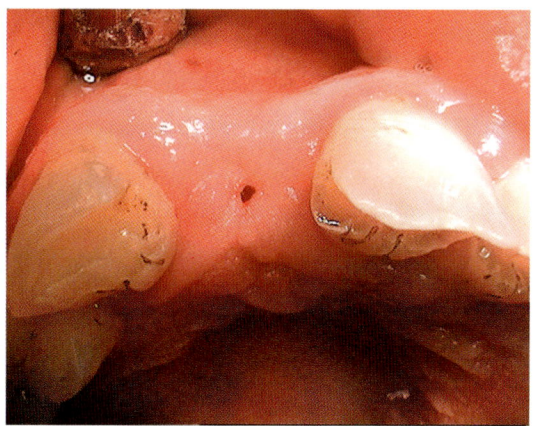
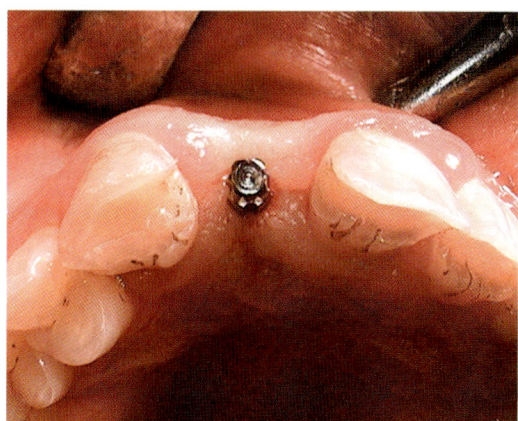

In the lower jaw in the most cases an additional 2.8 mm $\varnothing$ pilot hole for a 3.5 mm implant is required.

What do we do if we obtain no primary stability?

- ➢ insert an implant with a larger diameter
- ➢ insert more implants
- ➢ more solid splinting

Rule 2- Insert more implants

In the traditional implantology with costs for an implant of partly more than 500 € (net) this is only possible in exceptional cases.
With an implant price of under 100 € (gross) for a one-piece Champions® implant that is possible.

Let us have a look on the COSP (Critical Osseo Stabilisation Phase) graph. I call it the **„Champions' Bible"**. Here 5000 implants have been examined according to their stability during the proliferation and the remodelling phase.

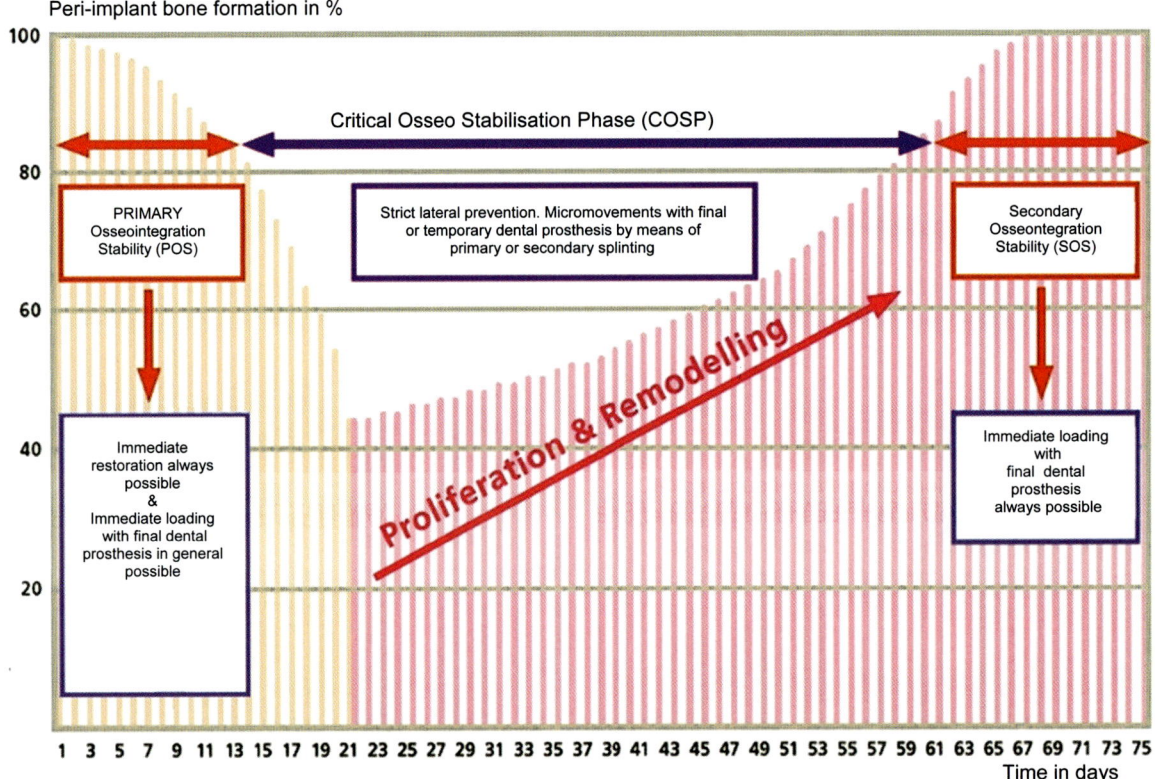

On the 21st day the most critical moment in the COSP is achieved! An implant that has been inserted with a torque of 70 Ncm could be removed with a torque of about 30 Ncm.
Since to this point in time nothing hurts any more, there is a danger that the patient will overload his teeth, and by doing so, his implants will loosen.

If we insert twice as many implants, we have a stability of 200%. It can easily sink to 50%. But in this case 100% stability of the nominal value remain.

and

Primary stability proceeds implant parallelism because *this* problem can be resolved with prep caps.

Example 1

When traditional implant methods are applied to a palatal free prosthesis, 6 implants are placed into the toothless upper jaw and fixed via a splint. Since ball head implants have no primary splinting, 8 implants are the minimum for a palatal free prosthesis after osseointegration.

If now, we also consider the problem that more than 50% of the stability is lost during the proliferation and remodelling phase (4th week), the dental prosthesis is retained by only around 4 implants within the difficult time frame. This can lead to a loosening of all implants!

For that reason and also with regard to some more risky immediate implant placements, we offer the alternative 8 +2 which is described in the chapter "comments".

Since the insertion of a 9th and 10t^h implant only takes some minutes, we only charge the material costs.

The chance to achieve an osseointegration of all implants is then extremely high.

  a) If 1 or 2 implants loosen we don't have to add any more implants to obtain a stable palatal free prosthesis.
  b) If all remain fixed, we have an unbeatable security buffer (e.g. material fractures, accidents and the like) for decades.

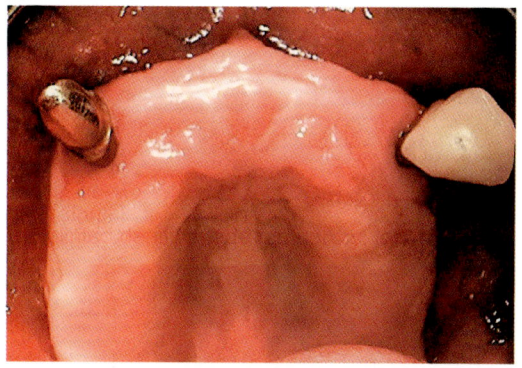
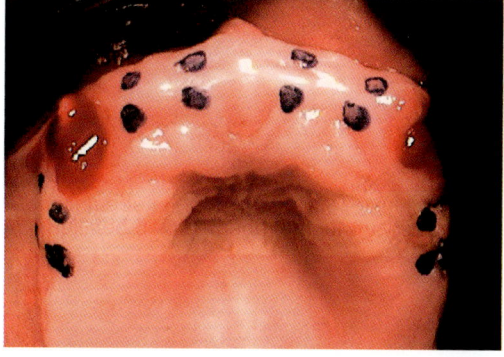
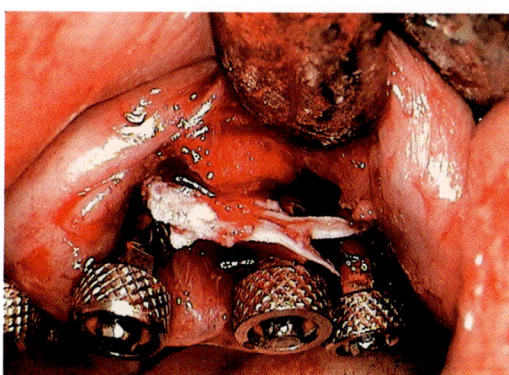
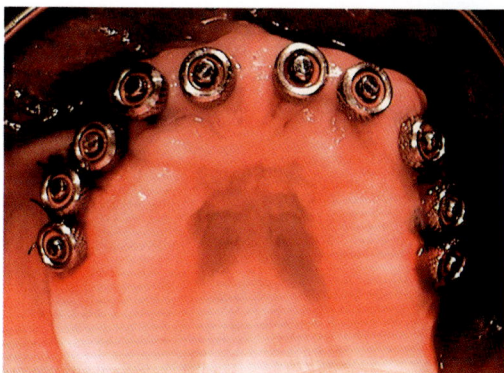

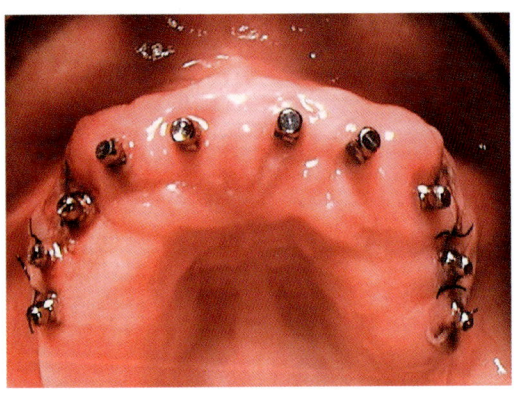 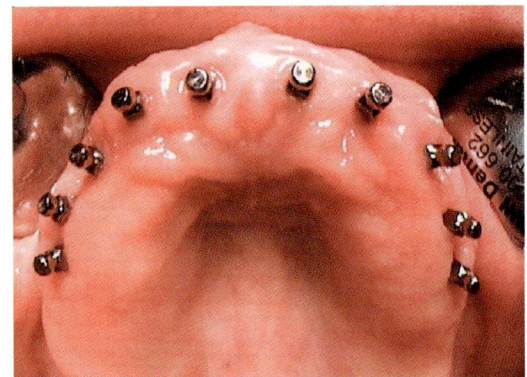

In *one* dental session the teeth were extracted, the 10 ball head implants inserted and an augmentation was performed. The clinical situation on the following day and the successful osseointegration after 8 weeks illustrate our theoretical approach.

Example 2

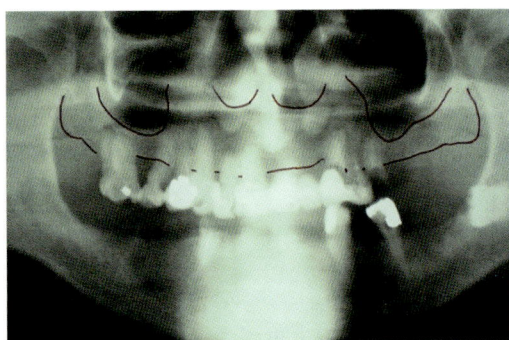 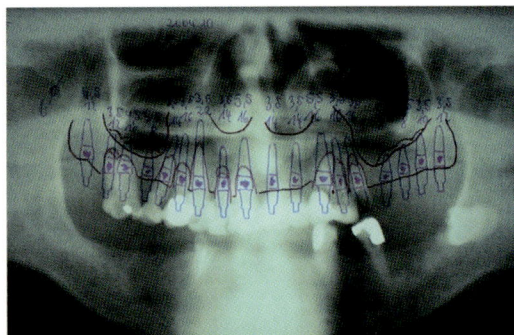

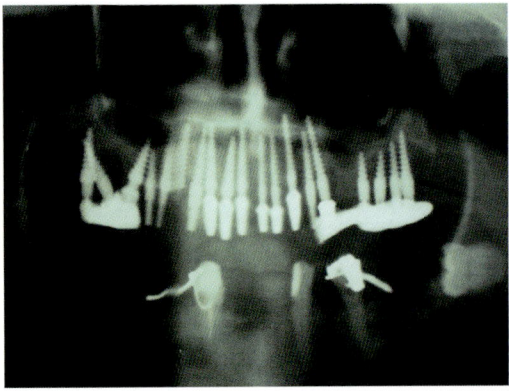 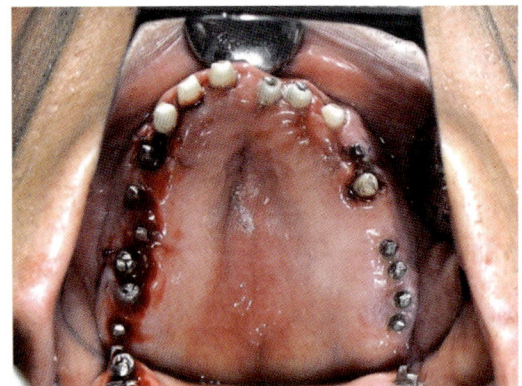

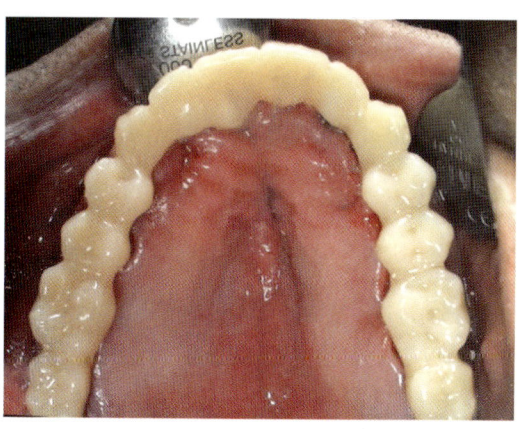 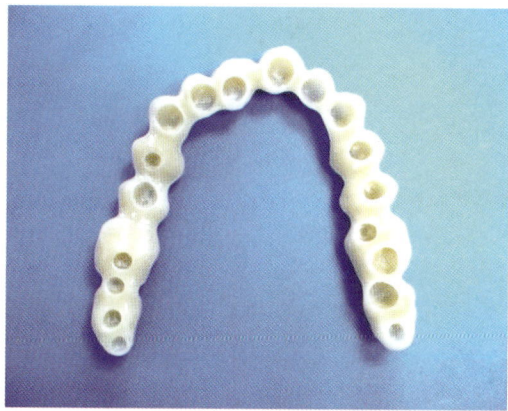

In *one* dental session all teeth were extracted, all implants inserted an restored with a dentist made temporary. On the following day a laboratory fabricated temporary was cemented and remained in place for the next 8 weeks.

What is the goal in this case where no more implants can be placed?

> more solid splinting
> Reinforce primary stability by using either: larger diameter and/or longer implants

Note:
The main factors for implant losses are:

1. **too few implants**
2. **use of two-piece implant systems**

because it leads to overloading and pumping effects, which in turn leads to bone loss, peri-implantitis and fractures.

Rule 3- Maximum splinting

Since there is a limit to the number of implants we can place, we splint

a) between the implants and/or

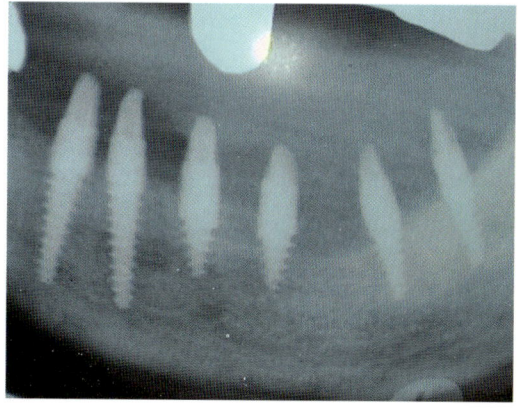 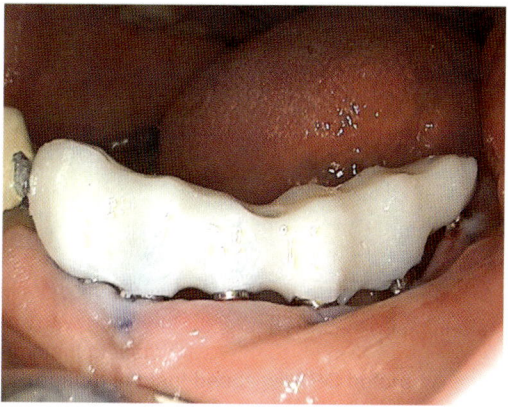

b) implants along with the neighboring teeth using resin materials.

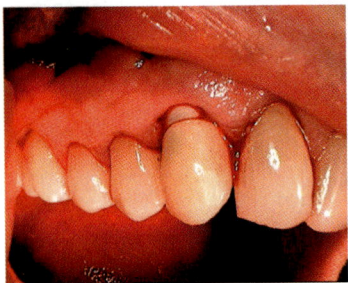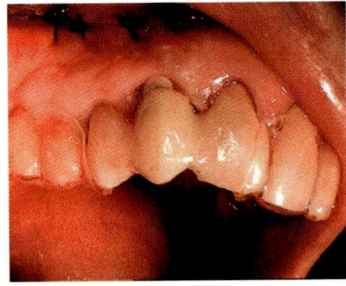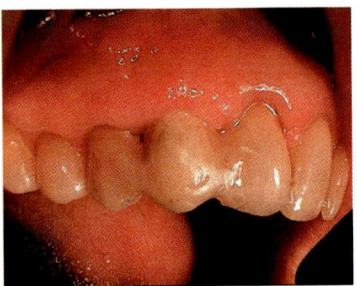

The right image shows clearly how the gingiva height "creeps" directly above the PrepCap during the osseointegration phase.

What are we doing, if we are not able to splint them or can only insufficiently splint them?

> insert more implants
> reinforce primary stability by using more thicker and/or longer implants

Note:
The combination of these rules is responsible for the success! In the case where primary stability and splinting is secured it is of course, not required to insert twice as many implants.

Rule 4 - Prevention of inflammatory processes

a) palatal or lingual "bypassing of the implant placement"

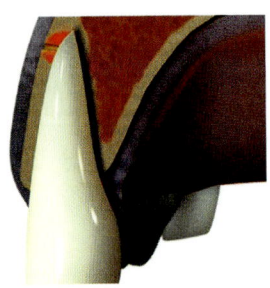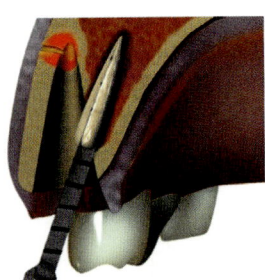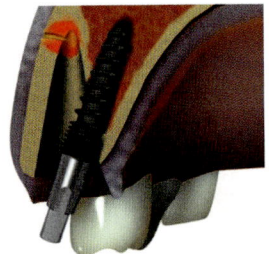

b) Curretage of the inflammatory tissue and debridement of the alveolus

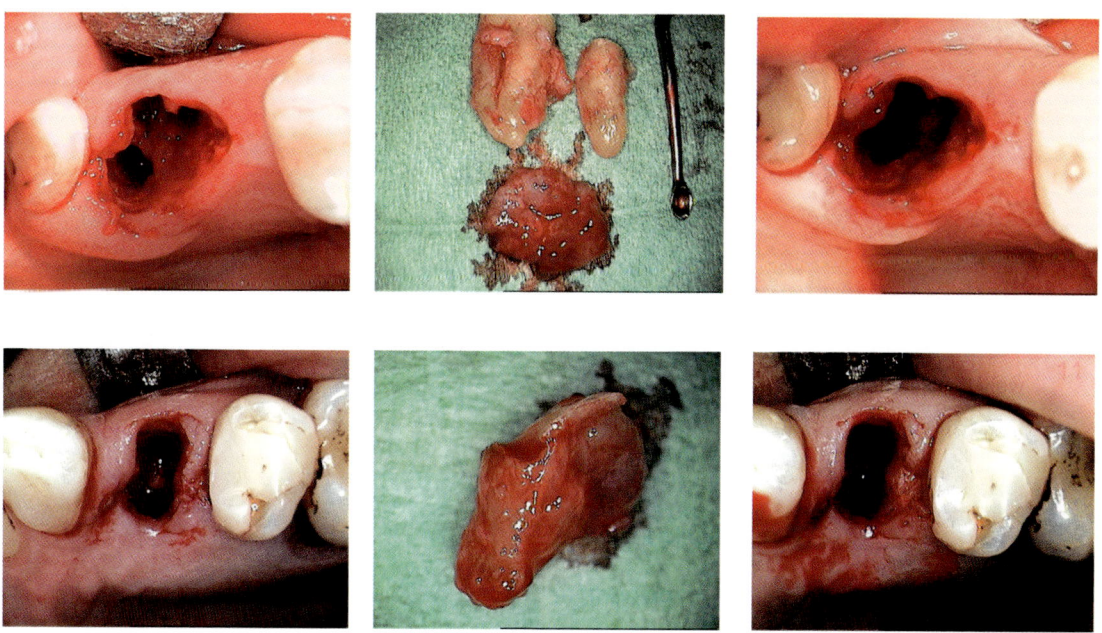

Rule 5 - Compensation for divergences

a) The use of straight and angled Prep-Caps that can be cemented and modified to achieve parallel abutments

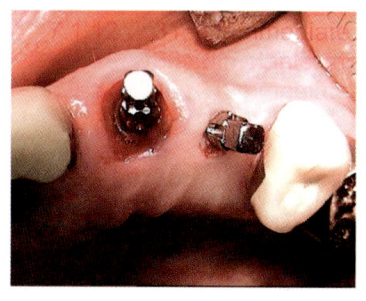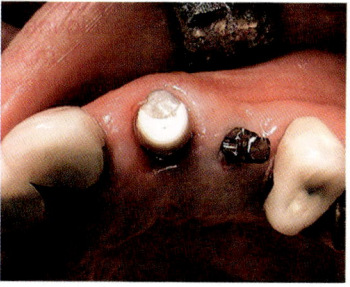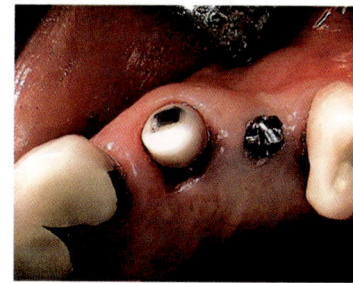

b) Grinding of the abutments

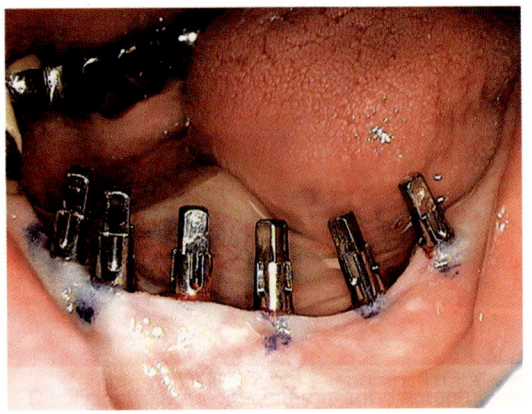 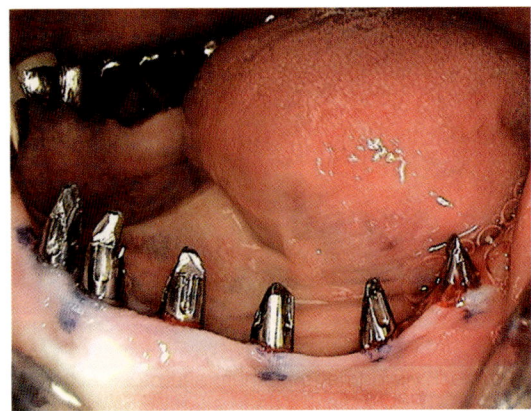

Rule 6 - Hygienic potential

We no longer use metal-ceramics!
Bone "loves" titanium and gingiva "loves" zirconium dioxide ceramics. As a consequence, we do not have to leave cleaning gaps.
Principles as for an upper jaw anterior tooth ceramic bridge apply. No bridge will be lost due to periodontitis being evoked by ceramics; in the most cases caries causes the loss. In no case, ceramic is the cause.

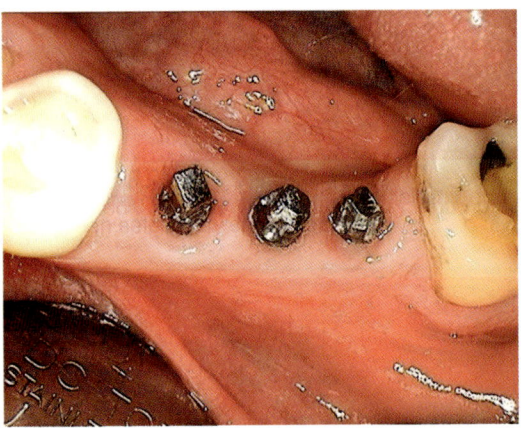 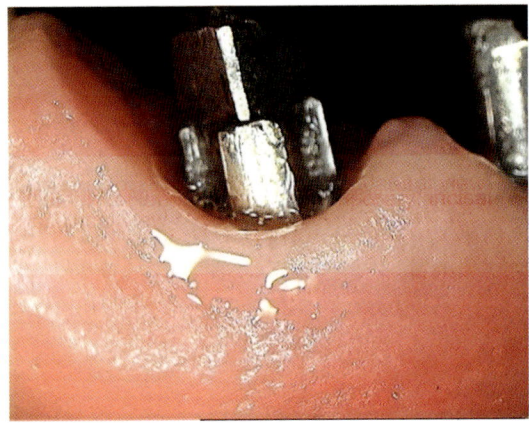

The cemented zirconium dioxide bridge loosened after 2 years. Everything is free of inflammation.

Rule 7 - Implant distance

The "key shaped" bone loss on two-piece implants is on the one hand, the result of the pump or suction characteristics at the contact point between the implant and the abutment and on the other hand, of the slot of 10 to 30 micrometres caused by production. Since bacteria have a size of 0.2 to 5 micrometers, this is like a wide opened barn door.
This difficulty does not occur with one-piece implants. For that reason there is no unphysiological bone loss, peri-implantitis and no defined minimum distance for the insertion of one-piece implants.

It should be noted that none of my colleagues has had a case where the loss of lower anterior teeth took place because there was less than 3mm between the implants?

Fixed teeth in one day

Motivated and full of energy we work to organize the gentle and comfortable treatment for each patient. We have worked tirelessly to achieve success in all steps in one session from implant placement to restoring or immediate loading.
By doing so, we naturally put the existing principles of the conventional "traditional" implantology into question!

But: Those who want something find ways, those who don't find reasons.   (Proverb)

That means:

1. By means of direct cementing of the matrices into the existing prosthesis ball head implants are **always immediately** loaded.

2. If a fixed dental prosthesis is planned, the patient **always** leaves our dental office with a cemented dentist made temporary. At your request or in case of a treatment in the anterior maxillary region, we integrate on the following day the laboratory made temporary. The final restoration takes place after one or eight weeks according to the situation.

In order to reach the source you have to swim against the current.   (Stanislaw Jerzy Lec)

1 - 2 Implants

7.1.1/Case 1

Patient: male, 65 years old

14 implants, 14/15 dental splinted crowns

05/05/2009	14	extraction
30/06/2009	14	Champions® implant Ø 4.5 x 16 mm, 40 Ncm
	15	tooth is prepared
	14/15	impression
		cemented dentist made temporary
07/07/2009	14/15	cemented zirconium dioxide splinted crown
Treatment period:		**1st week**
Remarks:	15	hypereruption, filling, hypersensitive
	13/14	the gap has been left since the opposite
		side also showed a gap
		early loading

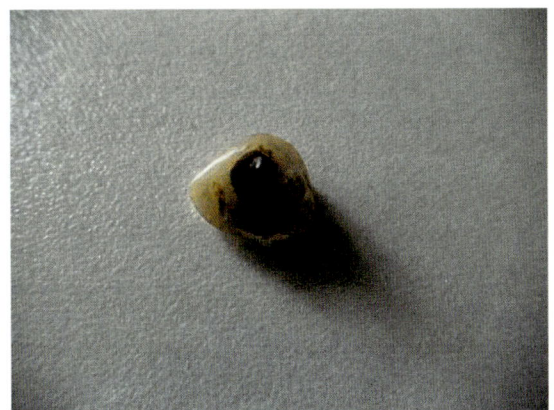

fractured crown...

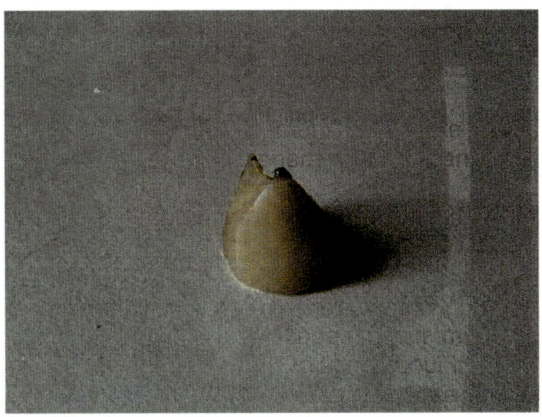

... in regio 14

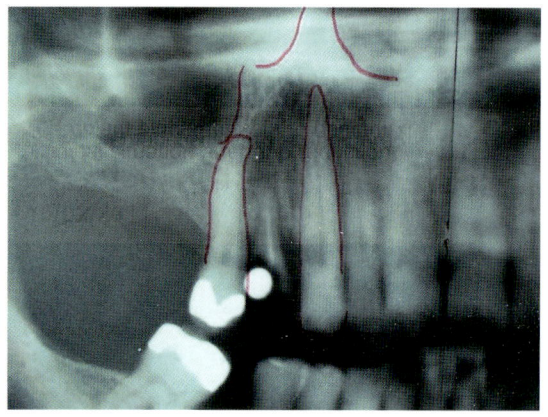

Radiograph of the initial situation,
panoramic radiograph

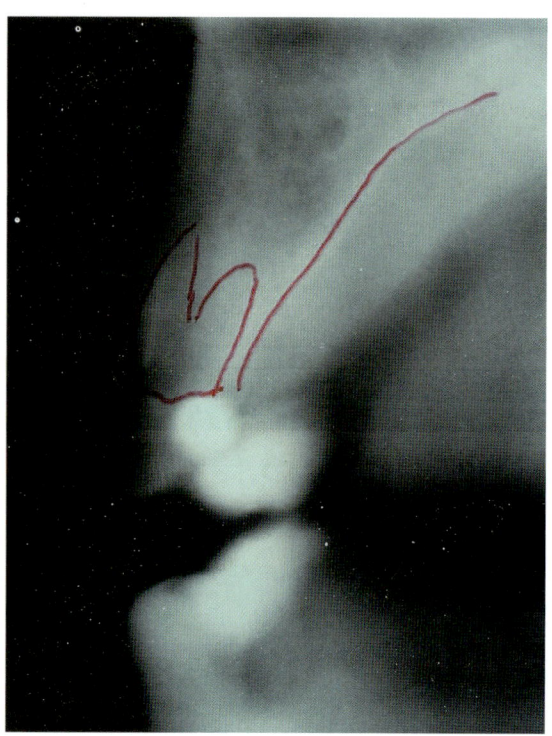

Initial situation,
cross-sectional image

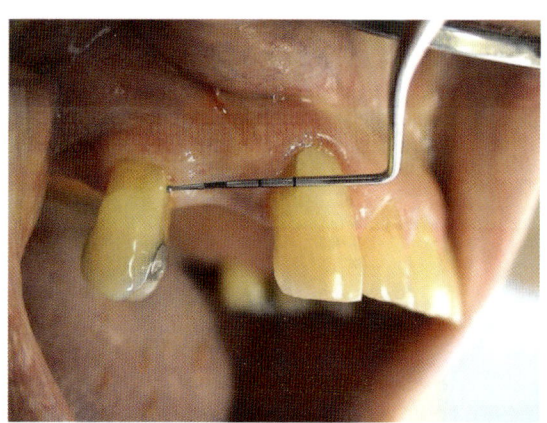

Clinical situation,
lateral view

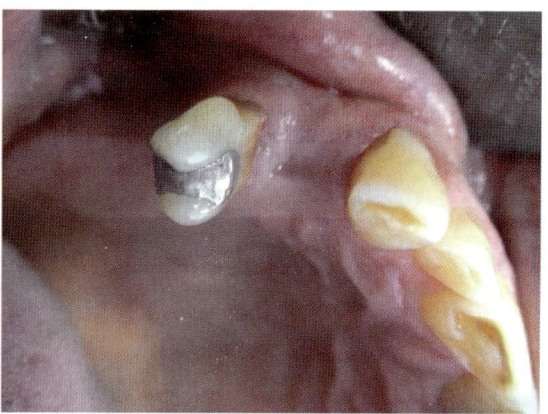

Clinical situation,
occlusal view

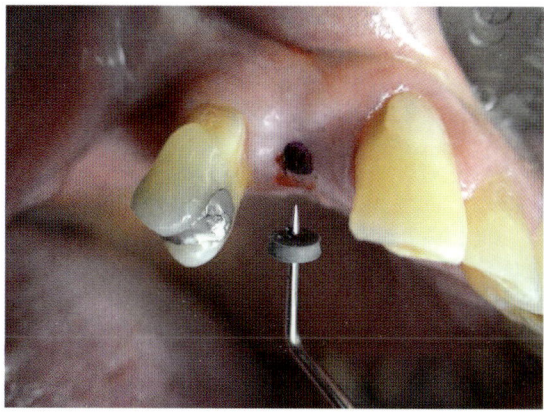

Measurement of the mucosal
thickness by using a probe

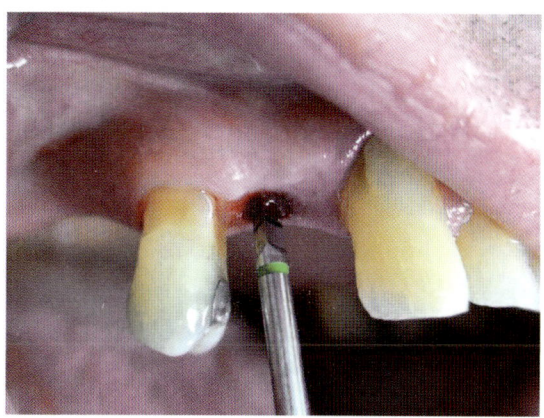

Pilot hole preparation

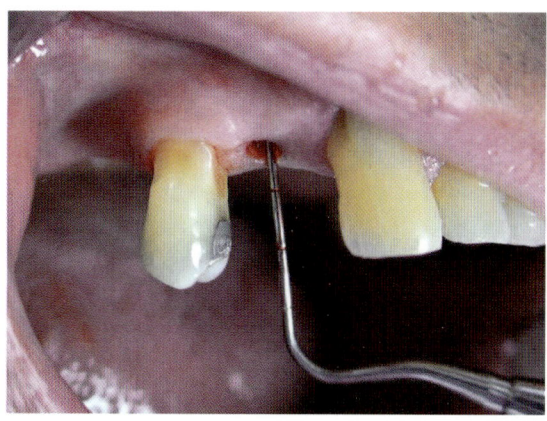

BCC- Bone Cavity Control

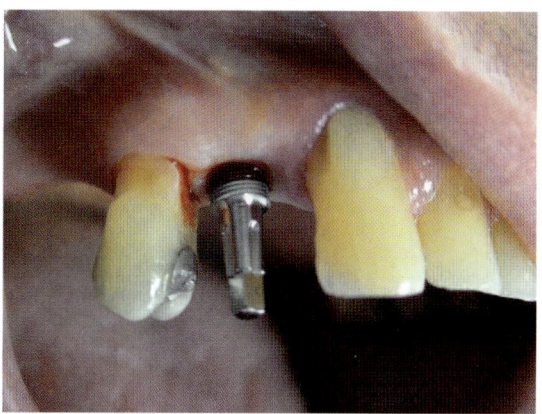

Almost completed implant placement

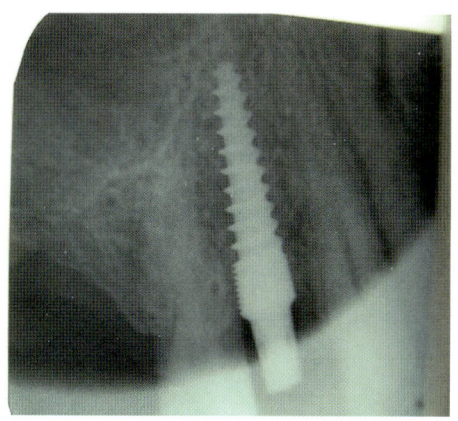

Radiographic control

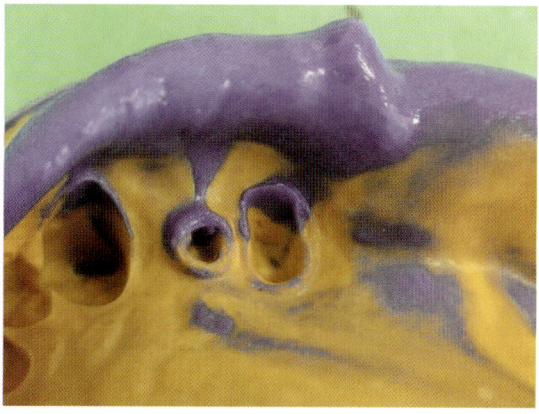

Impression

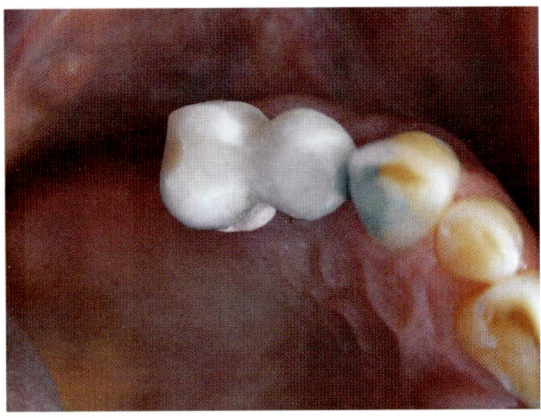

Dentist made temporary and
etching for the splinting

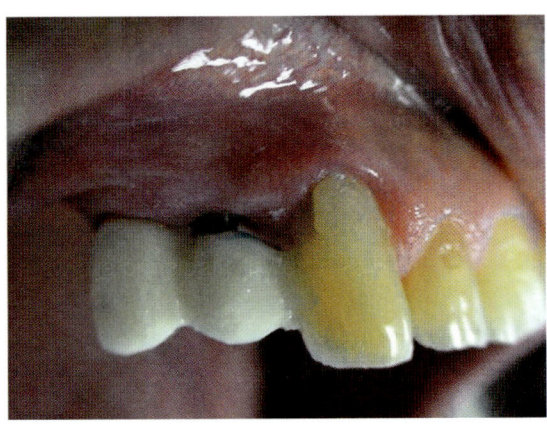

Splinted dentist made temporary

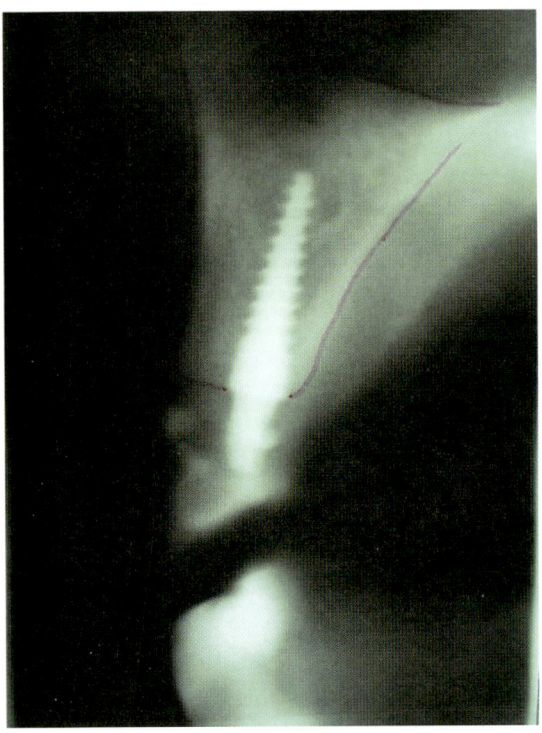

Radiographic control and cross-sectional image

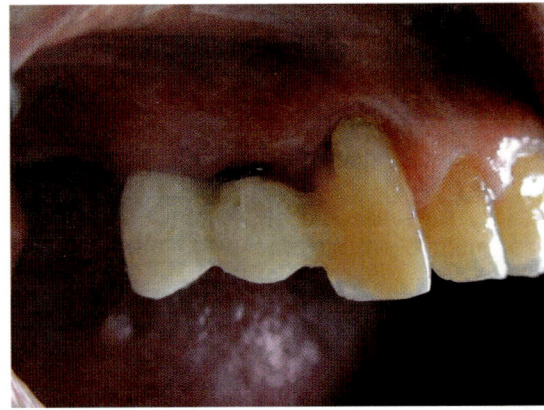

before impression taking

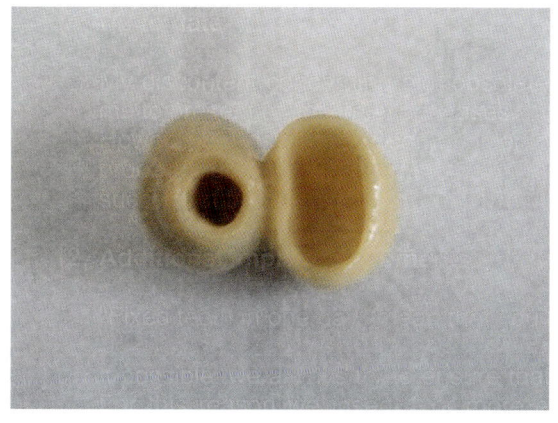

Zirconium dioxide splinted crown, basal view

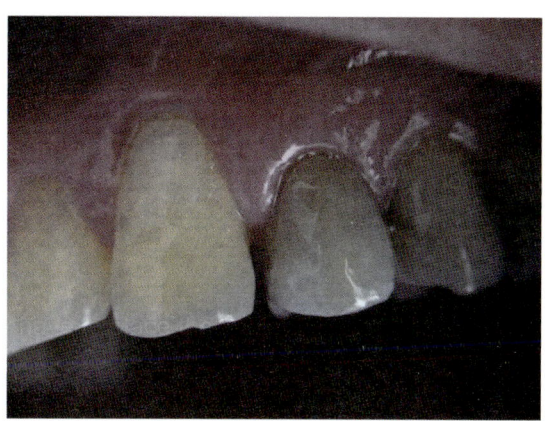

Gap between tooth 23 and 24

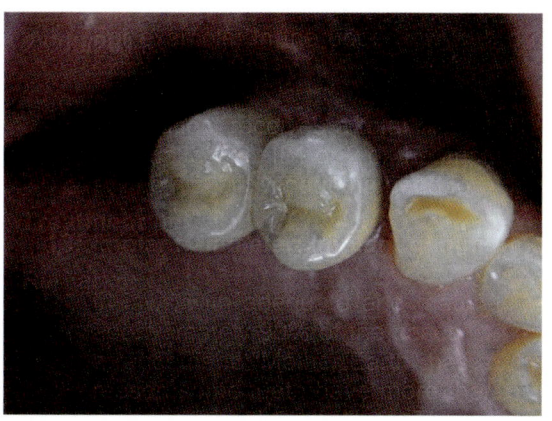

Final splinted crown, occlusal view; the patient wanted an equal look on both sides

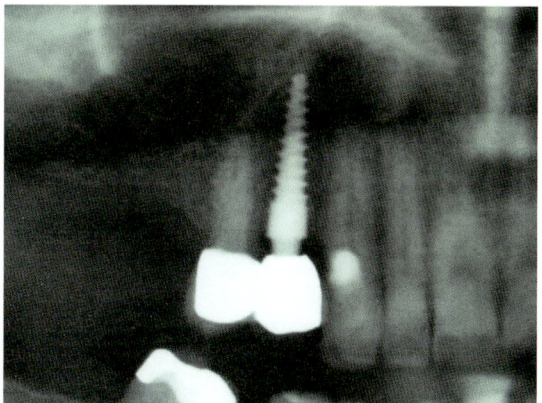

Panoramic radiographic control

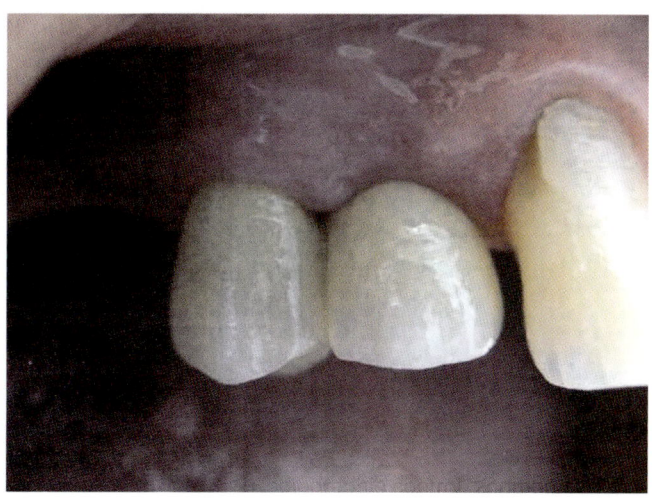

Final splinted crown, lateral view

7.1.2/Case 2

Patient: female, 47 years old

12,-21 surgical crown lengthening
2 implant placement
12, -22 2 splinted crowns

25/03/2010	22	extraction
	12-22	dentist made temporary
29/04/2010	22	Champions® implant Ø 3.5 x 14 mm, 80 Ncm zirconium Prep-Cap
	12,11,21	surgical crown lengthening
		excision of the labial frenulum
		dentist made temporary
30/04/2011	12-22	cemented laboratory made temporary
02/08/2011		Impression
11/08/2011	12/11,21/22	cemented zirconium dioxide splinted crown
Treatment period:		**3.4 months**
Remarks:		Indirect sinus lift
		Surgical crown lengthening
		Excision of the labial frenulum

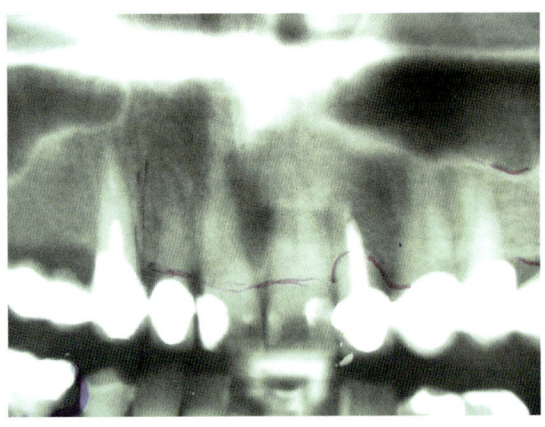

22 periodontitis

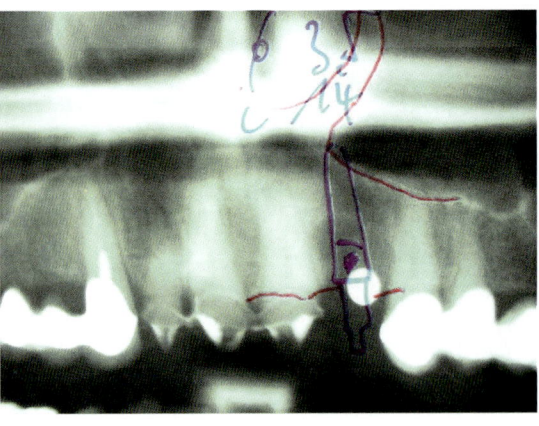

22 planned implant placement after extraction and preparation of regios 12,11,21

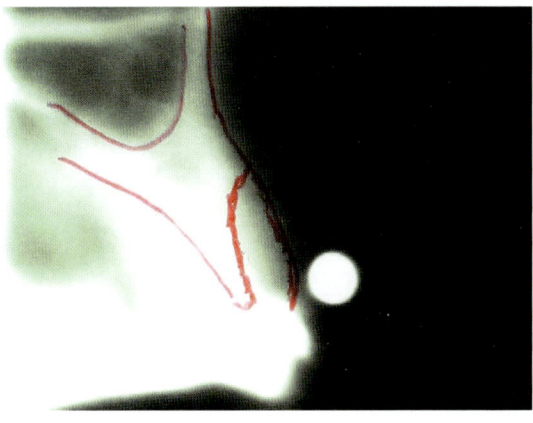

22 cross-sectional image illustrating bone loss

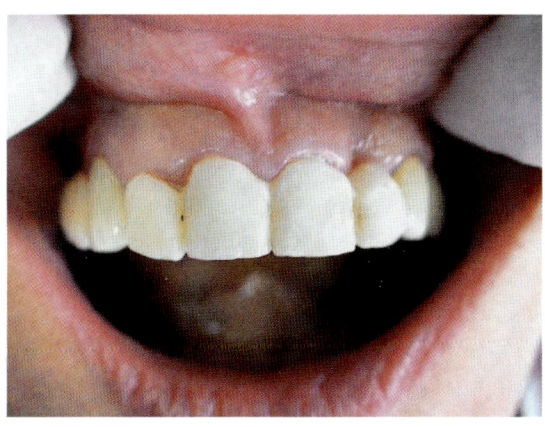

Dentist made temporary after extraction of tooth 22

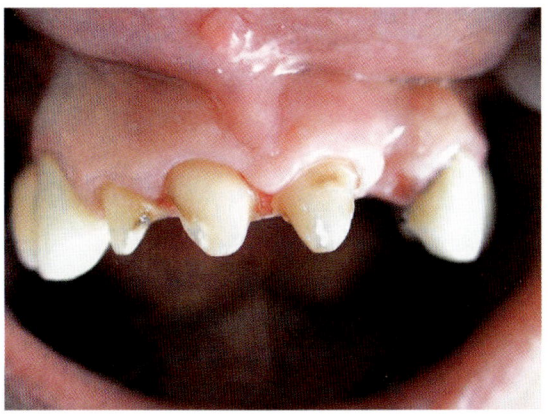

Situation before implant placement

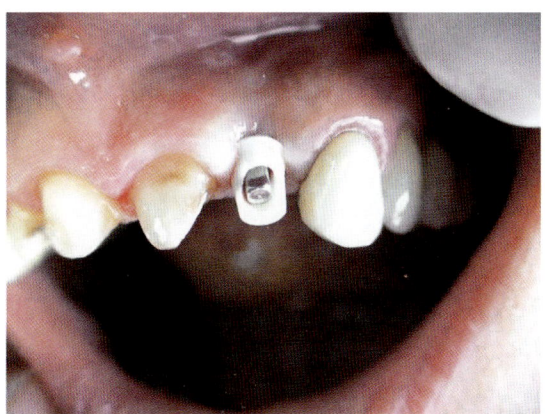

Implant with PC

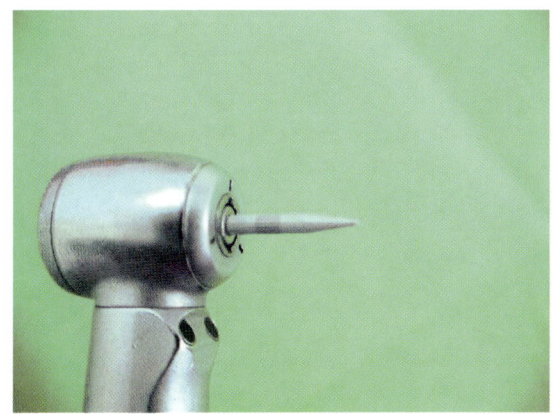

Gingival Margin Trimmer

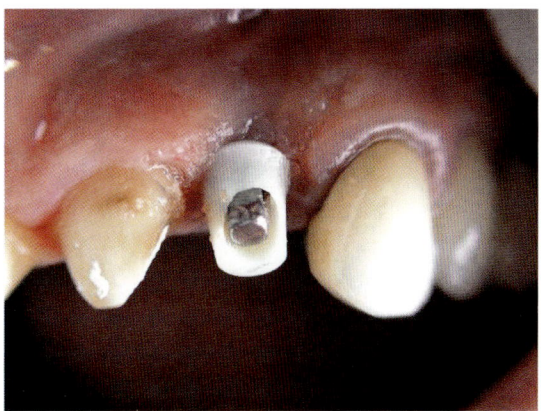

22 mesial trimming of the gingiva

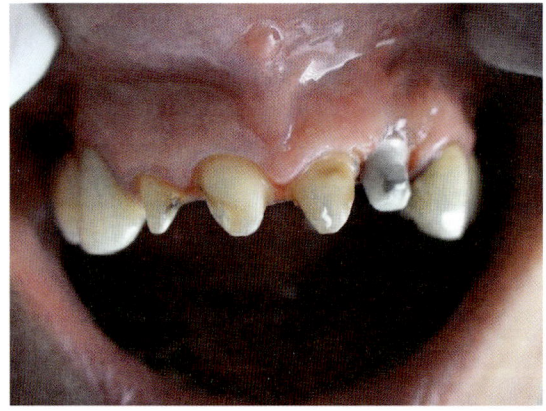

Cemented PC

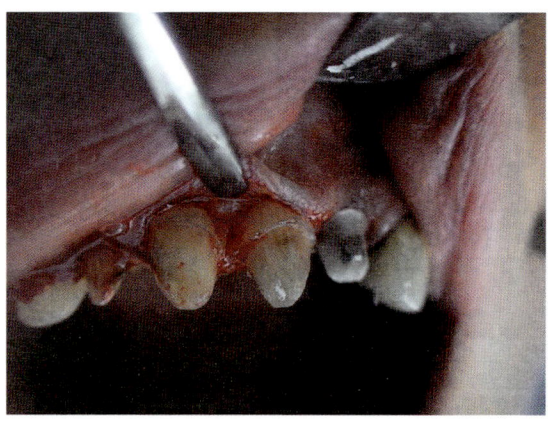

Surgical crown lengthening

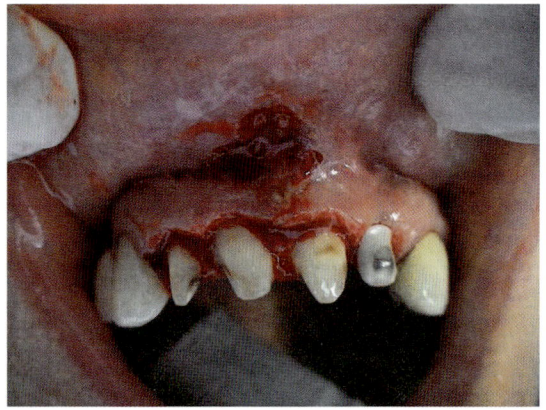

Labial frenulum excision

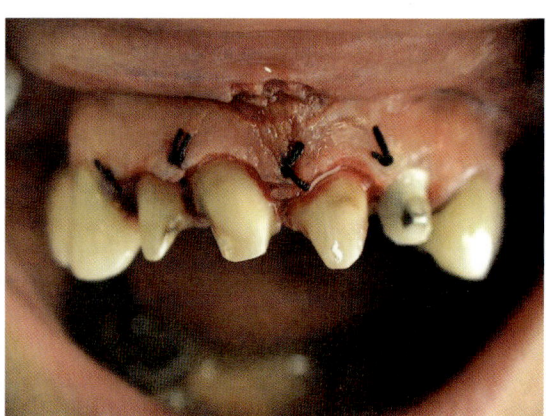

Wound closure

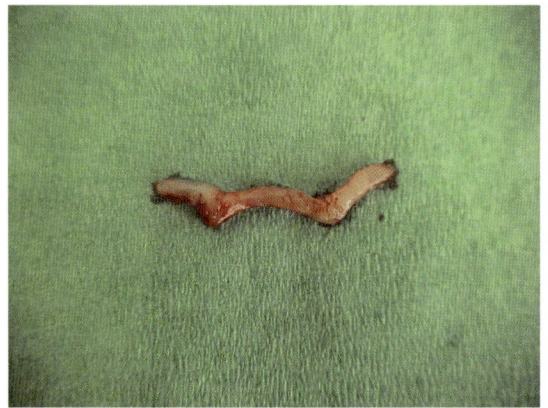

Excised gingiva from regio 12-21

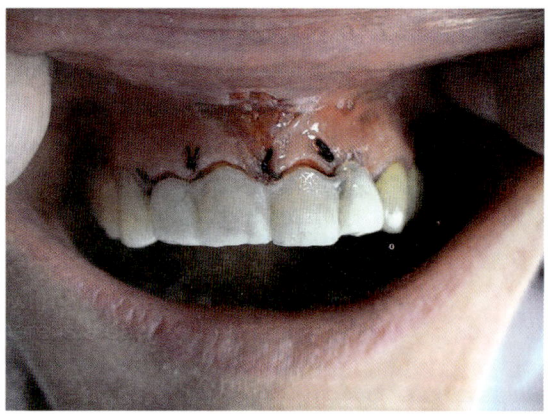

New dentist made temporary

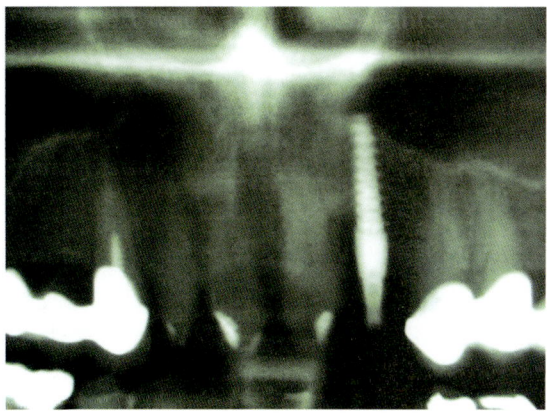

Radiographic implant control, panoramic radiograph

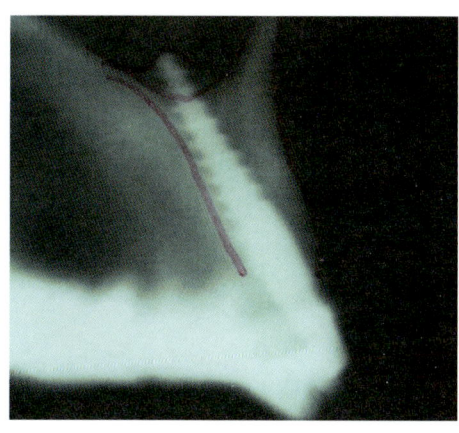

Cross-sectional image after implant placement

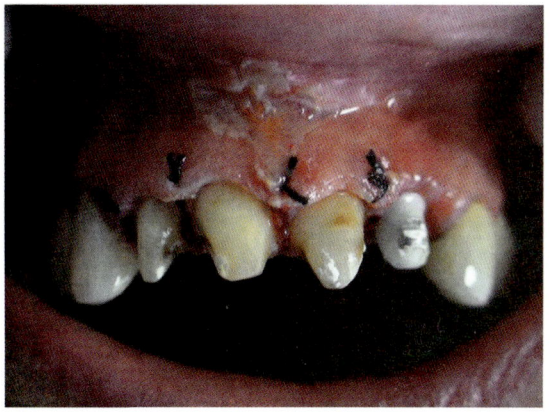

Clinical situation, 1st postoperative day

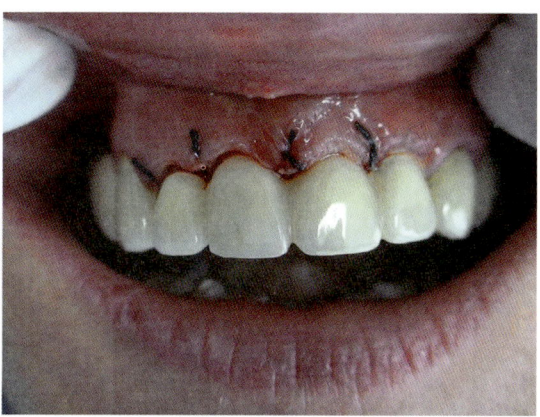

Laboratory made temporary, 1st postoperative day

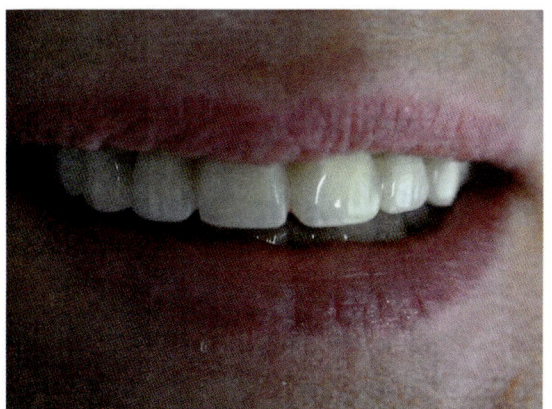

Labial view, 1st postoperative day

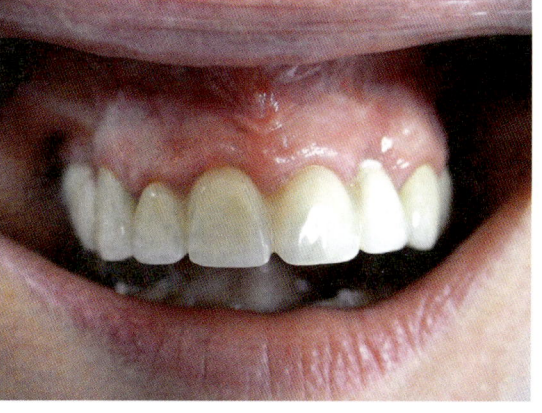

Clinical situation on the day of impression taking

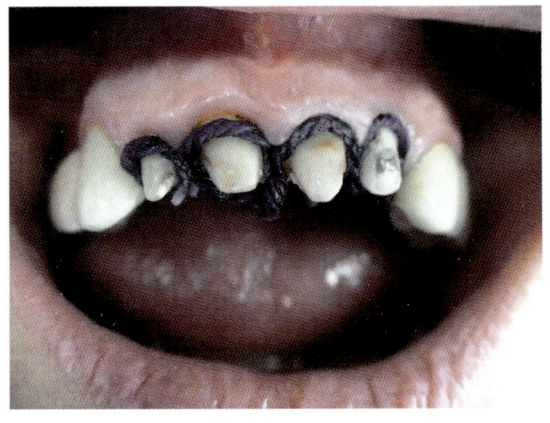

Retraction sutures before impression taking

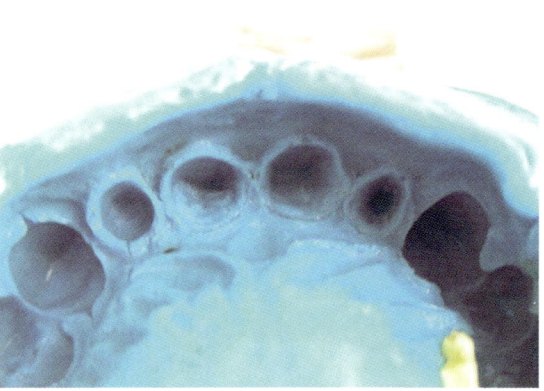

Final impression

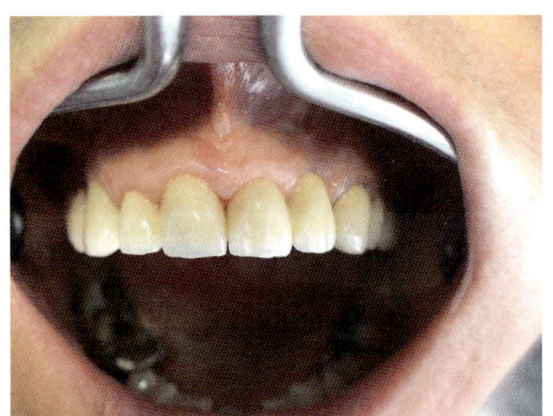

Final image

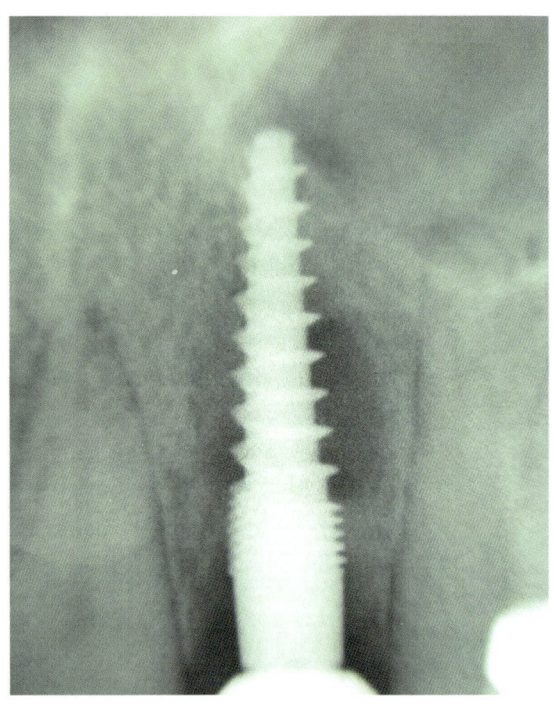

Radiographic control, zooming

7.1.3/Case 3

Patient: female, 49 years old

11 preparation with surgical crown lengthening
21 immediate implant placement
11/21 splinted crown

21/06/2011	11	preparation, surgical crown lengthening
	21	extraction, curretage
		Champions® implant Ø 4.5 x 16 mm
		>40 Ncm, PT +8
	11,21	cemented dentist made temporary
22/06/2011	11,21	cemented laboratory made temporary
30/08/2011	11.21	impression, Periotest +7
07/09/2011	11,21	cemented zirconium dioxide splinted crown
Treatment period:		**2.5 months**
Remarks:	11	surgical crown lengthening
	21	partial loss of the vestibular layer

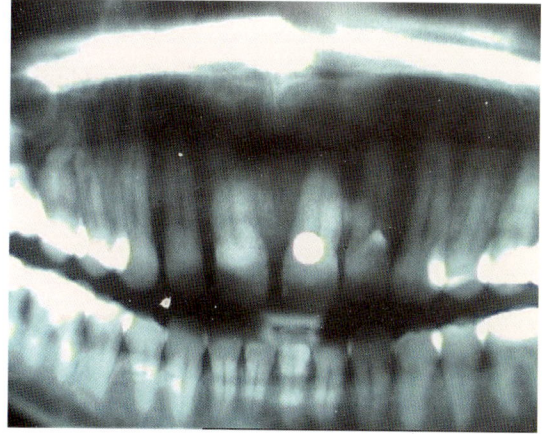

Initial situation, panoramic radiograph

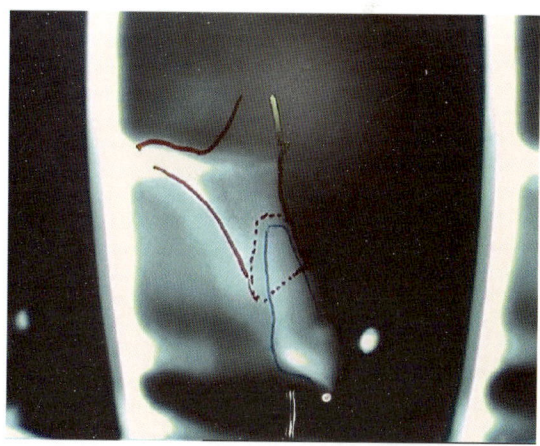

Initial situation, cross-sectional image

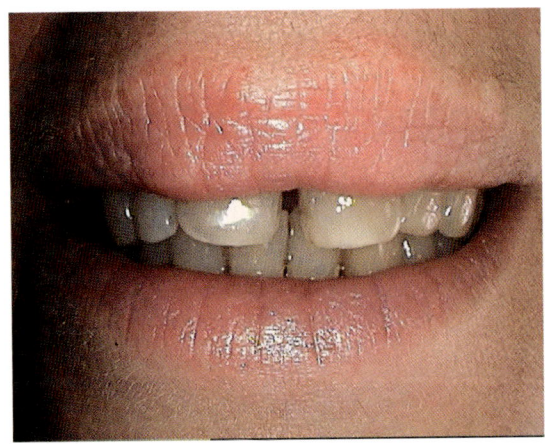

Initial situation, smile line

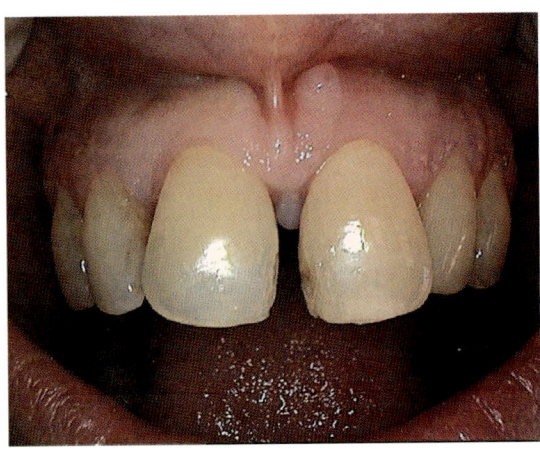

Clinical initial situation, anterior view

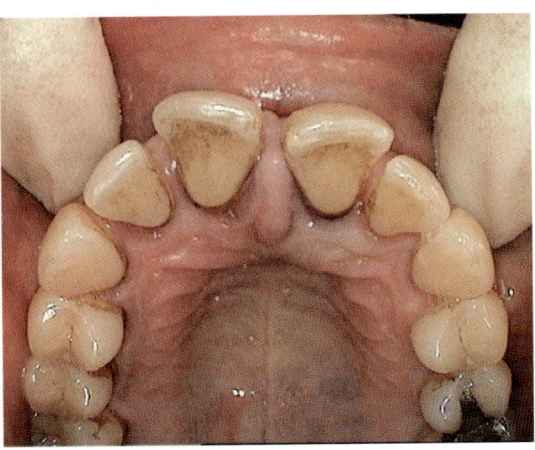

Clinical initial situation, occlusal view

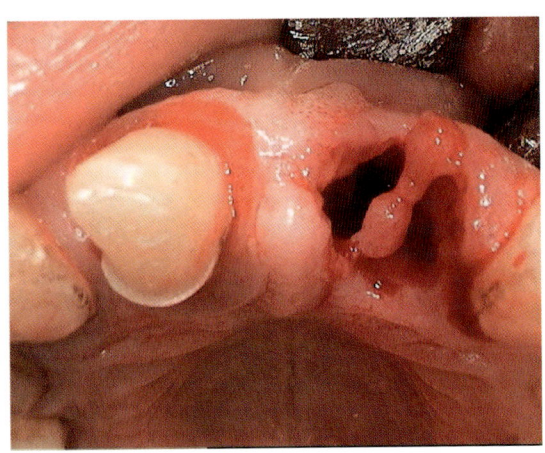

Alveolus after extraction

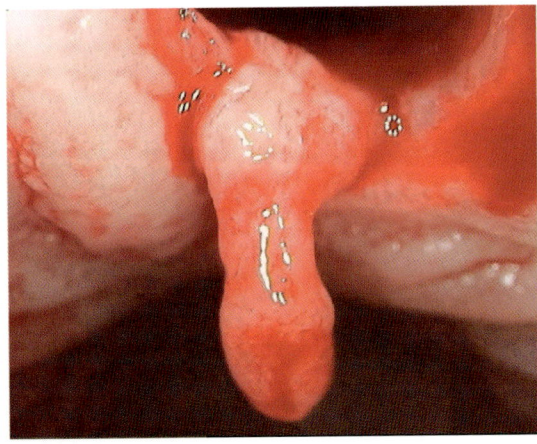

Inflammatory tissue, macro image

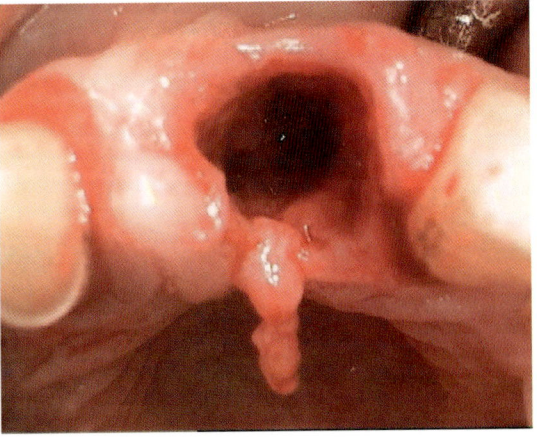

Situation of the alveolus, overview image

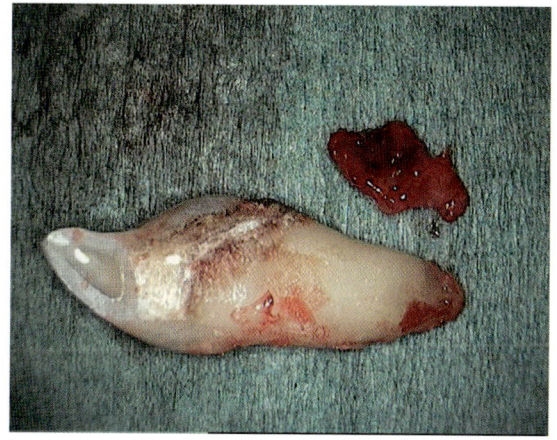

Extracted tooth, retrieved inflammatory tissue

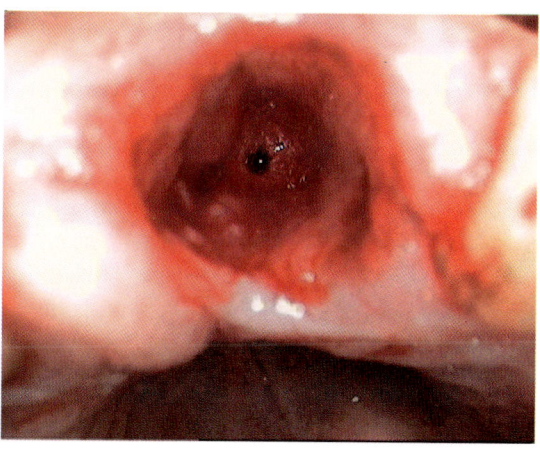

Pilot hole

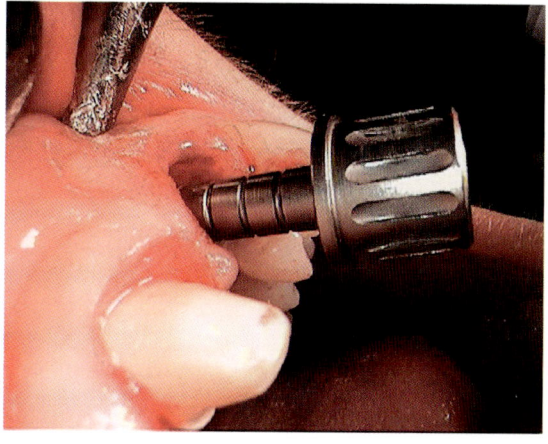

Bone spreading with bone condenser

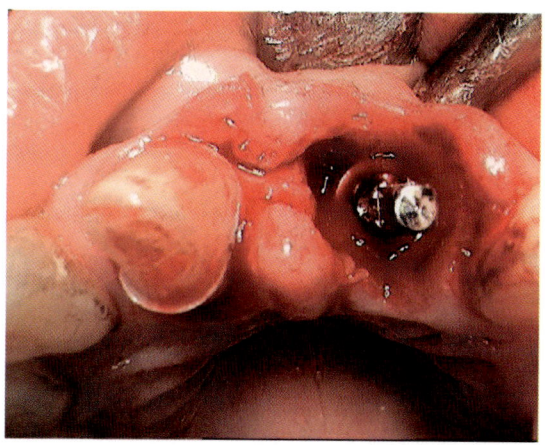

11 preparation, 21 implant placement

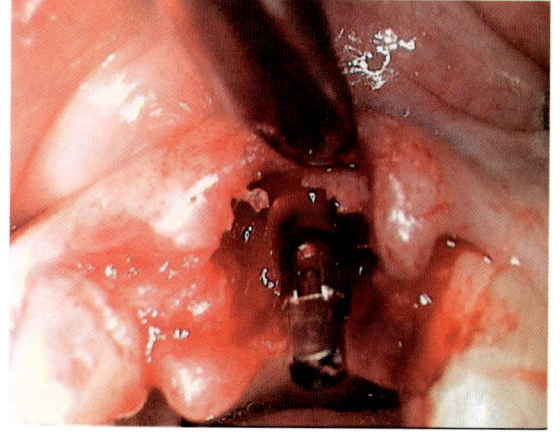

21 macro image

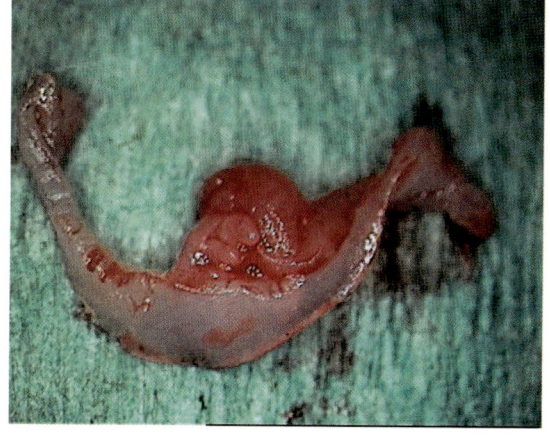

Excised gingival tissue from regio 11, vestibular

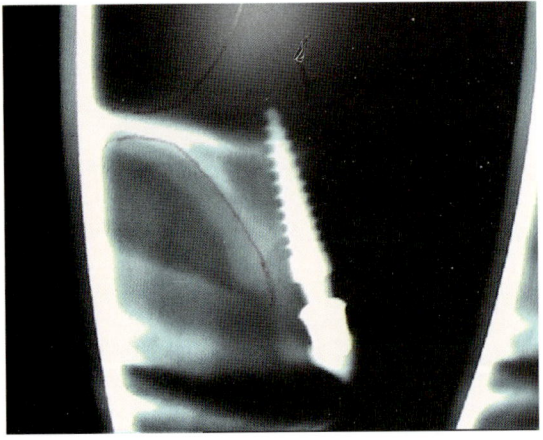

Radiographic control, cross-sectional image

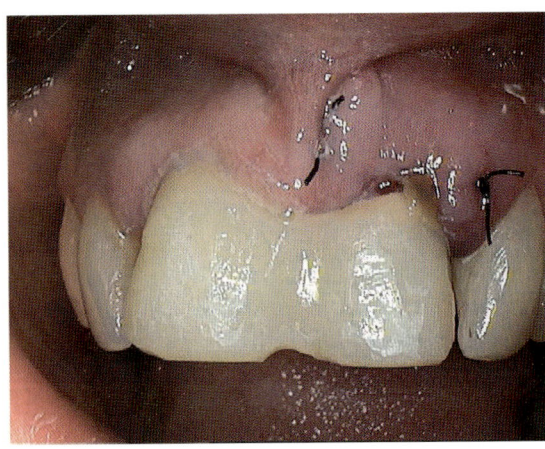

Cemented dentist made temporary

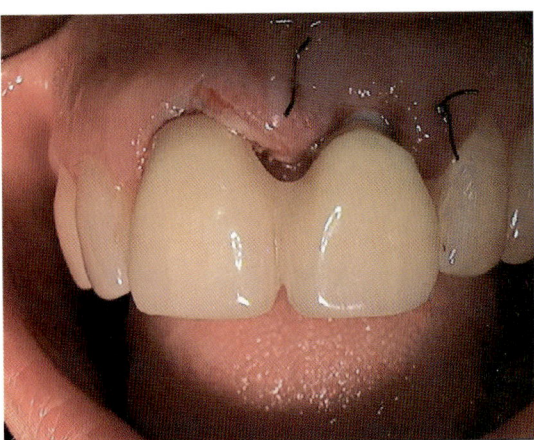

Cemented laboratory made temporary, anterior view

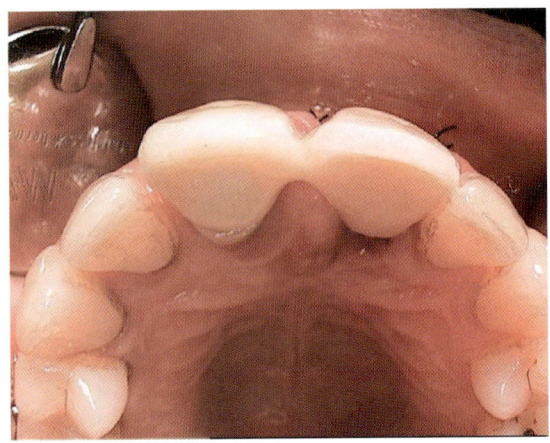

Cemented laboratory made temporary, incisal view

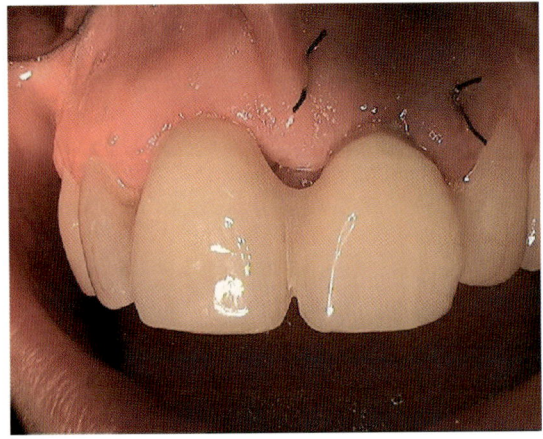

Situation before suture removal, anterior view

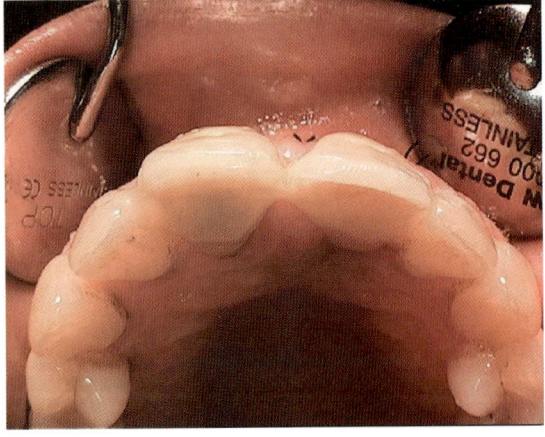

Situation before suture removal, incisal view

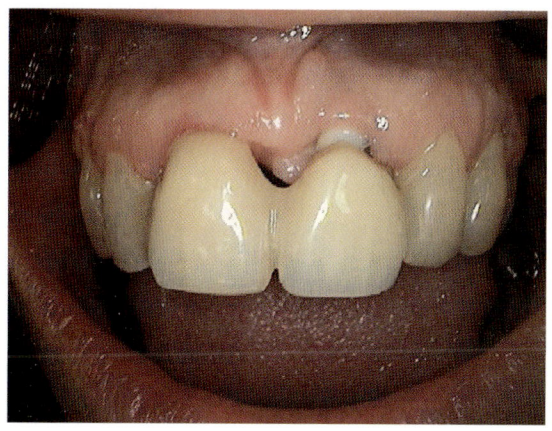

Clinical situation before impression taking

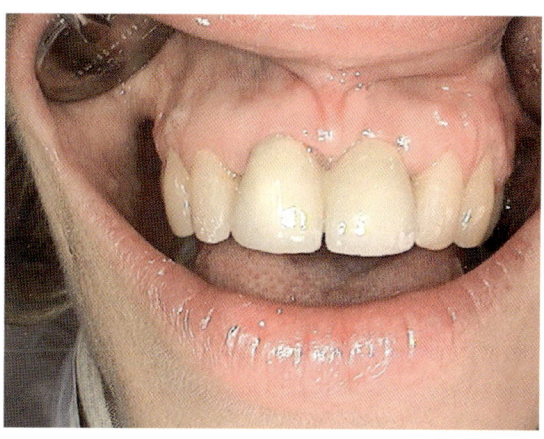

splinted crown after final integration, anterior view

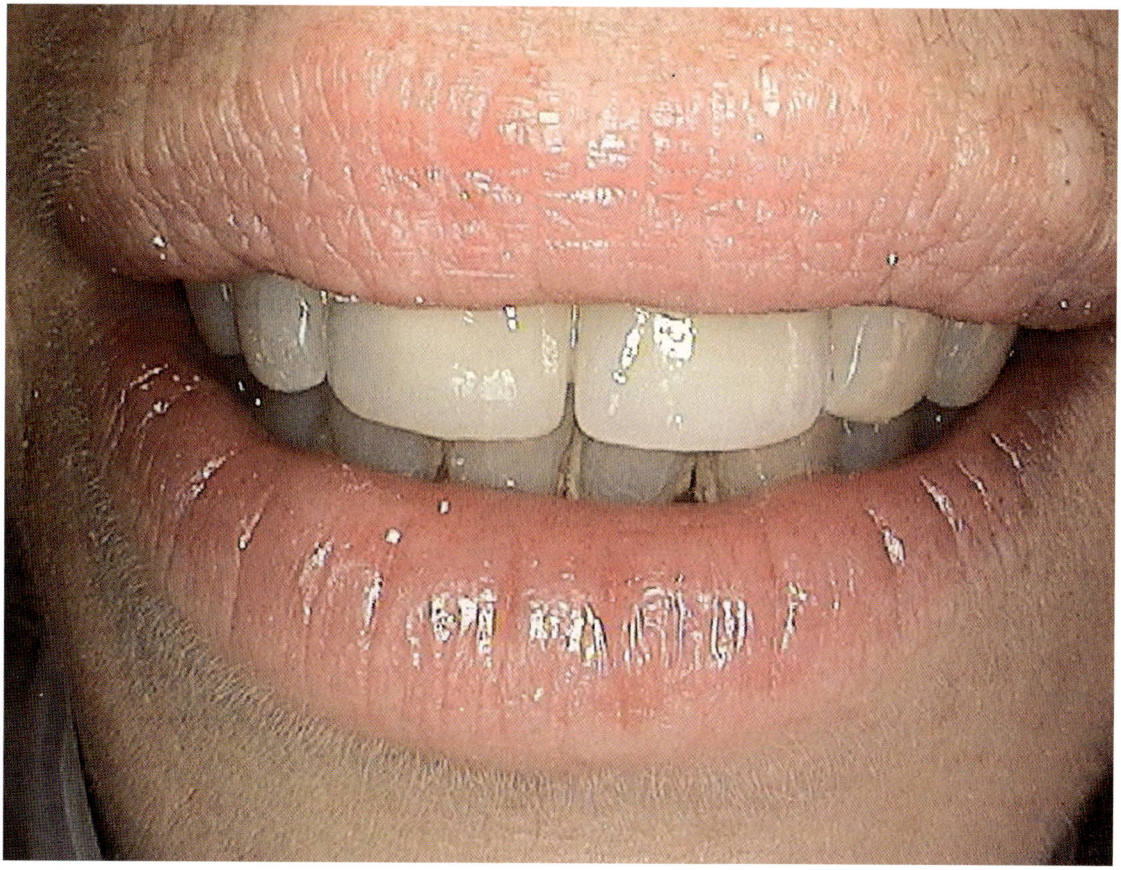

splinted crown after final integration, smile line

7.1.4/Case 4

Patient: male, 49 years old

31,41 extraction, gap narrowing with orthodontic plate
1 implant, augmentation, crown

13/07/2009	31,41	extraction orthodontic device to reduce gaps
22/09/2009	31,41	flap reflection Champions® implant Ø 3.5 x 20 mm, 40 Ncm augmentation with non-reactive beta-tricalcium phosphate, autologous bone and an absorbable membrane cemented dentist made temporary, splinting
08/01/2010		impression
22/01/2010	41	cemented zirconium dioxide crown
Treatment period:		**4 months**
Remarks:		Bone spreading, augmentation Orthodontic device in order to narrow gaps on teeth 31, 41 Due to the unfavourable bite position no orthograde integration could be achieved. Today, we only use in exceptional cases extraneous grafts, if no autologous bone is

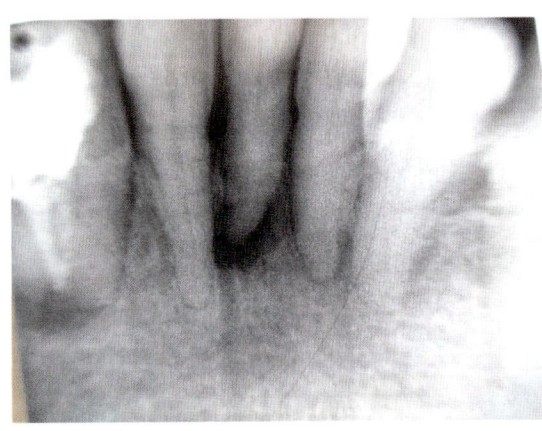

Radiological initial situation

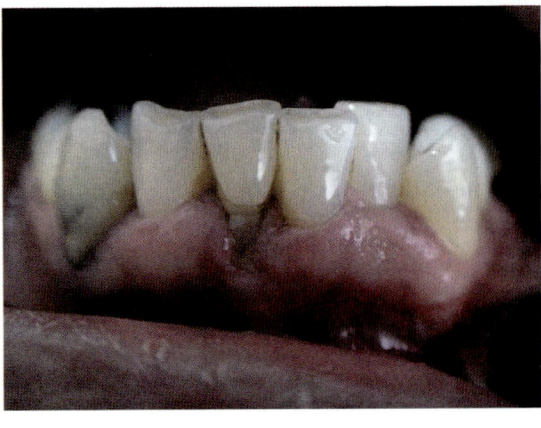

Clinical initial situation, anterior view

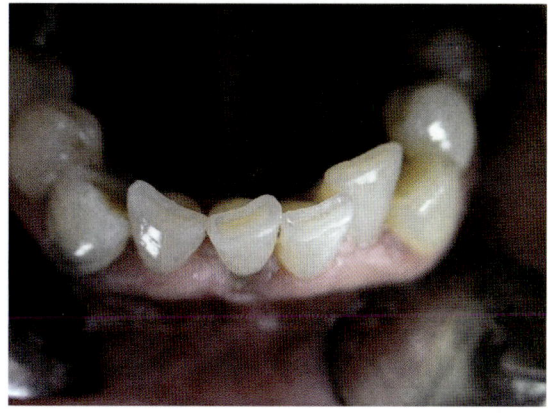

Clinical initial situation, incisal view

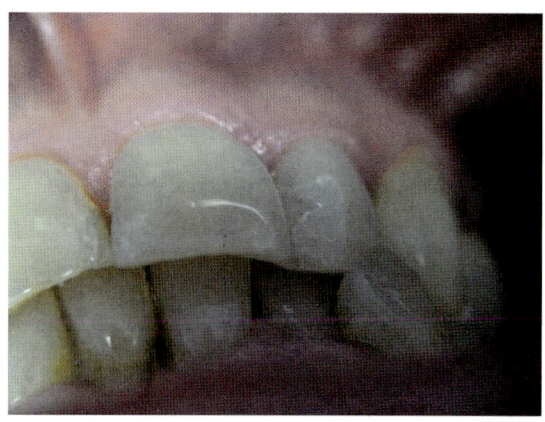

Unfavourable habitual occlusion

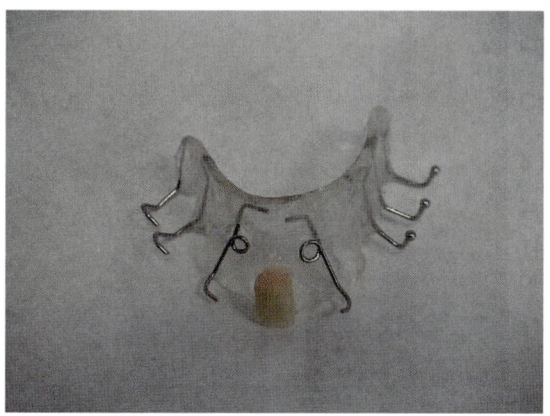

Orthodontic device to close gaps

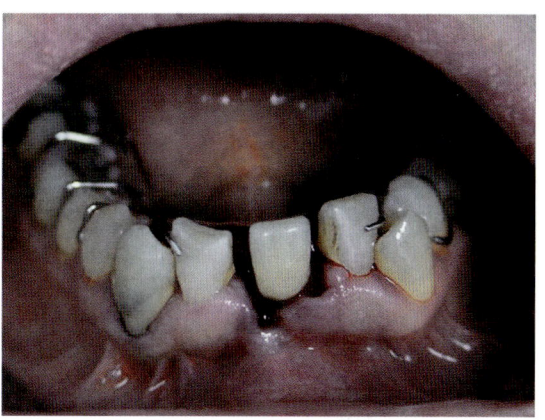

Gap closing at the beginning

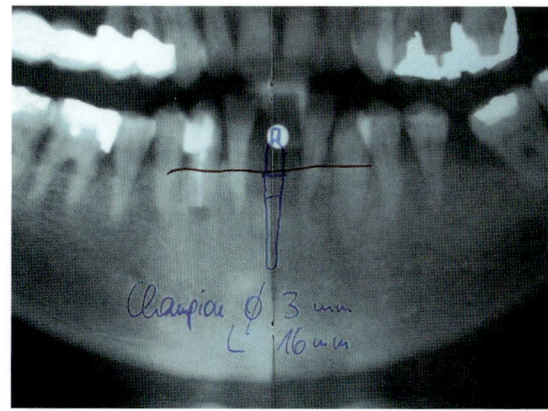

Panoramic radiograph for planned treatment

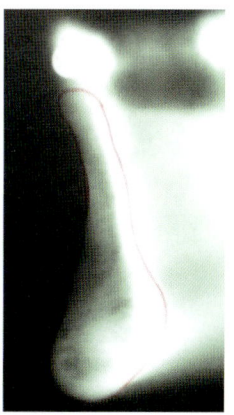

Cross-sectional image

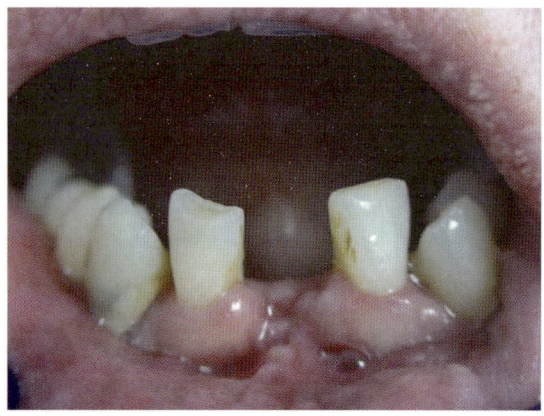

Clinical situation after gap reduction

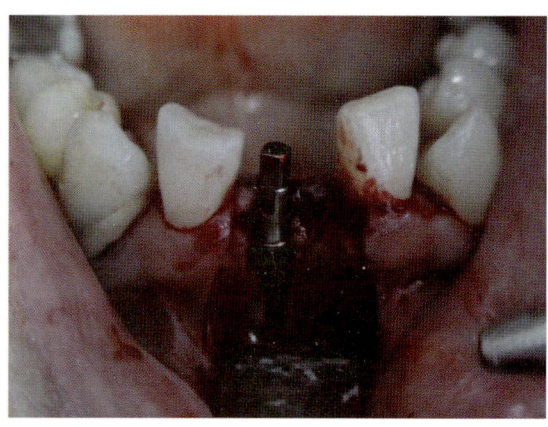

Implant placement

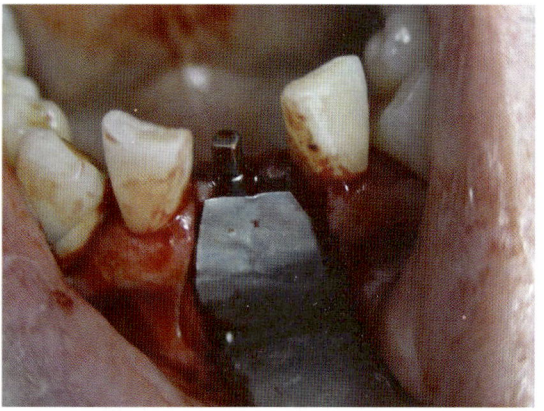

Try-in of the membrane template

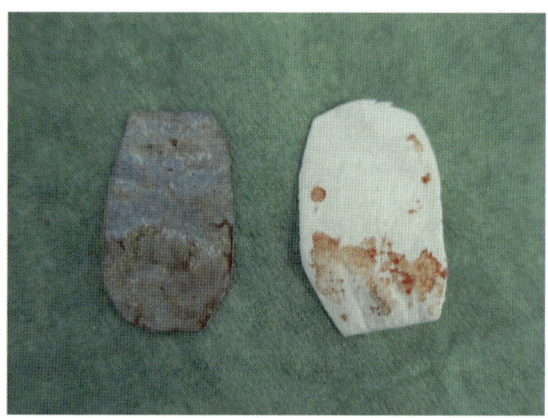

Customisation of an absorbable membrane

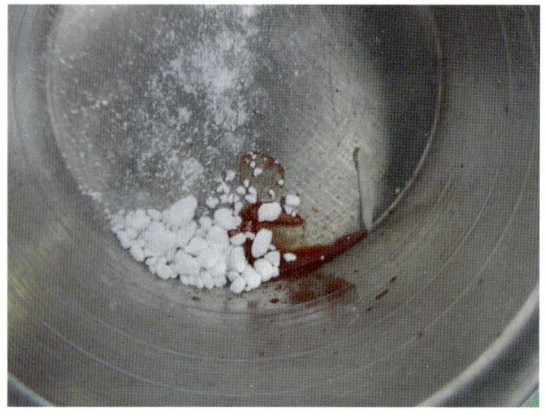

Non-reactive beta-tricalcium phosphate

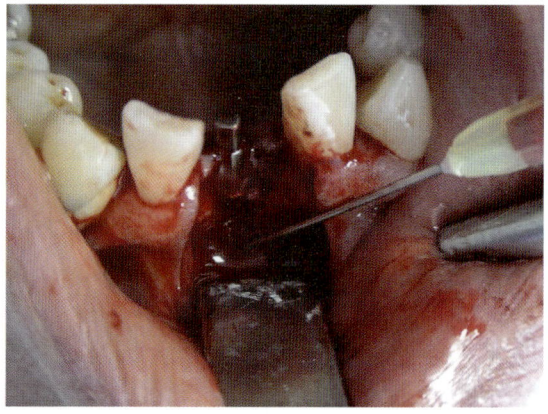

Autoblood withdrawal

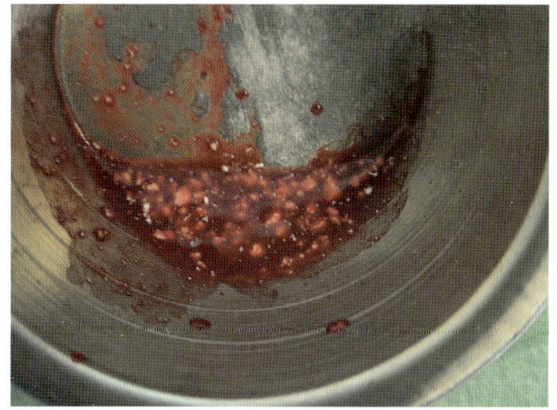

Prepared graft

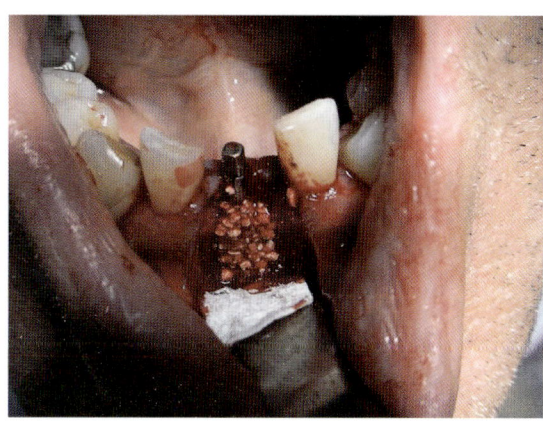

Graft in situ

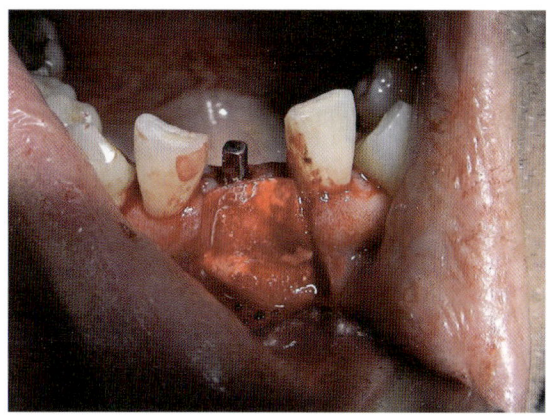

Membrane coverage

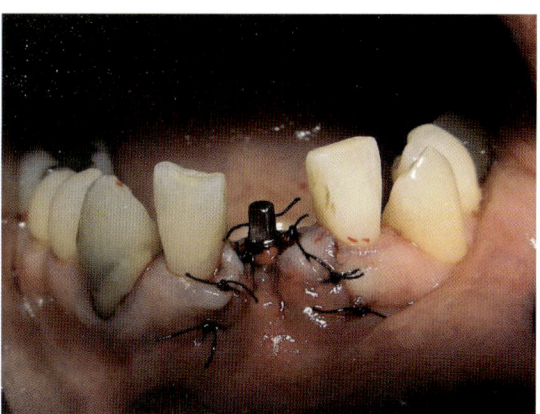

Wound closure

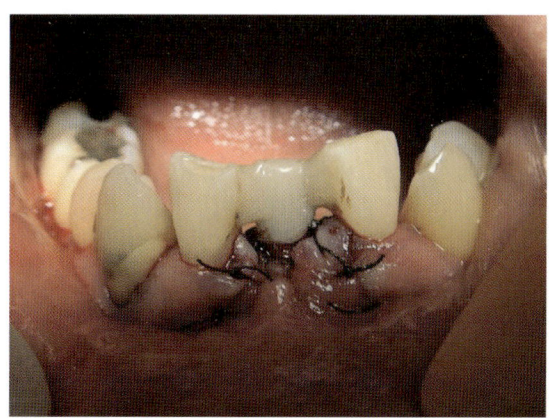

Temporary crown with splinting

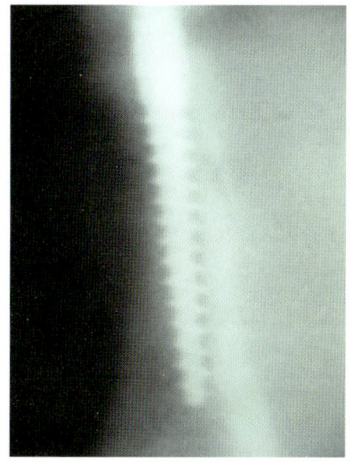

Radiographic control and cross-sectional image

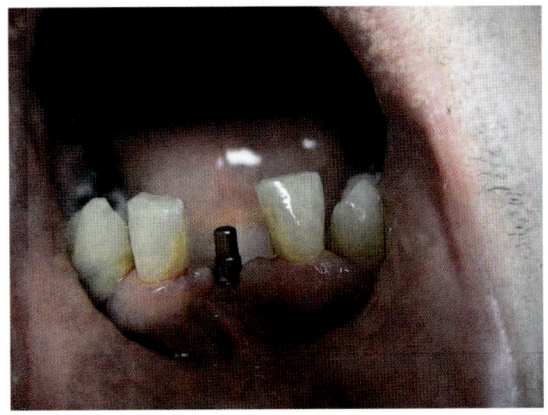

Before impression taking

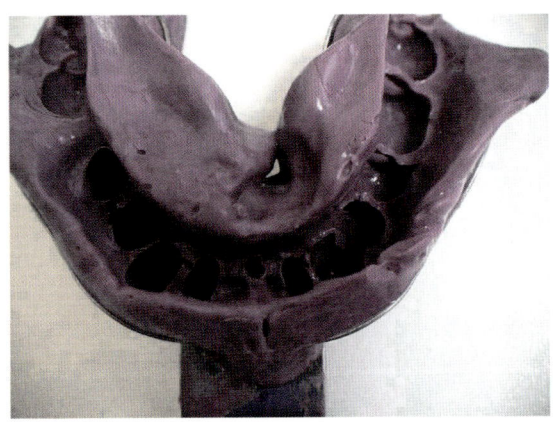

Final impression

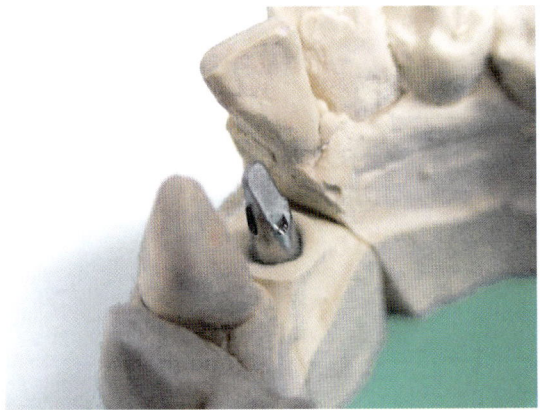

Cast

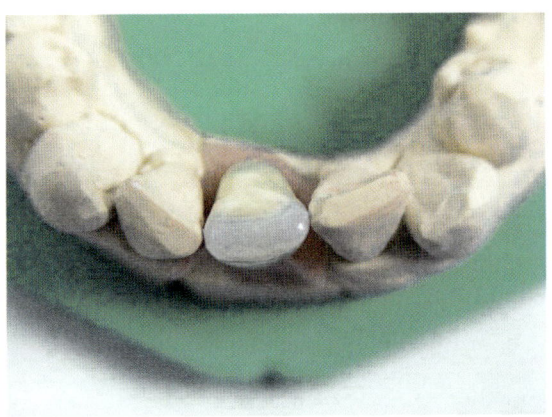

Crown

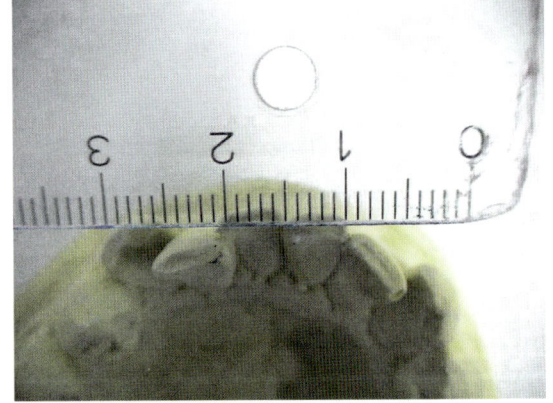

Gap reduction from 10 mm...

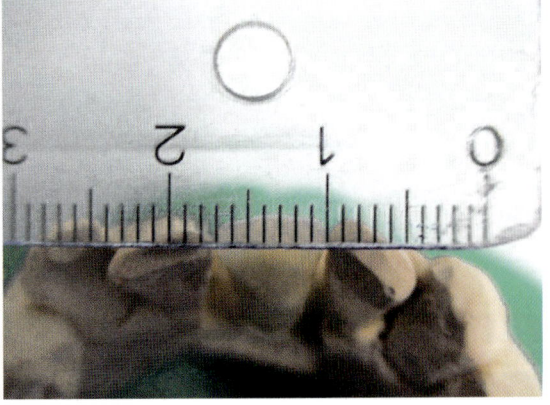

...to 7 mm

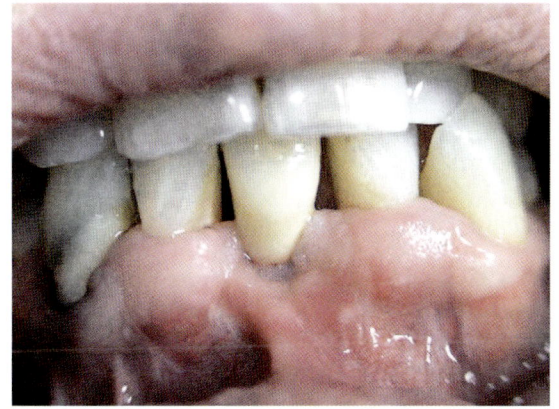

Cemented crown

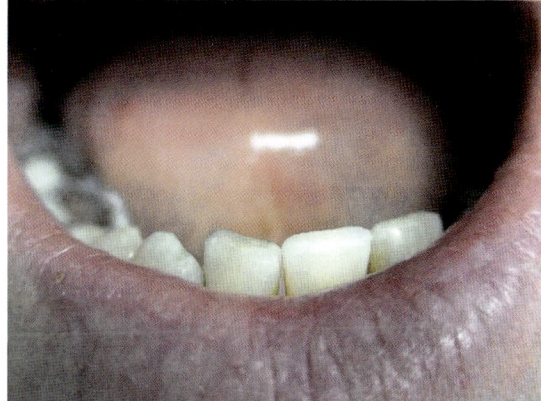

View of the crown

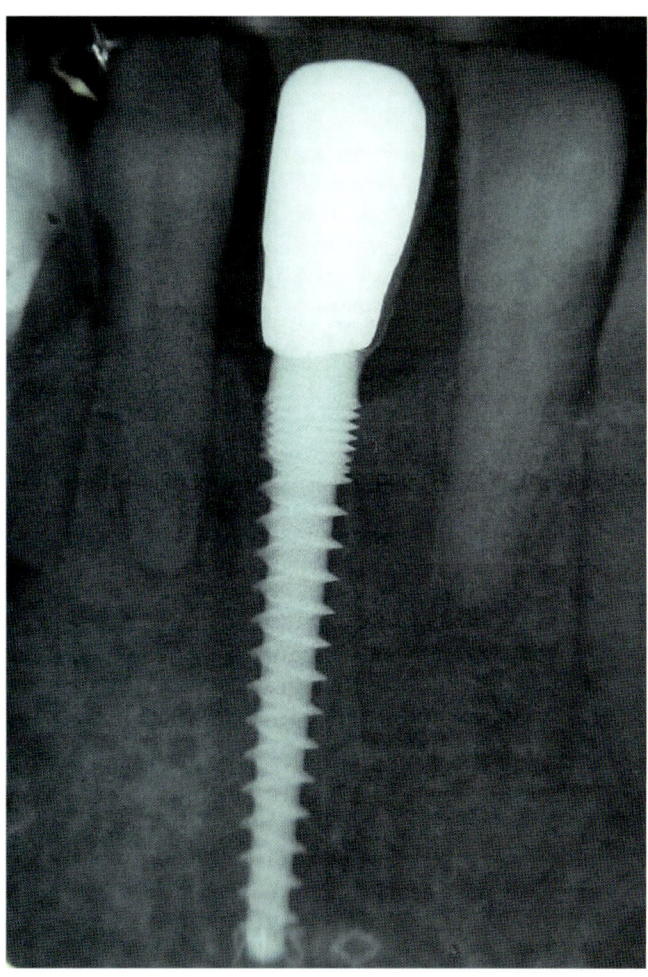

Radiographic control, zoomed dental X-ray

7.1.5/Case 5

Patient: female, 42 years old

24 immediate implant placement, zirconium dioxide crown

29/11/2010	24	extraction Champions® implant Ø 5.5 x 12 mm, >40 Ncm, Periotest -2 cemented dentist made temporary, splinted
10/01/2011		fraction of the temporary, implant is fixed new dentist made temporary with stronger splinting
14/02/2011		Impression, Periotest -5
19/02/2011	24	cemented zirconium dioxide crown
Treatment period:		**2.6 months**
Remarks:		Indirect sinus lift Extremely short implant stump Extension of the slot

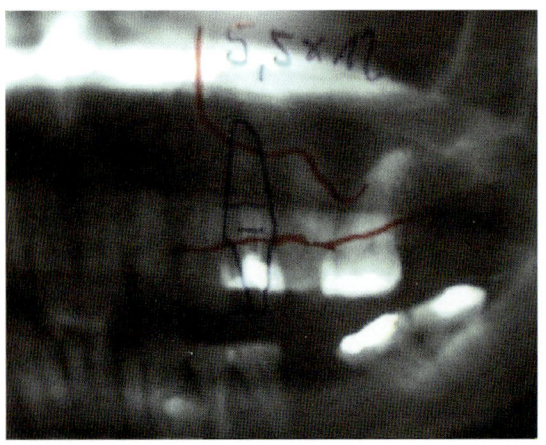

Planned treatment, initial situation, panoramic radiograph

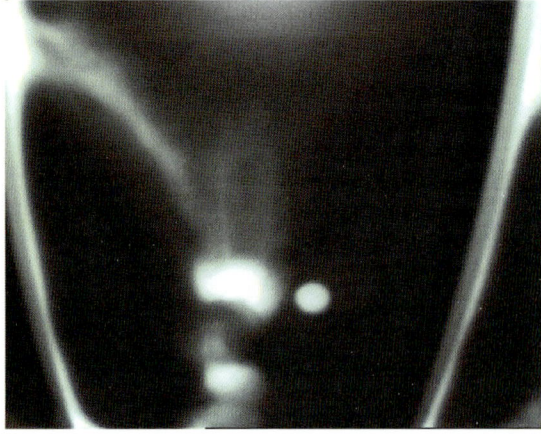

Cross-sectional image

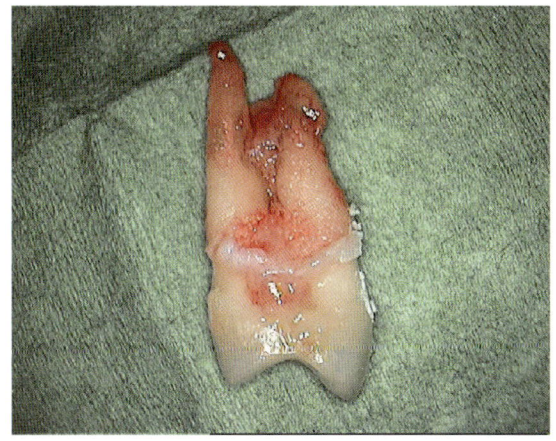

Extracted tooth 24

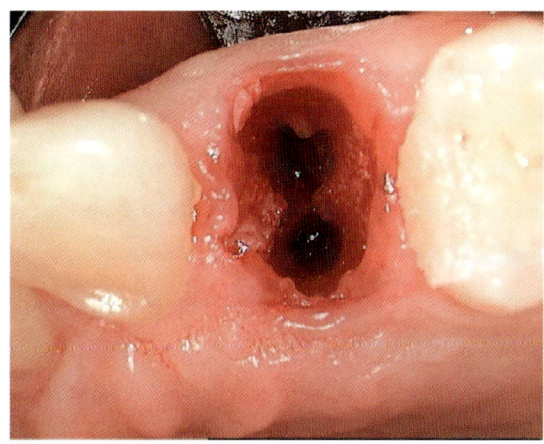

Alveolus after extraction, occlusal view

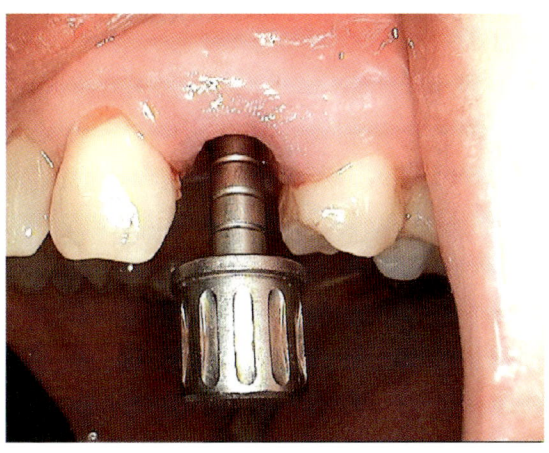

Condenser, lateral view

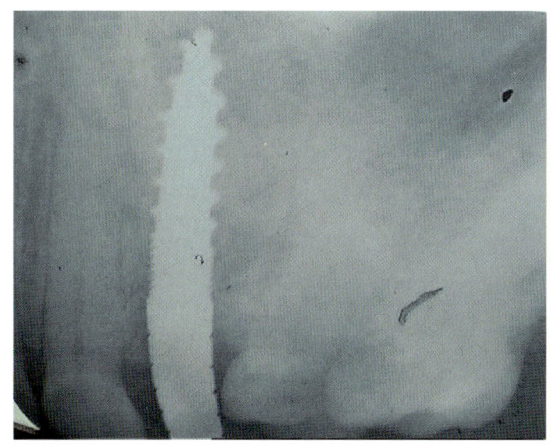

Condenser in the X-ray image, zoomed detail

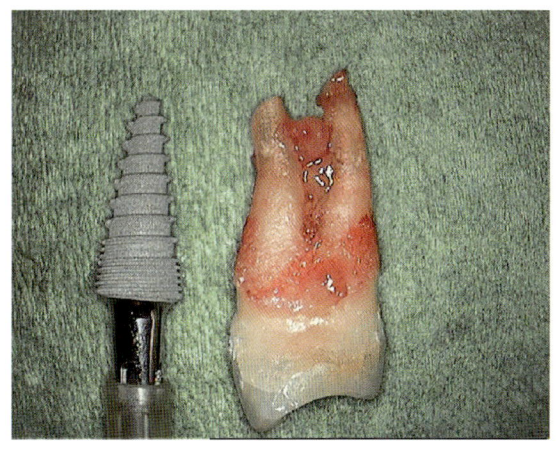

Implant selection

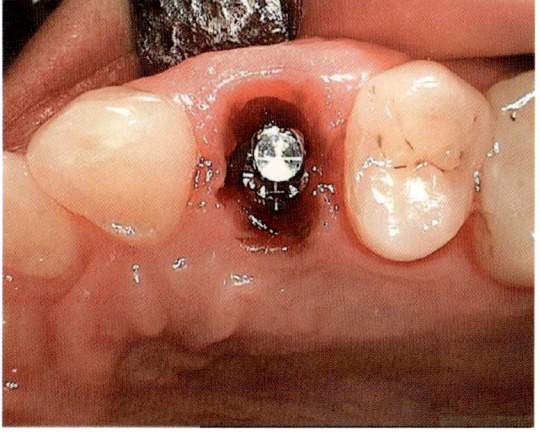

Inserted implant, occlusal view

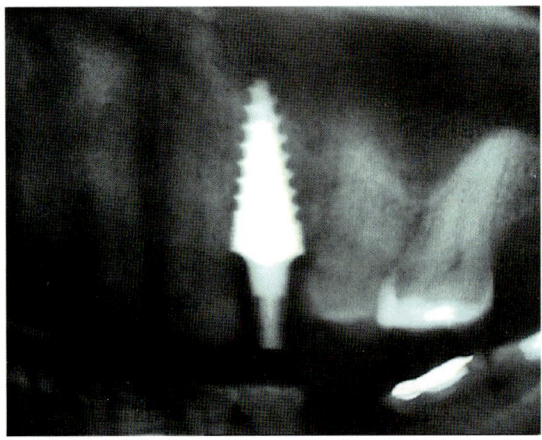

Radiographic control, zoomed panoramic radiographic detail

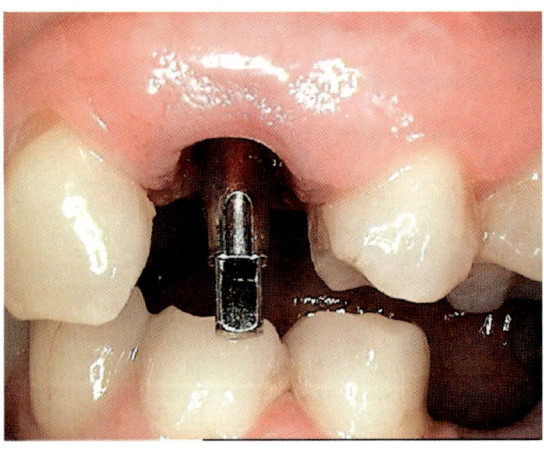

Implant in situ, without shortening no habitual occlusion is possible

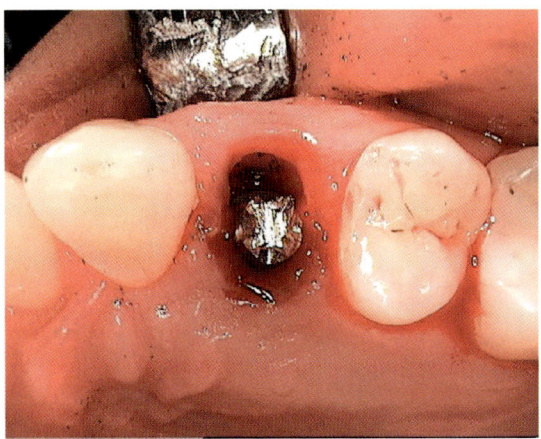

Shortened implant head, occlusal view

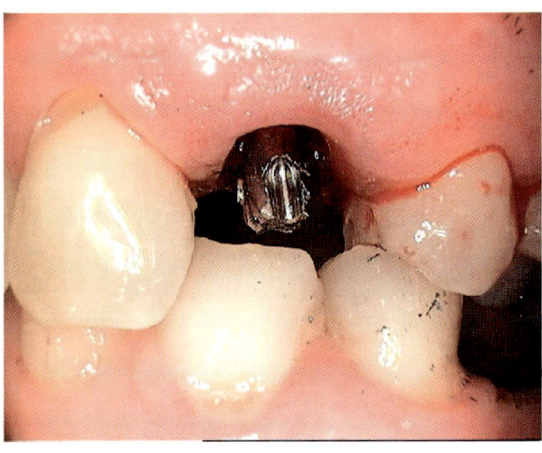

Shortened implant head, lateral view

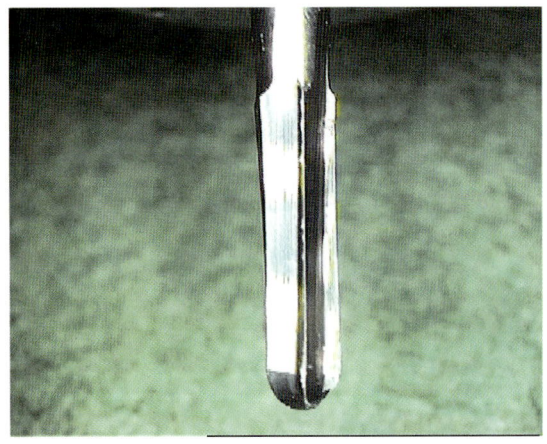

Used drill

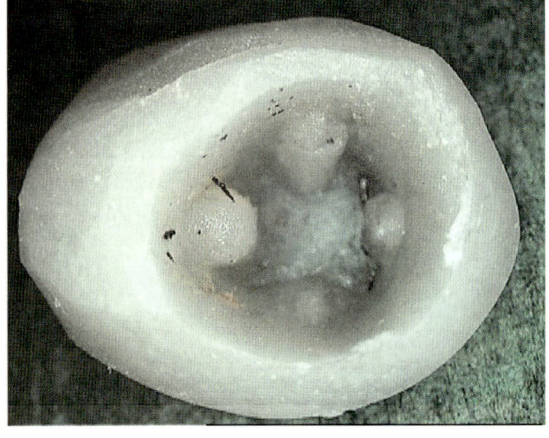

Dentist made temporary

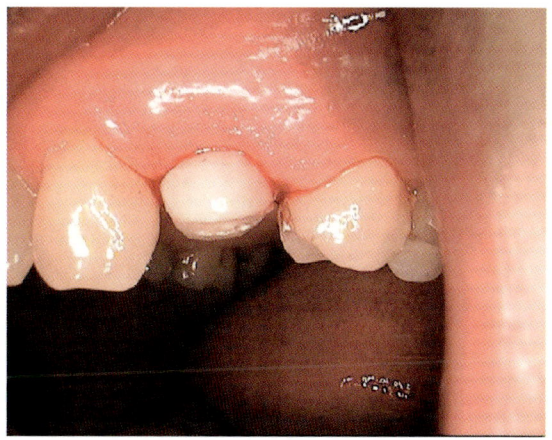

Cemented dentist made temporary

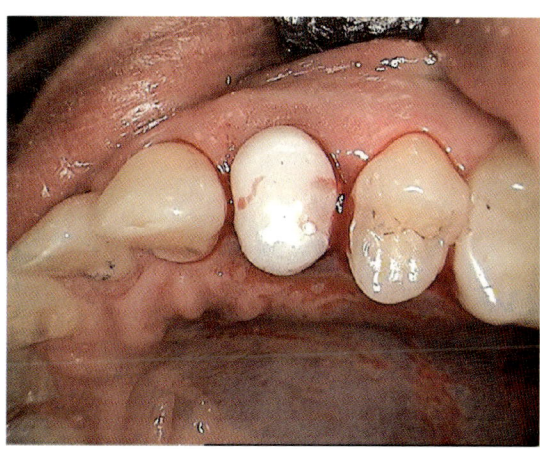

Cemented dentist made temporary, occlusal view

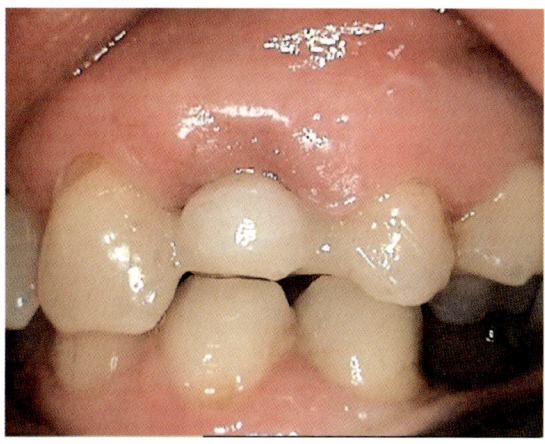

Splinted dentist made temporary, lateral view

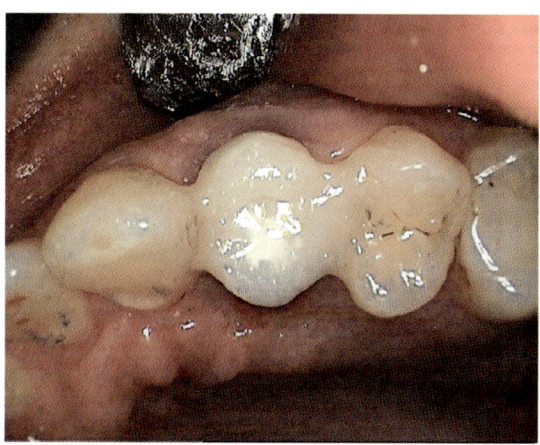

Splinted dentist made temporary, occlusal view

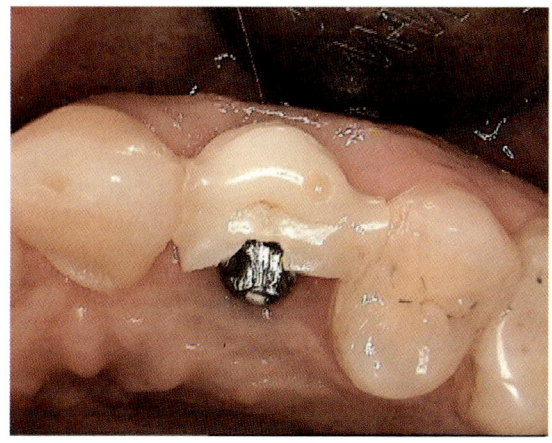

Fracture of the temporary

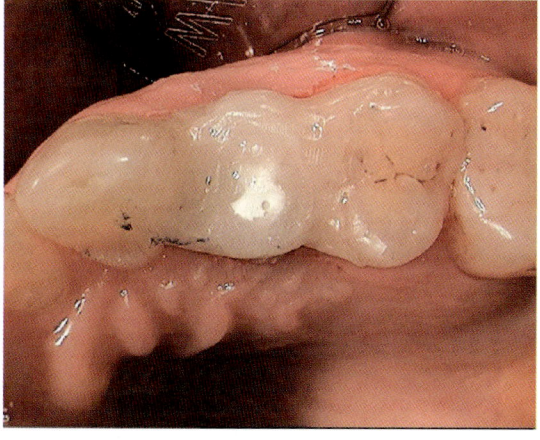

New temporary with stronger splinting

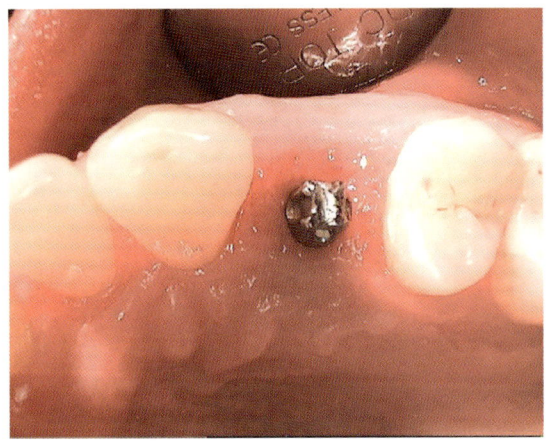

Clinical situation before impression taking

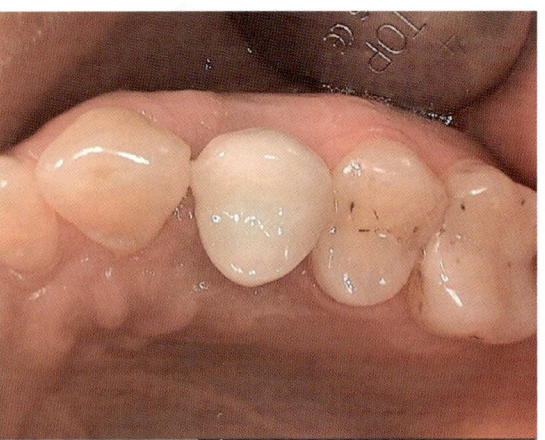

Cemented crown, occlusal view

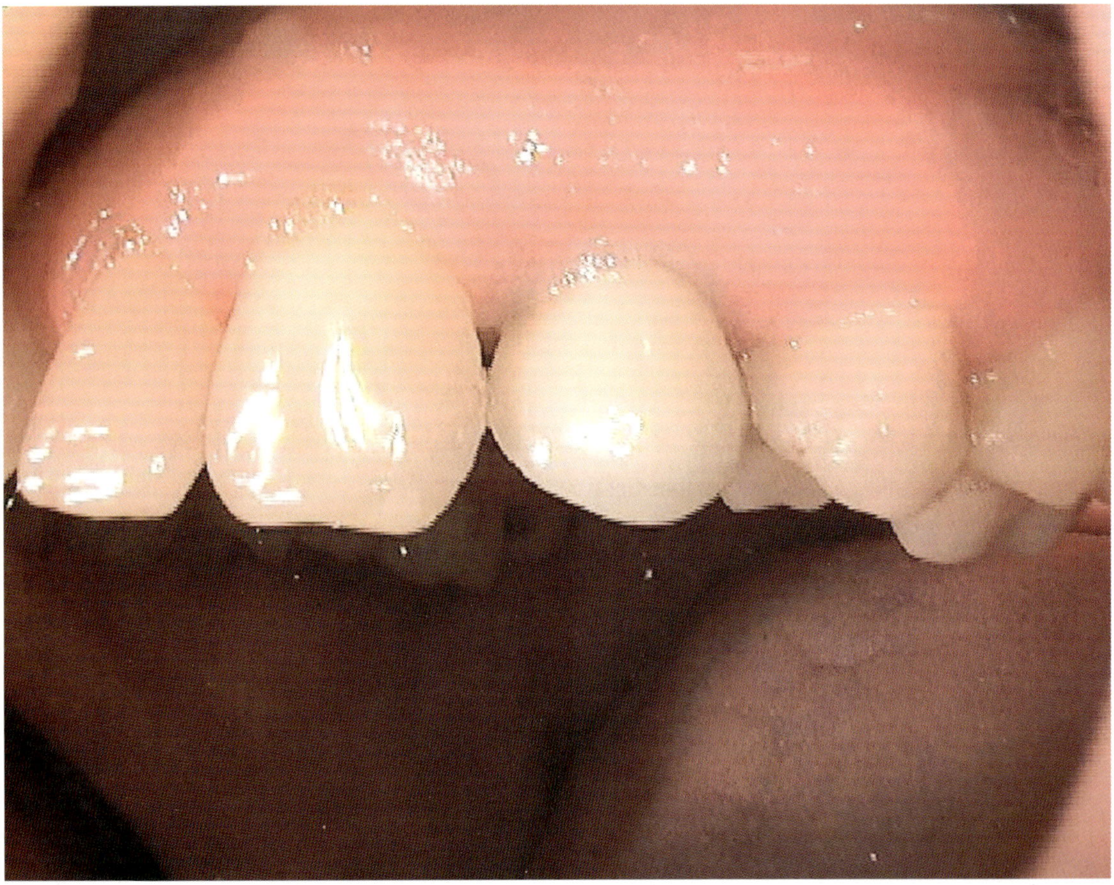

Cemented crown, lateral view

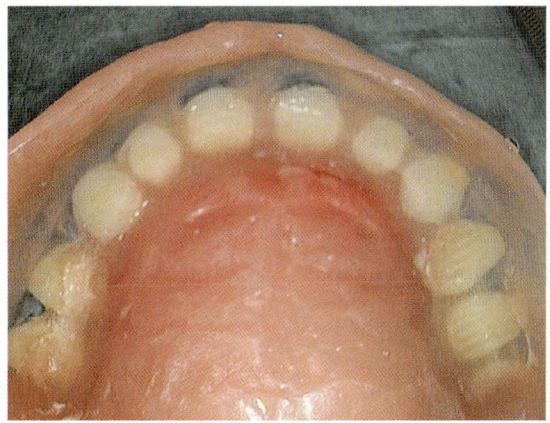

Reworked prosthesis on the day of the surgery session

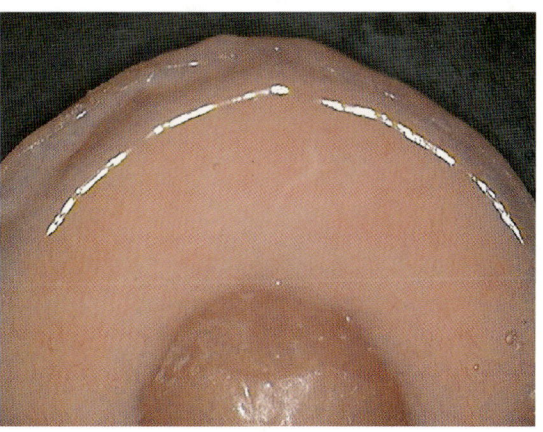

Injected cold-cured polymer

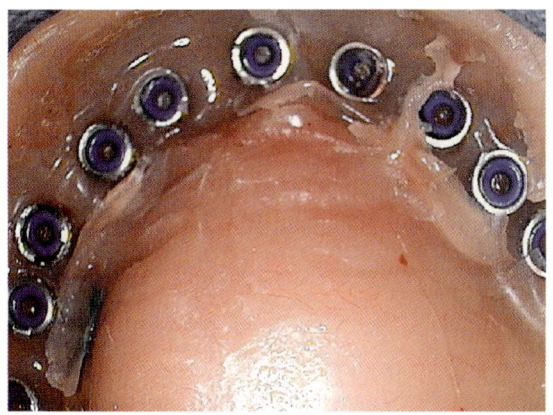

Cured cold-cured polymer

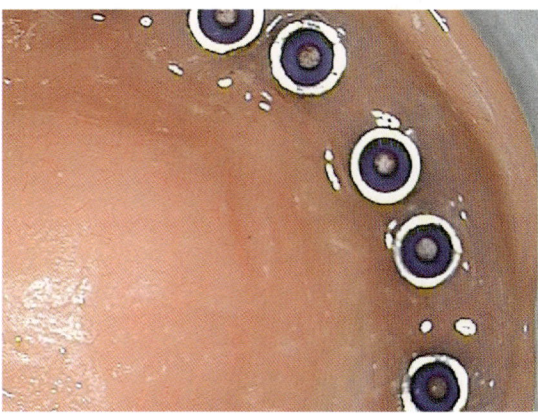

Prepared and polished prosthesis

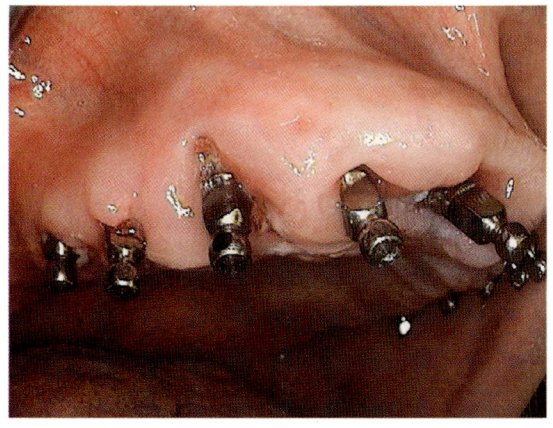

5 days after surgical procedure, right side

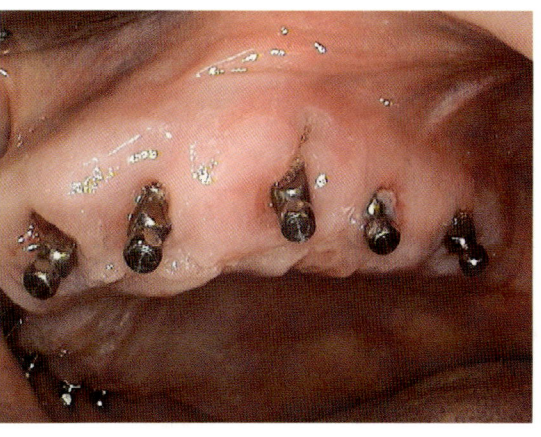

5 days after surgical procedure, left side

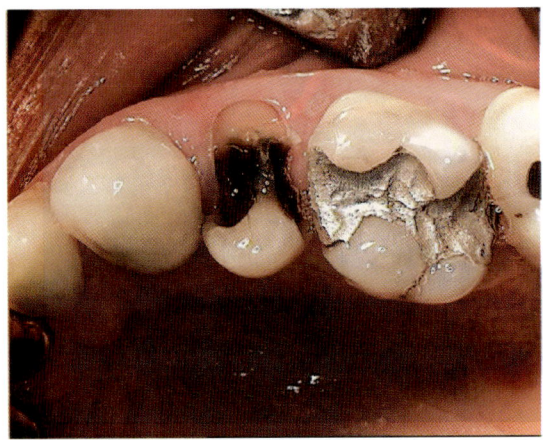

Clinical initial situation, occlusal view

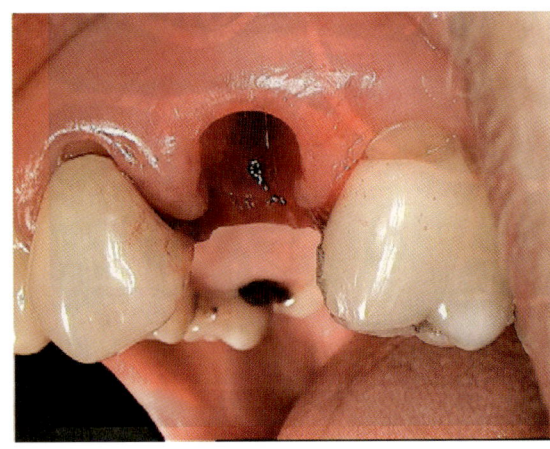

Alveolus after extraction, vestibular view

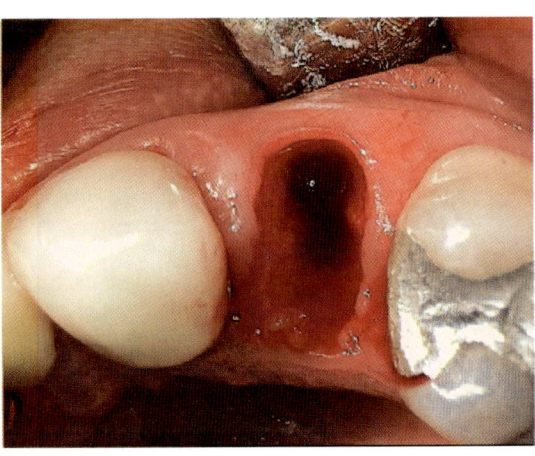

Alveolus after extraction, occlusal view

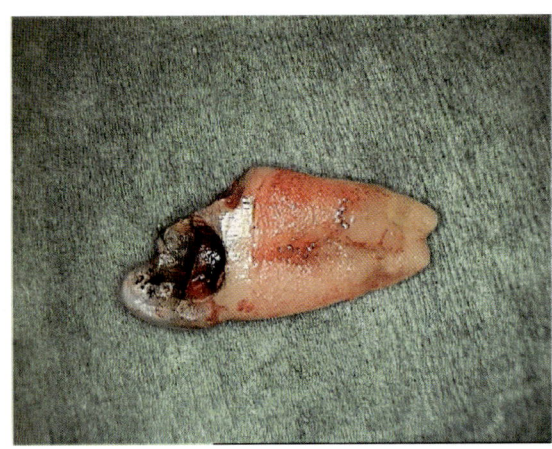

Extracted tooth

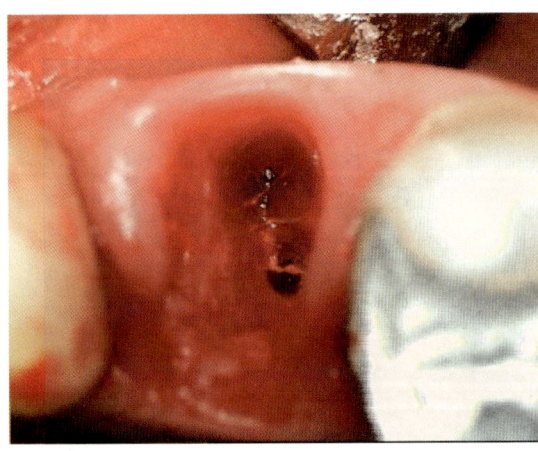

Palatal pilot hole preparation

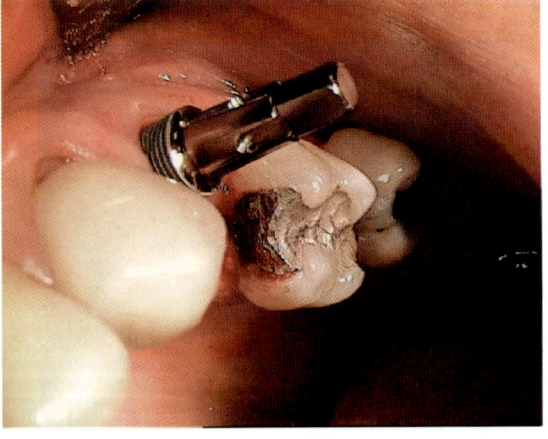

Insertion at the beginning, vestibular view

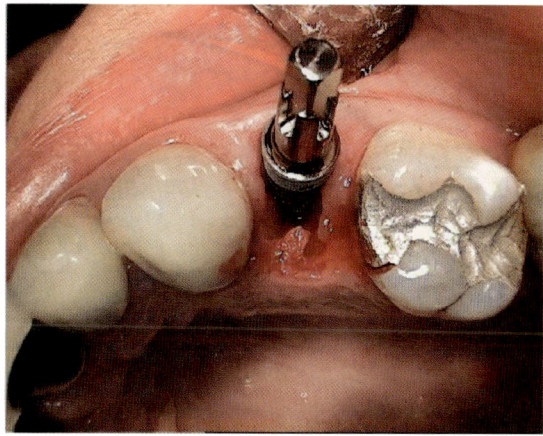

Insertion at the beginning, occlusal view

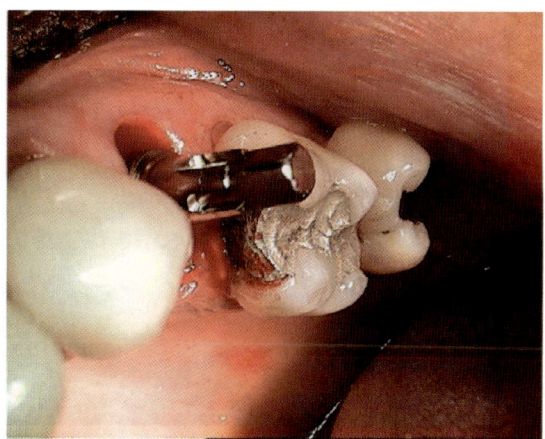

Axial change of the direction at the beginning, vestibular view

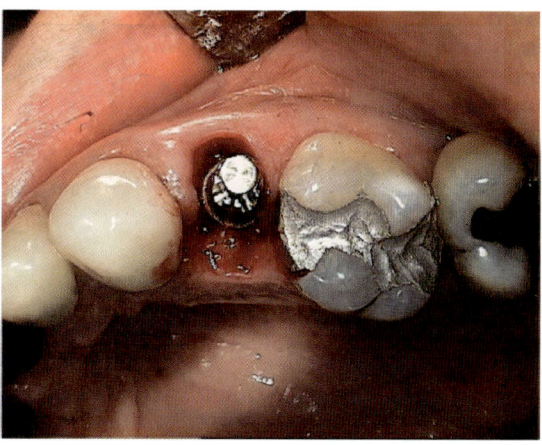

Axial change of the direction at the beginning, occlusal view

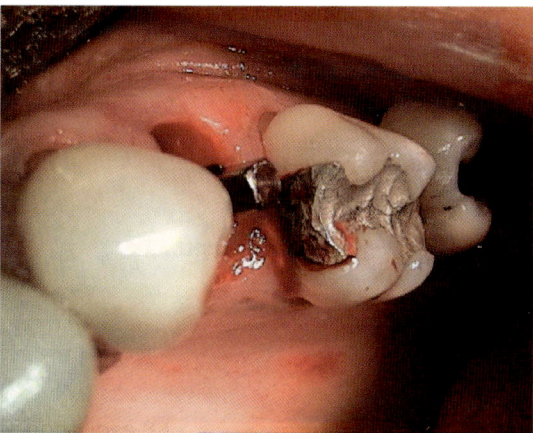

Axial change of the direction at the end, vestibular view

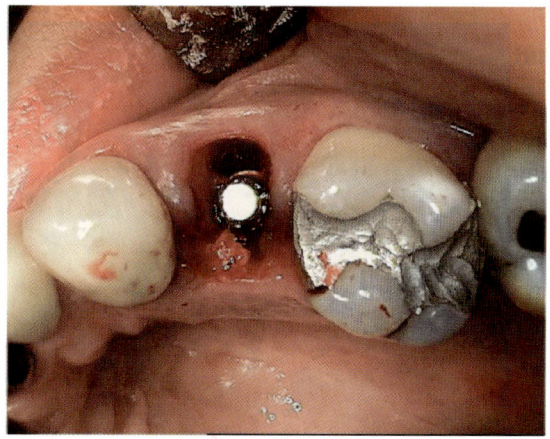

Axial change of the direction at the end, occlusal view

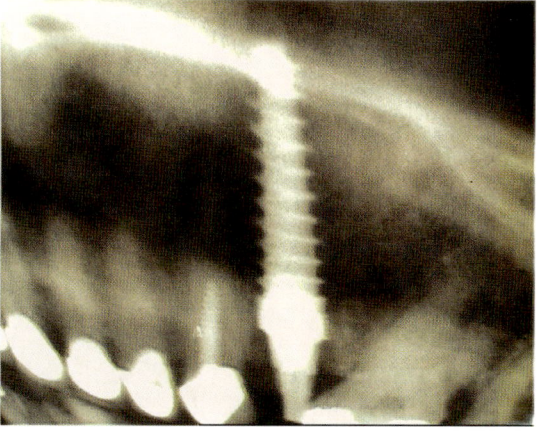

Panoramic radiographic control,

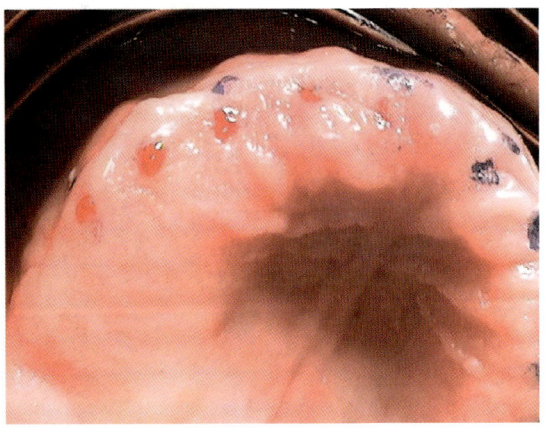

Upper jaw right side, pilot hole preparation

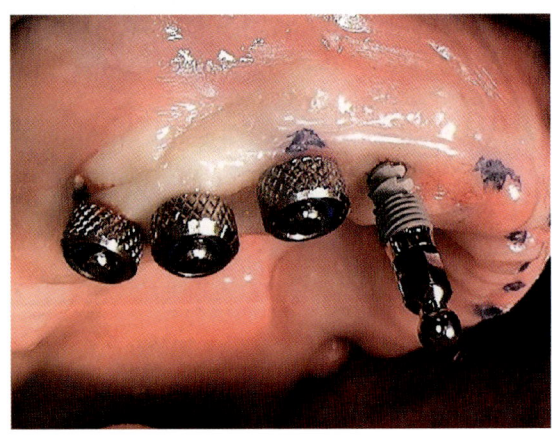

Implant placements

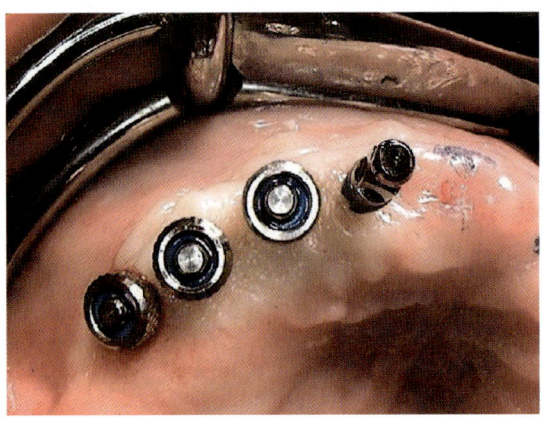

12- Insertion at the beginning...

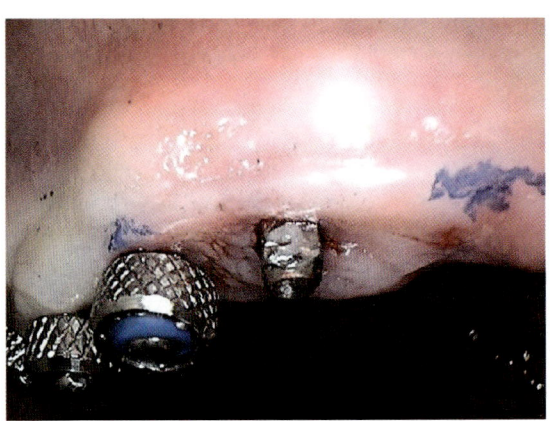

...implant fracture...

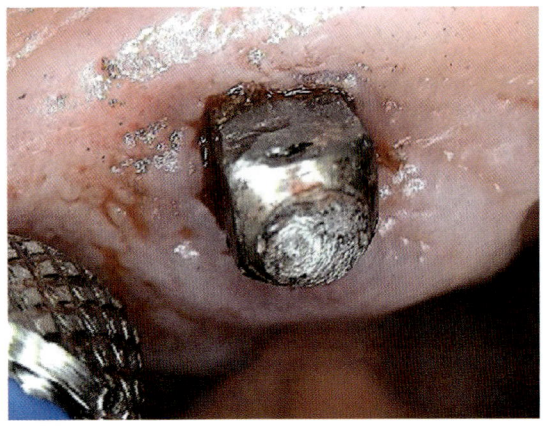

...in macro view...

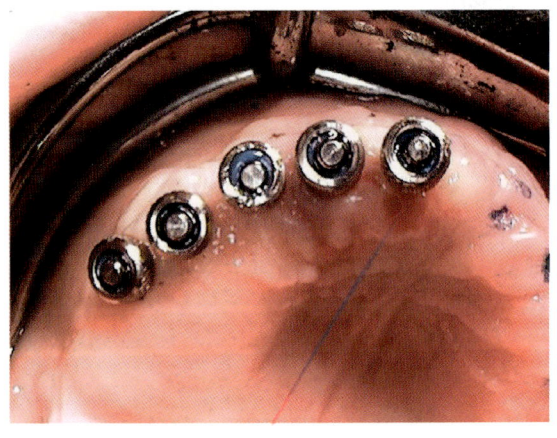

explantation, additional implant placement

7.5.11/Case 49

Patient: female, 70 years old

15-25 10 tulip head implants with early loading

28/09/2011	Upper jaw	Extension to a metal-free overdenture with gaps in regio 16-26 for matrices
29/09/2011	15	Champions® implant Ø 3.0 x 8 mm, 20 Ncm, Periotest 0
	14	Champions® implant Ø 3.0 x 8 mm, 30 Ncm, Periotest +6
	13	Champions® implant Ø 4.0 x 10 mm, 40 Ncm, Periotest +1
	12	Champions® implant Ø 3.0 x 12 mm, 40 Ncm, Periotest +1
	11	Champions® implant Ø 3.0 x 12 mm, >40 Ncm, Periotest +4
	21	Champions® implant Ø 3.0 x 12 mm, >40 Ncm, Periotest +3
	22	Champions® implant Ø 3.0 x 10 mm, >20 Ncm, Periotest +6
	23	Champions® implant Ø 4.0 x 10 mm, >40 Ncm, Periotest -3
	24	Champions® implant Ø 3.0 x 10 mm, > 30 Ncm, Periotest +3
	25	Champions® implant Ø 3.0 x 8 mm, 20 Ncm, Periotest -3
		10 matrices (blue) cured into the denture resin

04/10/2011		Post-control, images
Treatment period:		**2 hours**
Remarks:		After osseointegration followed the palatal free creation of the prosthesis. Due to financial reasons the patient refused a fixed restoration. Immediate implant placement Immediate loading

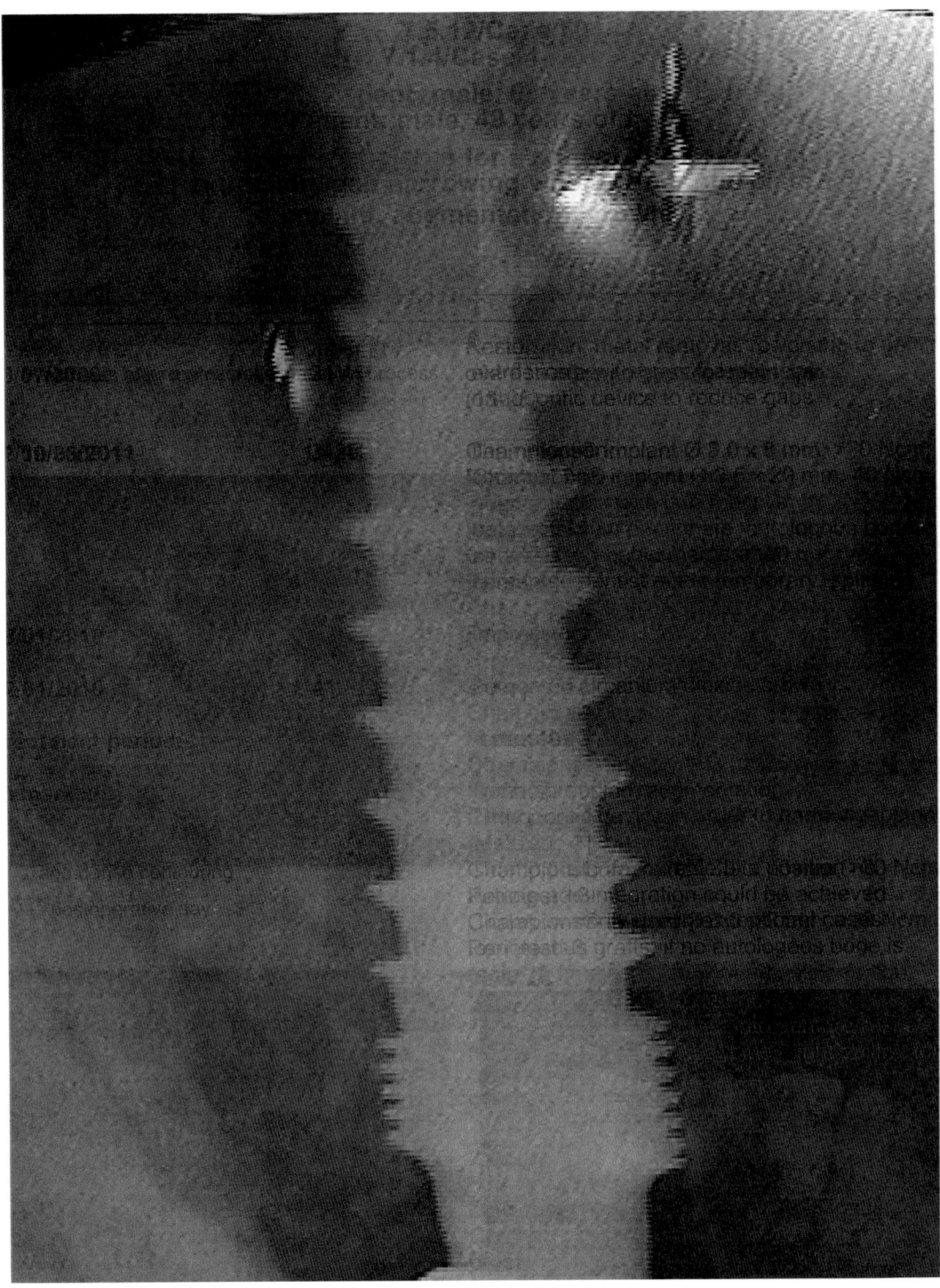

Radiographic control X-ray

7.1.7/Case 7

Patient: male, 43 years old

31 cystectomy, implant placement, crown

07/09/2010	31 32,41	extraction, cystectomy due to an alveolus positive vitality test
01/11/2010	31 31	Champions® implant Ø 3.5 x 22 mm, 40 Ncm cemented and splinted dentist made temporary
19/01/2011	31	cemented zirconium dioxide crown
Treatment period:		**2.5 months**
Remarks:		Big cyst Biocortical implant support Before implant placement the gap was not restored.

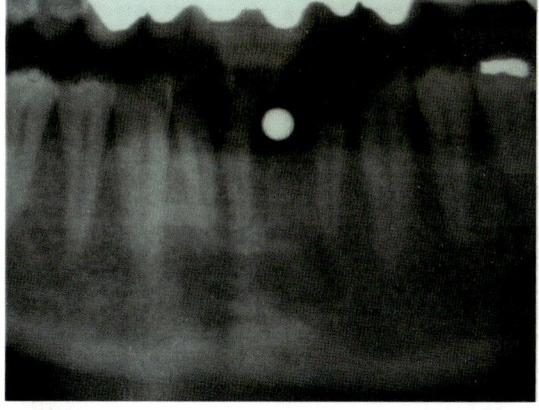

Initial panoramic radiograph

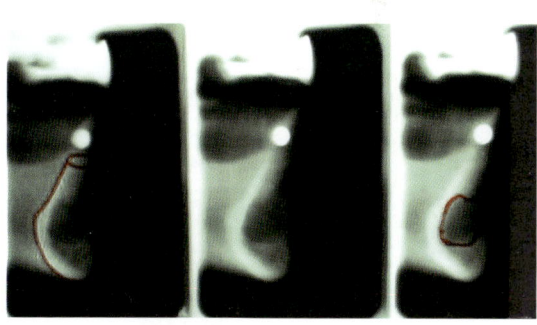

Spiral computed tomography

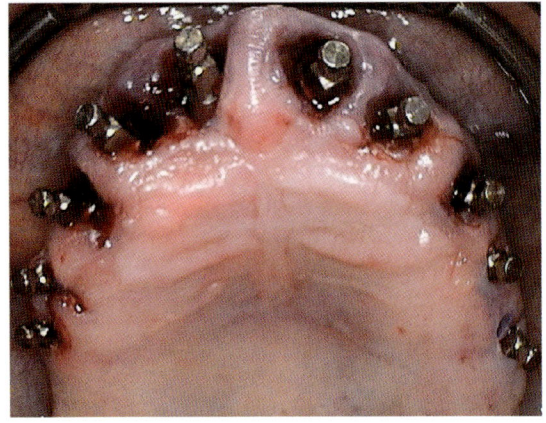

Overview image after implant placement, occlusal view

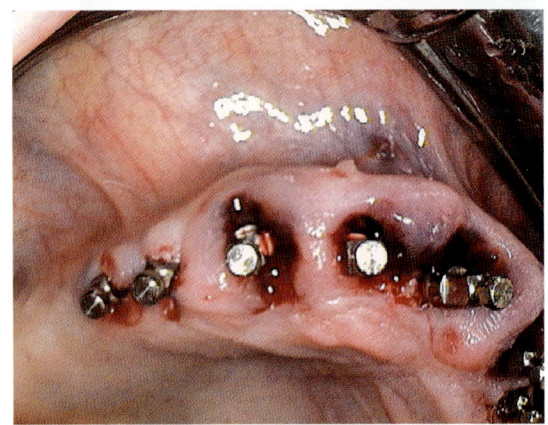

Detailed image, right side

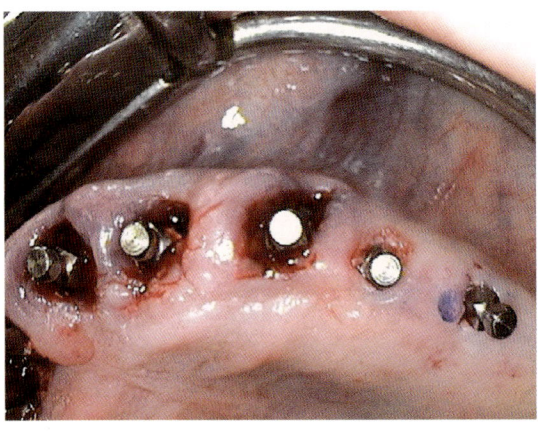

Detailed image, left side

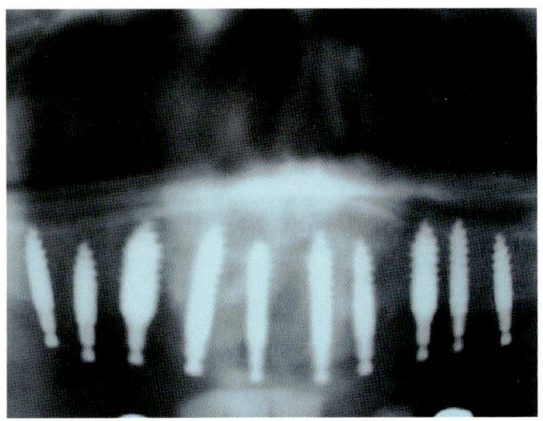

Panoramic radiographic control

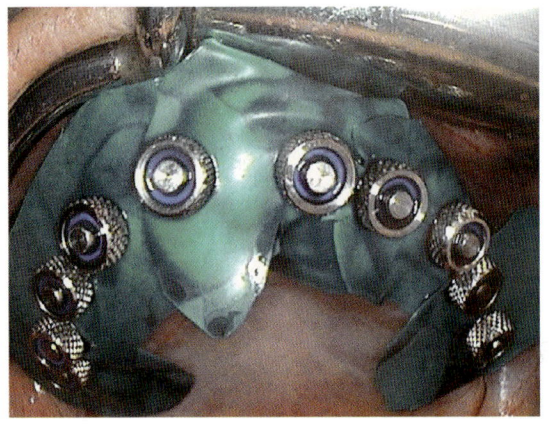

Preparation of the implanted region with rubber dam for the polymerisation process of the matrices

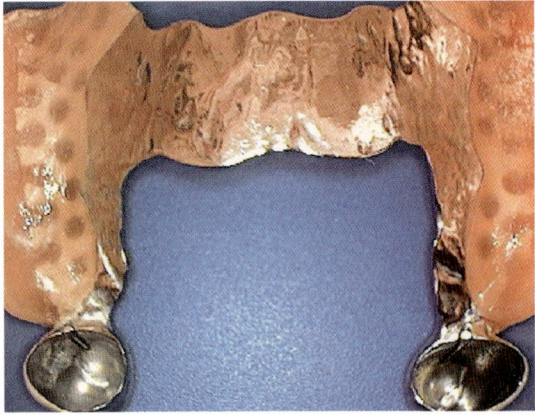

Former prosthesis from the previous day

Additional literature

Nikellis I, Levi A, Nicolopoulus C.Immediate loading of 190 endosseous dental implants:a prospective oberservational study of 40 patient treatments with up to 2-year data. Int J Oral Maxillofac Implants.19 (1):116-23.

Henry PJ, van Steenberghe D, Blombäck U, Polizzi G, Rosenberg R, Urgell JP, Wendelhag I. Prospective multicenter study on immediate rehabilitation of edentulous lower jaws according to the Branemark Novum protocol. Vlin Implant Dent Relat Res.2003; 5(3):137-42.

Degidi M, Nardi D, Piatelli A. Immediate versus one-stage restoration of small-diameter implants for a single missing maxillary lateral incisor:a 3-year randomizied clinical trial. J Periodontol.2009 Sep;80 (9):1393-8.

DegidiM, Piattelli A, Shibli JA, Perrotti V, Iezzi G.Early bone formation around immediately restored implants with and without occlusal contact: a juman histolgic and histomorphometiric evaluation. Case report: Int J Oral Maxillofax Implants. 24(4): 734-9.

Cannizzaro G, Torchio C, Leone M, Esposito M. Immediate versus early loading of flapless-planced implants supporting maxillary full-arch prostheses: a randomised controlled clinical trial. Eur J Oral Implantol.2008; 1 (2):127-39.

Chiapasco M. Early and immediate restoration and loading of implants in completely edentulous patients.Int J Oral Maxillofax Implants.2004;19 Suppl:76-91.

Ioannidou E, Doufexi A. Does loading time affect implant survival? A metaanalysis of 1.266 implants. J Periodontol.2005 Aug; 76(8):1252-8.

Misch CE, Wang HL, Misch CM, Sharawy M, Lemons J, Judy KW. Rationale for the application of immediate load in implnat dentistry: Part I. Implant Dent.2004 Sep; 13(3): 207-17.

Misch CE, Wang HL, Misch CM, Sharawy M, Lemons J, Judy KW. Rationale for the application of immediate load in implnat dentistry: Part II. Vlin Implant Dent Relat Res.2004; 13(4):310-21.

Romanos GE, Toh CG, Siar CH, Swaminathan D. Histologix and histomorphometric evaluation of peri-implant bone subjected to immediate loading: an experimental study with Macaca fascicularis. Int J Oral Maxillofac Implants.17 (1):44-51.

Testori T, Del Fabbro M, Galli F, Francetti L, Taschieri S, Weinstein R. Immediate occlusal loading the same day or the after implant placement: comparison of 2 different time frames in total edentulous lower jaws. J Oral Implantol.2004;30(5):307-13.

Urive R, Penarrocha M, Balaguer J, Fulfueiras N. Immediate loading in oral implants. Present situation. Med Oral Patol Oral Cir Bucal. 2005.

Ryser MR, Block MS, Mercante DE. Correlation of papilla to crestal bone levels around single tooth implants in immediate or delayed crown protocols. J Oral Maxillofac Surg.2005 Aug;63(8): 1184-95.

Tarnow DP; Emtiaz S, Classi A. Immediate loading of threaded implanta at stage 1 surgery in edentulous arches: ten consecutive case reports with1-to 5-year data. Int J Oral Maxillofac Implants.12(3): 319-24.

7.1.8/Case 8

Patient: male, 40 years old

11 extraction with Benex, immediate implant placement, crown

11/04/2011	11	extraction with Benex Champions® implant Ø 4.5 x 16 mm, >60 Ncm, Periotest 0 zirconium Prep-Caps, preparation dentist made temporary
12/04/2011	11	cemented laboratory made temporary, splinting
09/06/2011	11	post-preparation impression, Periotest -1
23/06/2011	11	cemented zirconium dioxide crown

Treatment period: **2.5 months**

Remarks: Immediate implant placement
Extraction with Benex
Direction change of the implant axis during the
implant placement

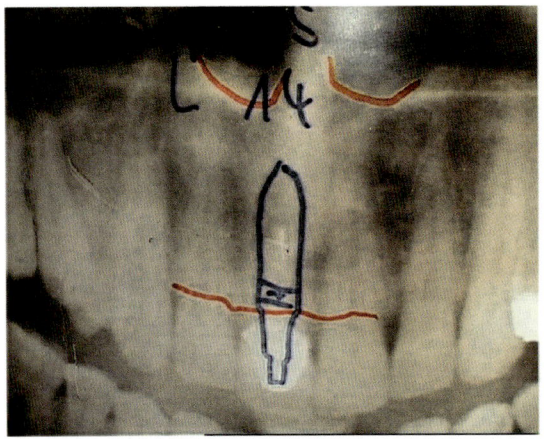

Planned treatment, initial panoramic radiograph

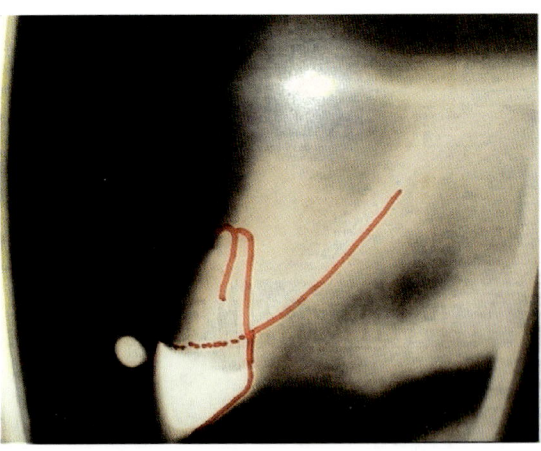

11 cross-sectional image

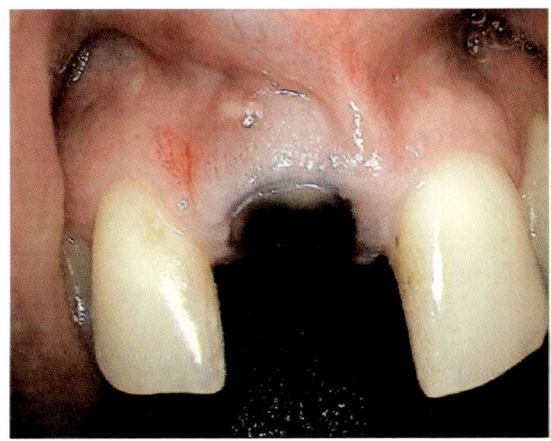

Decapitation, anterior view

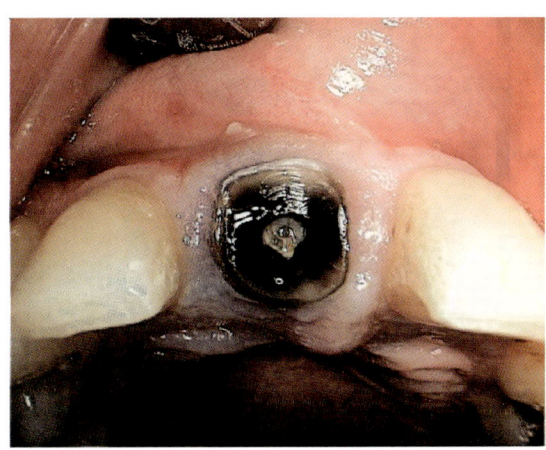

Decapitation, occlusal view

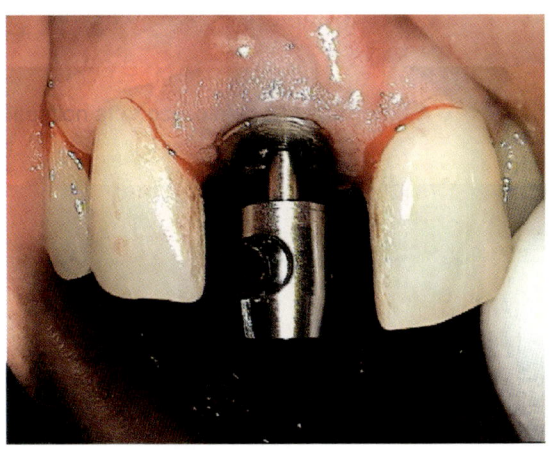

Inserted extraction screw

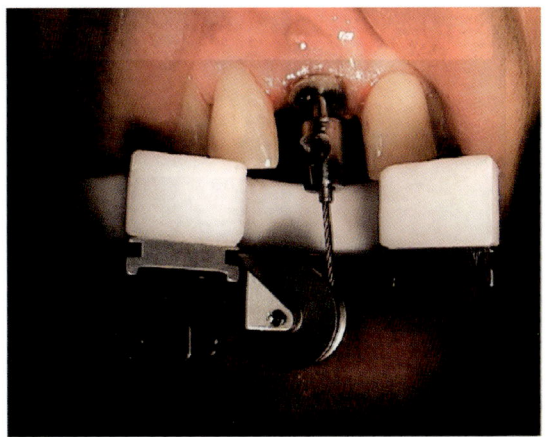

Positioned extractor tool

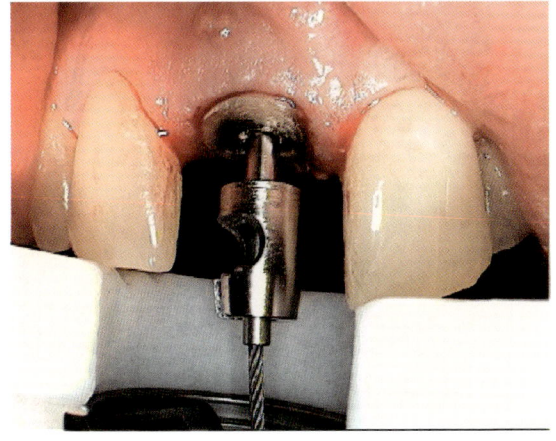

By means of controlled and slow turning...

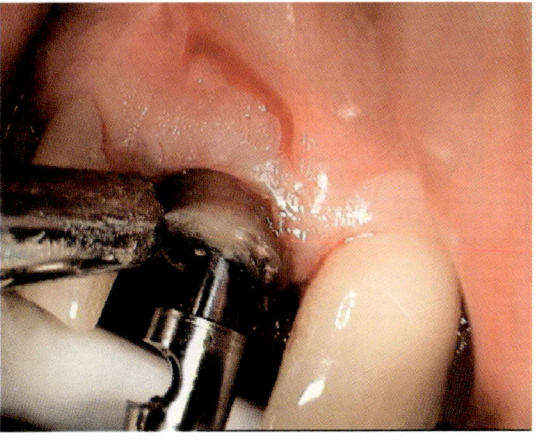

...the tooth is luxated...

57

The author

DS Frank Schrader, Albertstr. 33, D-39261 Zerbst/Anhalt

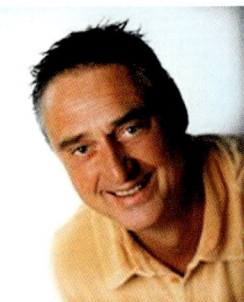

1981–86
- Studies of dental medicine at the Martin-Luther-Universität in Halle-Wittenberg in Germany

1986
- State examination
- Diploma thesis with a Master's degree in Stomatology

1991
- own dental office in Zerbst

1998
- Member of the German Association for Dental, Oral and Orthodontic Medicine (Deutsche Gesellschaft für Zahn-, Mund-, und Kieferheilkunde, DGZMK)

1999
- Member of the Implant Association for Dentists (IGfZ eG, Implantologische Genossenschaft für Zahnärzte)
- Member of implant associations: German Association of Dental Implantology (Deutsche Gesellschaft für Implantologie, DGI), Middle German State Association for Dental Implantology (Mitteldeutsche Landesverband für Zahnärztliche Implantologie, MVZI)
- Presentations for patients
- Presentations and training for dentists
- National and International publications in the field of implantology

2007
- Foundation of an Implantology continuing education centre
- Live- surgical procedures
- Hands-on courses
- Live-broadcast from the operating room into the conference room
- Dental training for dentists
- More than 700 implants per year
- Reference and training practice for the German company CHAMPIONS®-IMPLANTS-GMBH

2012
- Publishing of the implant book „Teeth in a day" part I

2013
- Publishing of the implant book „Teeth in day" part II

Fon +49(0)3923/2097
Fax +49(0)3923/612521
info@zahnarzt-zerbst.de

www.zahnarzt-zerbst.de
www.teethinaday.de
www.implantologisches-zentrum-zerbst.de

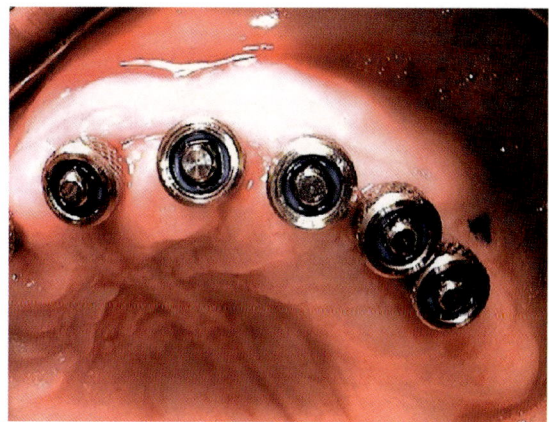

Implant placement, upper jaw and left side

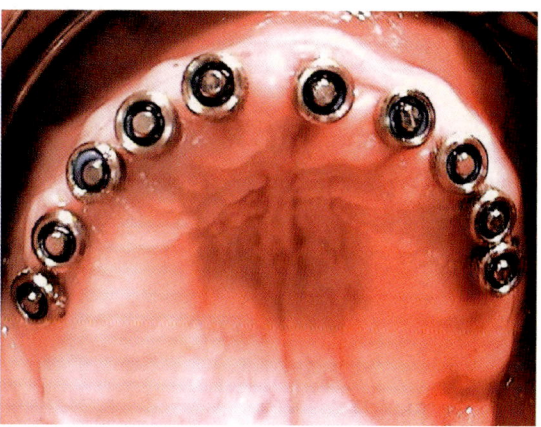

Completed implant placement, with attached metal matrices

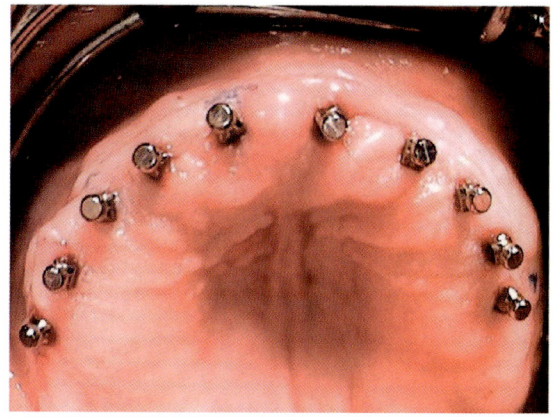

Completed implant placement, without matrices

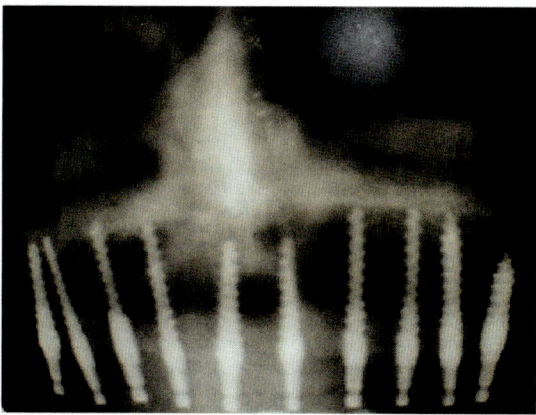

Panoramic radiographic control

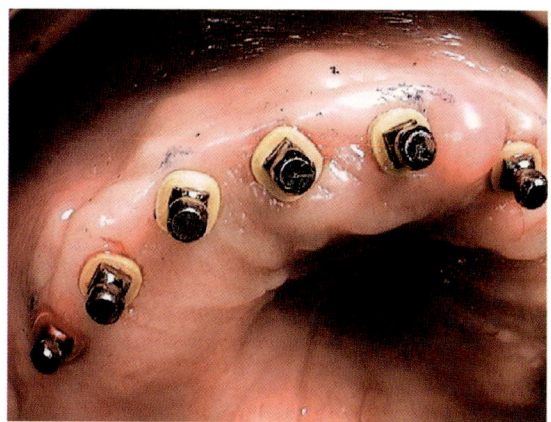

Rubber rings to prevent non-removal of the prosthesis after the cementing of the matrices into the prosthesis

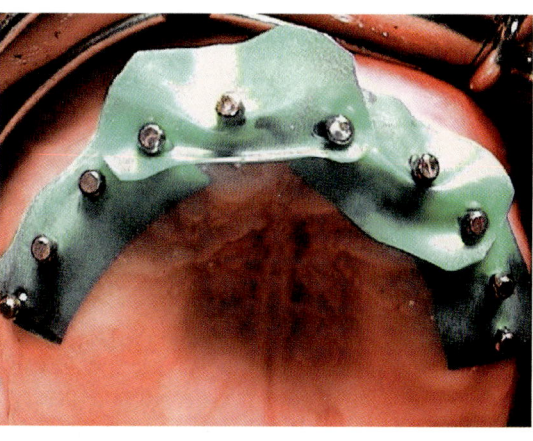

Rubber dam to protect the gingiva and the implants

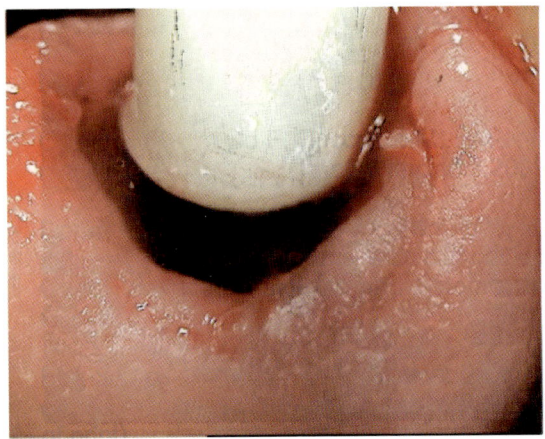

On the day of surgery, palatal view

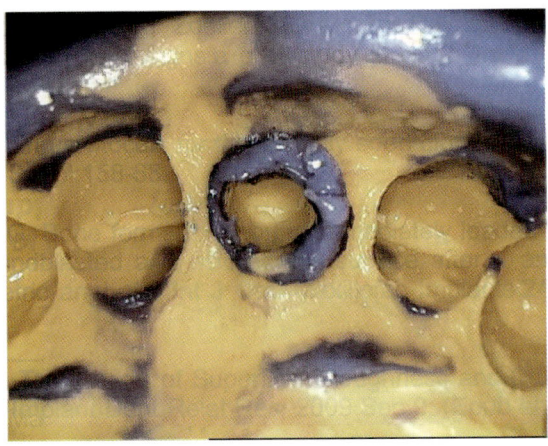

Impression taking for laboratory made temporary

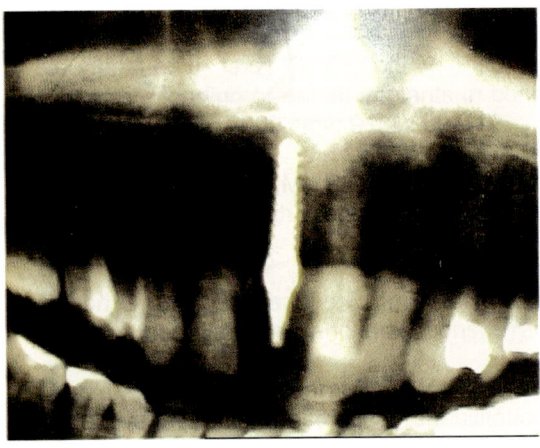

Final radiographic control, panoramic radiograph

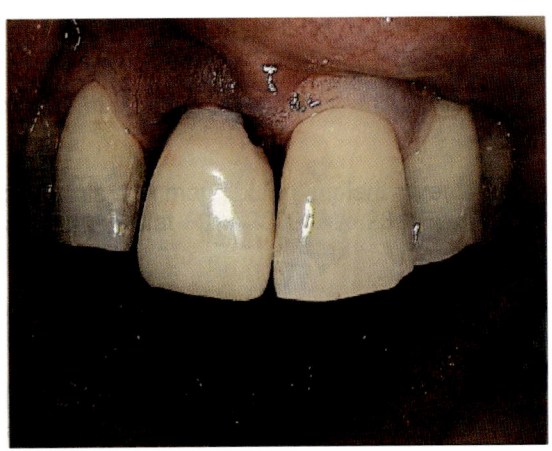

Dentist made temporary

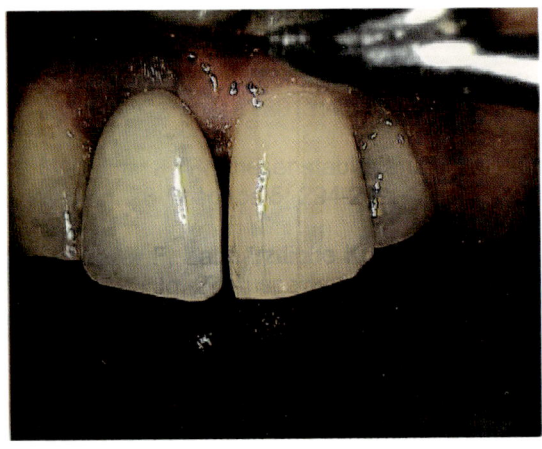

Laboratory made temporary, gingival contact is too strong

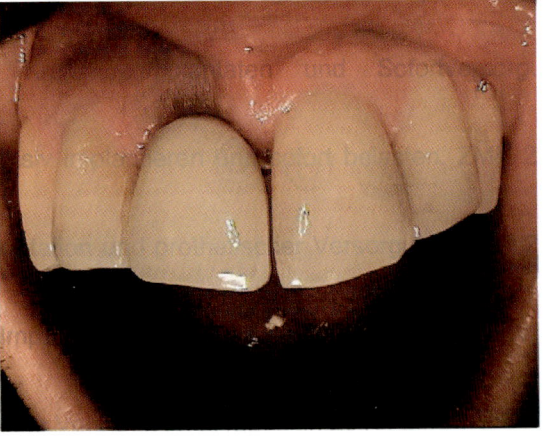

Laboratory made temporary, shortened and adapted

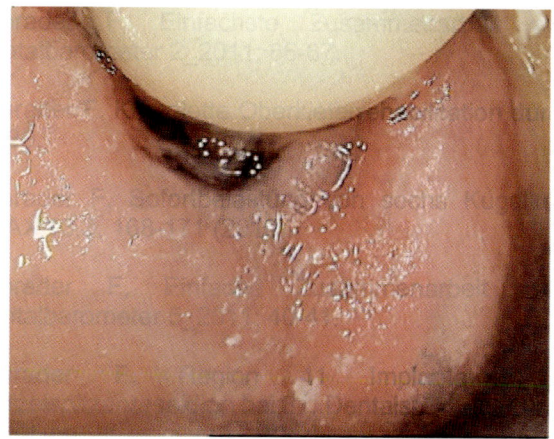

1st postoperative day, palatal view

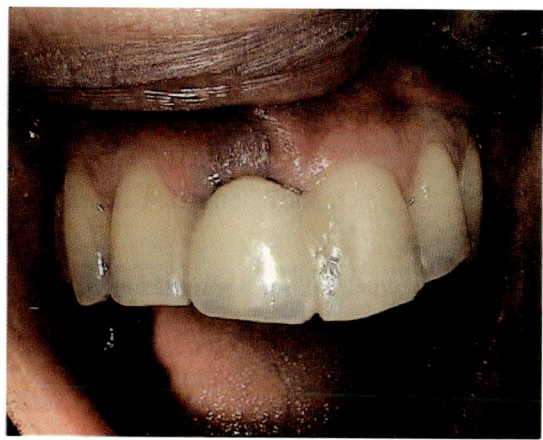

Splinted laboratory made temporary, 1st postoperative day...

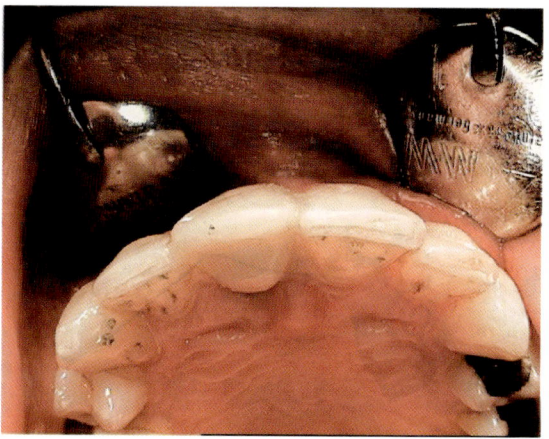

...and incisal view

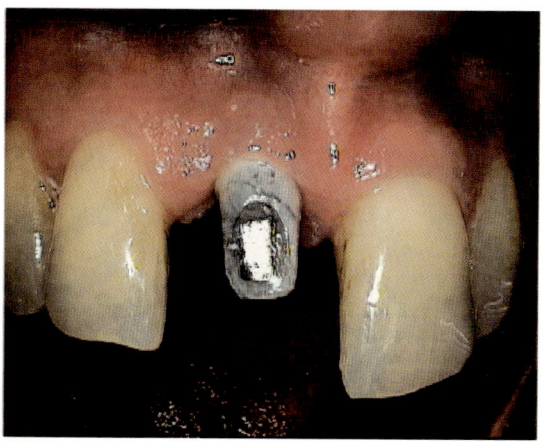

Clinical situation before impression taking...

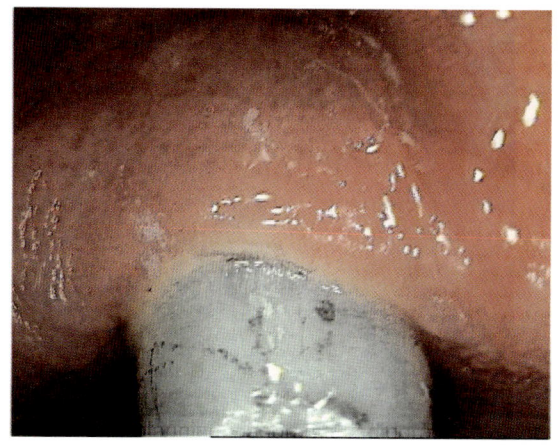

...and close-up view

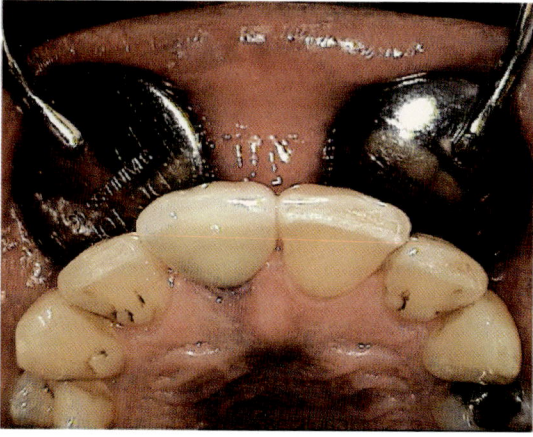

Final cemented crown

Acknowledgement

Oh my dear,

So many people helped me.

My first thanks go to my team who had and still has to handle the daily stress with me. Even though if the journey is the reward - you had to struggle through "our perfectionism".
Permanently in weekly half-our lasting team meetings you were challenged to implement the constantly changing parameters and working procedures.
Thank you so much!

I wish to thank my long-term mate Bert Siegemund, who has not only produced DVDs on traditional implant placements with me, but who also has brought this book forward to you. Thanks for burning the midnight oil, so it looks like you like me, really like me.

I thank Dr. Armin Nedjat the "Champions inventor" who has the substance of a genius in the Champions implantology for providing me with his illustrations.

I thank Dr. Ulrich Brause for his meticulous proofreading and his advice.
For all the time you sacrificed.
Seriously: Thanks a lot for doing a great job.

I also thank all the other many "Champions" who ensured suggestions and improvements.

I thank both my dental laboratories (Dentaltec Michael Schmidt and Dentallabor Thomas Reckrühm) for their professional denture works and in particular you, Thomas for your efforts to fulfil my ambitious expectations.

I thank my parents who raised me to be the person that I am today.

I thank my sweetheart for her patience to do without me in the small hours..
For her affectionate willingness to endure my impatience and for her calmness to tolerate without complaints my daily shoptalk as a dental layman.

Most of all I wish to thank you, who read my first book. For the fact that you hopefully let me know what I have forgotten or what I have done wrong in order to maybe quench your thirst for knowledge in "Implantology 2 - immediate implant placement forever."

Yours,
Frank Schrader

7.1.9/Case 9

Patient: male, 36 years old

21 immediate implant placement, Prep-Cap, crown

20/05/2011	21	extraction Champions® implant Ø 4.5 x 14 mm, >40 Ncm, Periotest 0 cemented zirconium Prep-Cap preparation cemented dentist made temporary
21/05/2011	21	cemented laboratory made temporary, splinted
02/08/2011	21	Impression, Periotest -3
16/08/2011	21	cemented zirconium dioxide crown

Treatment period: **3 months**

Remarks: Palatal pilot hole preparation of the implant cavity
Leaving a ledge to easier adapt
the mucous layer after extraction.

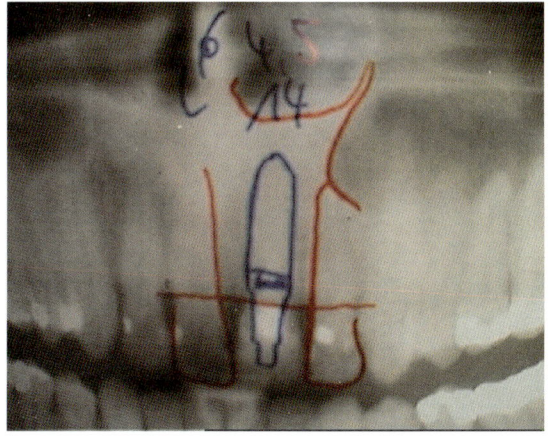

Panoramic radiograph for planned treatment

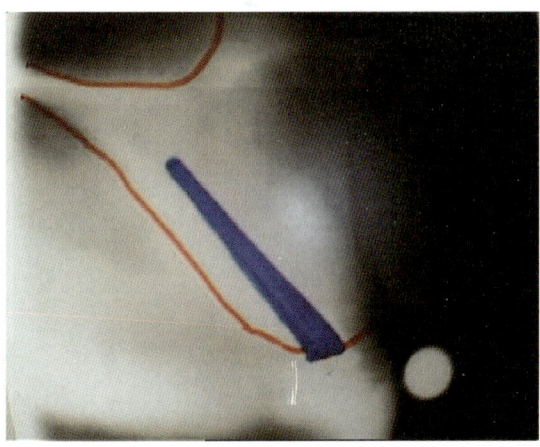

Cross-sectional radiography, including planned implant placement...

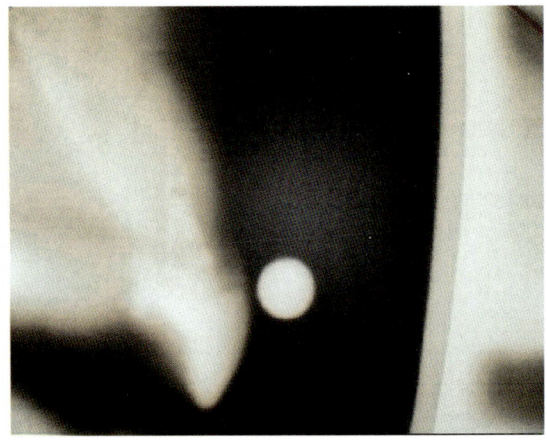

...and without planned implant placement

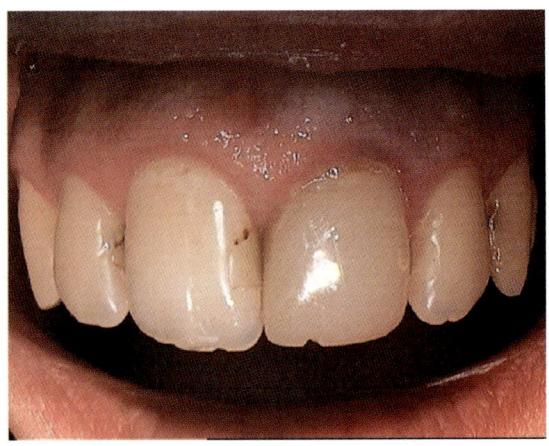

Clinical initial situation, anterior view

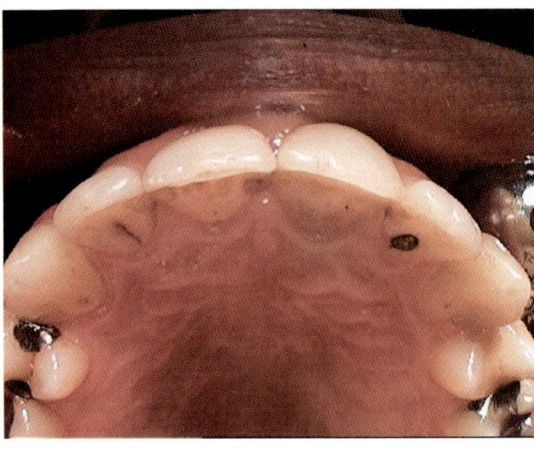

Clinical initial situation, palatal view

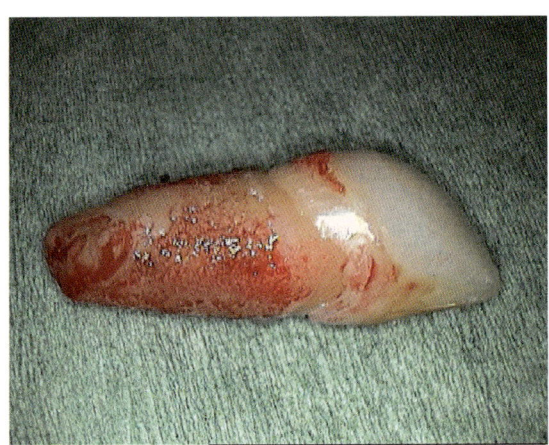

Extracted tooth 21

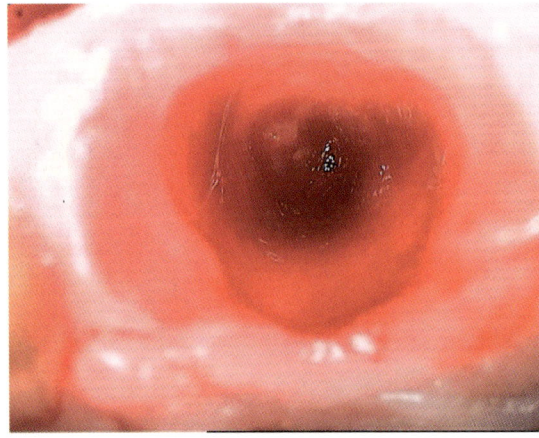

Alveolus after extraction...

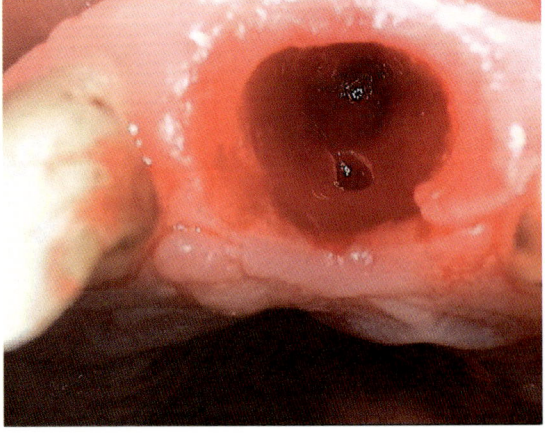

...with palatal pilot hole preparation

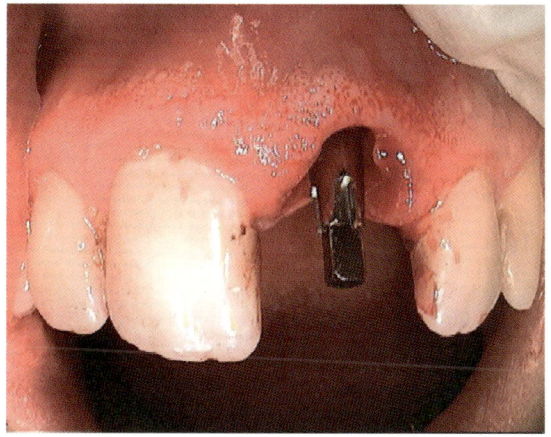

Completed implant placement, anterior view

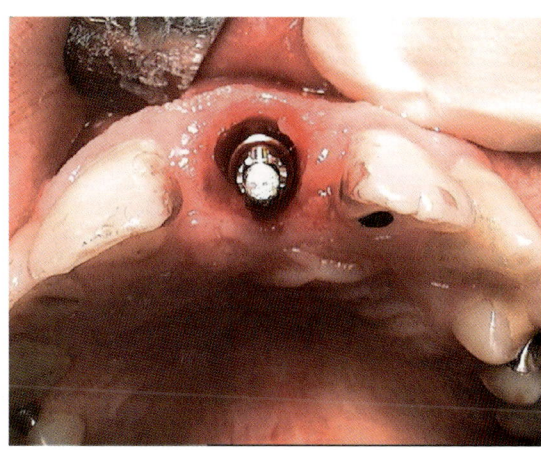

Completed implant placement, incisal view

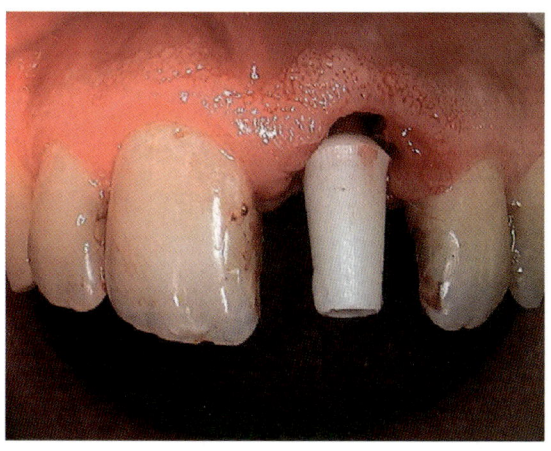

Cemented PC, anterior view

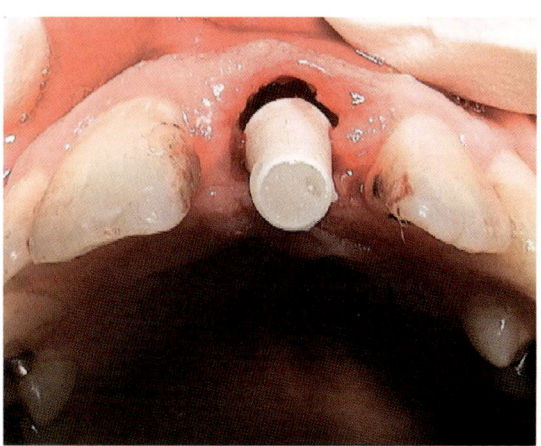

Cemented PC, incisal view

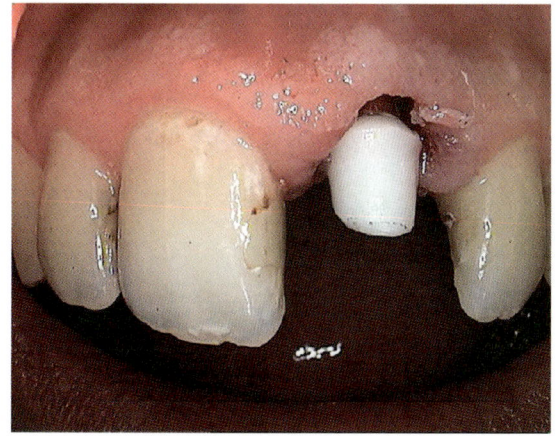

Prepared PC, anterior view

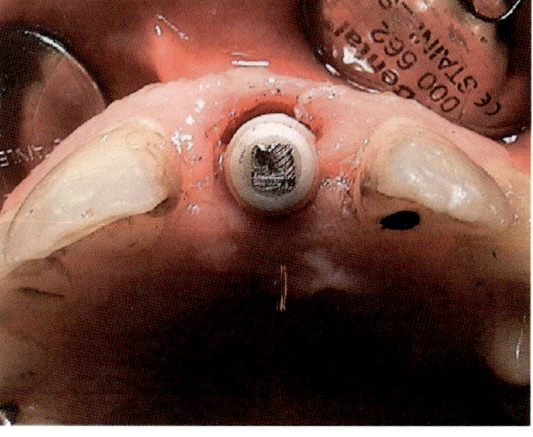

Prepared PC, incisal view

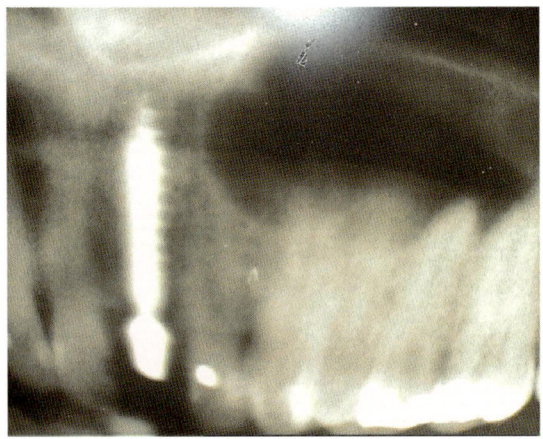

Radiographic control, panoramic radiograph

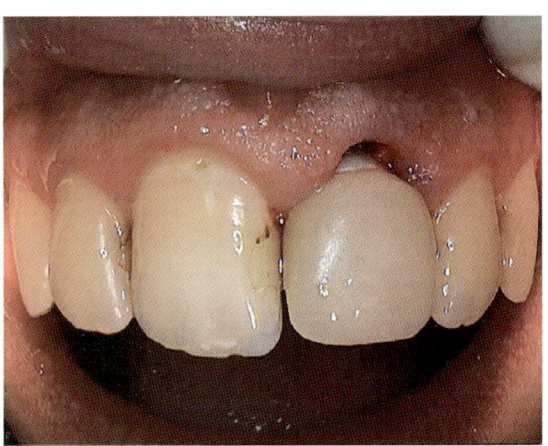

1st postoperative day, laboratory made temporary extends up to the PC ledge

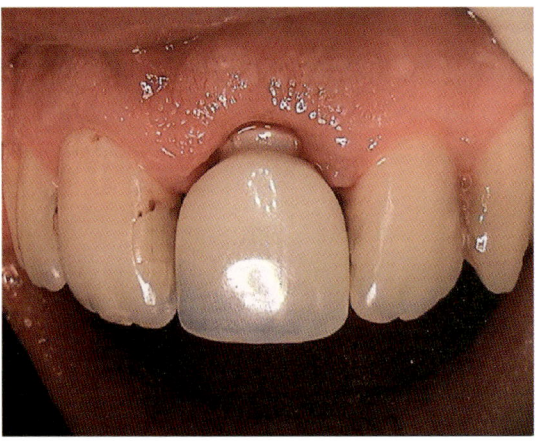

1st postoperative day, laboratory made temporary has been selectively shortened

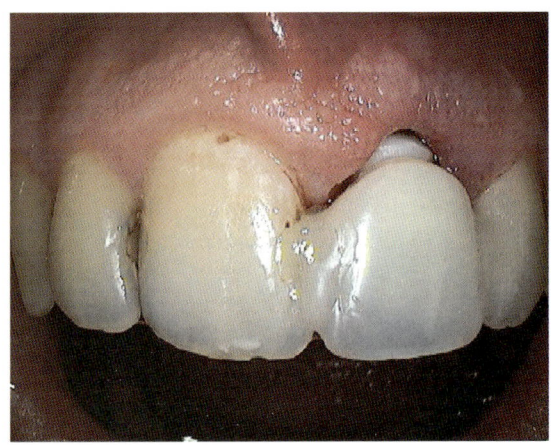

Splinted laboratory made temporary

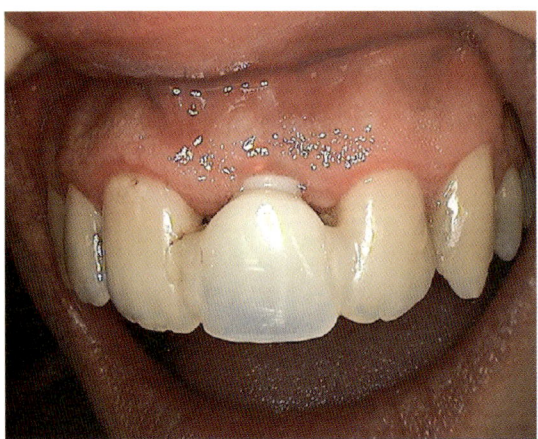

Clinical situation after osseointegration

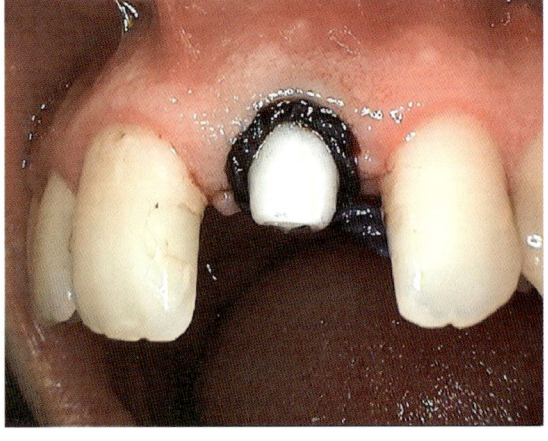

Retraction suture in regio 21, before impression taking

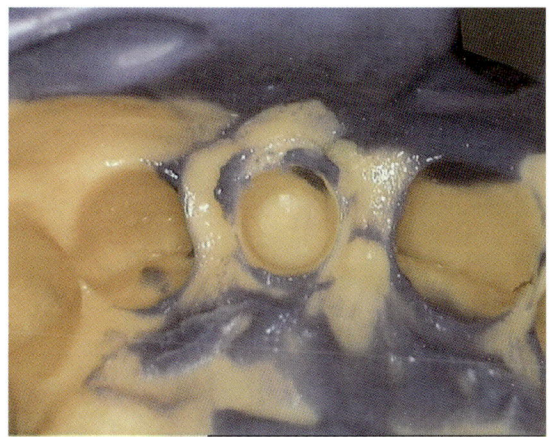

Impression taking

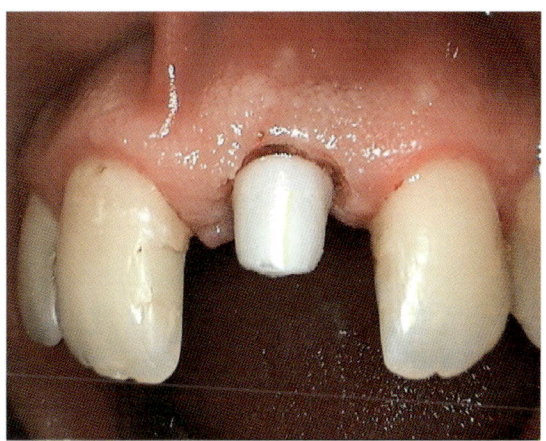

Before insertion of the crown in regio 21, anterior view

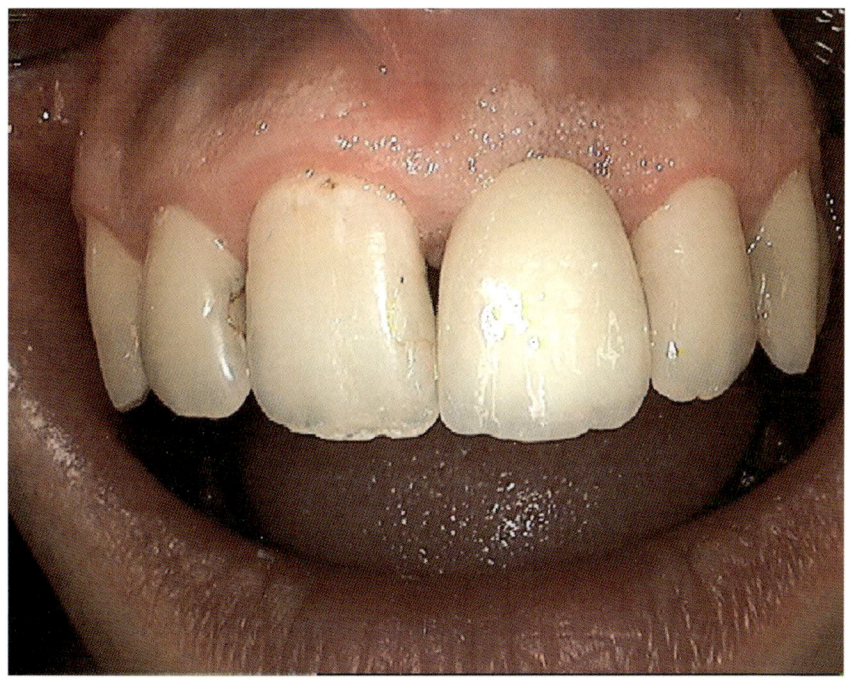

After insertion of the crown in regio 21, anterior view

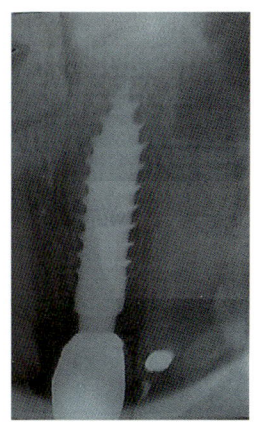

Final radiographic control

7.1.10/Case 10

Patient: male, 30 years old

15 immediate implant placement, Prep-Cap, crown

17/03/2011	15	extraction Champions® implant Ø 5.5 x 10 mm, 50 Ncm, Periotest -1 zirconium Prep-Cap cemented with GlasIonomer based cement and prepared cemented frasaco crown, splinted
30/05/2011		impression, Periotest -1 new cemented dentist made temporary
16/06/2011		Cemented zirconium dioxide crown
Treatment period:		**3 months**
Remarks:		Indirect sinus lift Protection of the "holy" vestibular layer Maximum gingival retention by leaving a blank for the ledge on the PC.

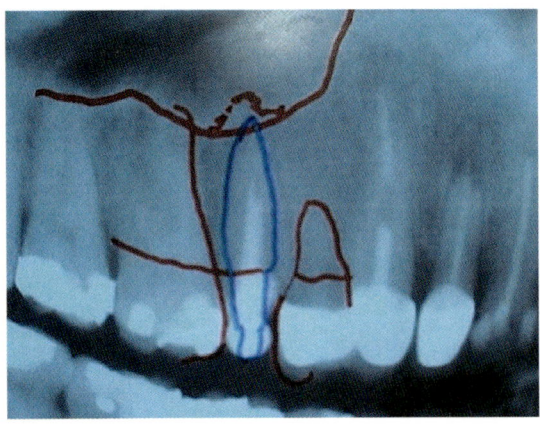

Planned treatment, initial panoramic radiograph

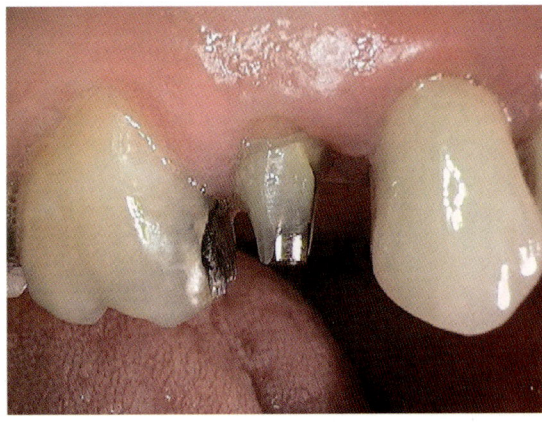

Clinical situation with...

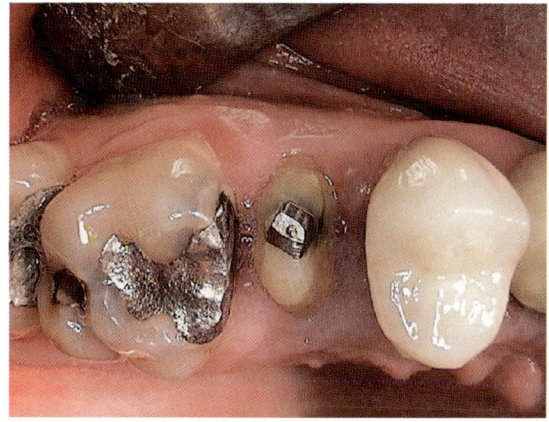

...fractured tooth

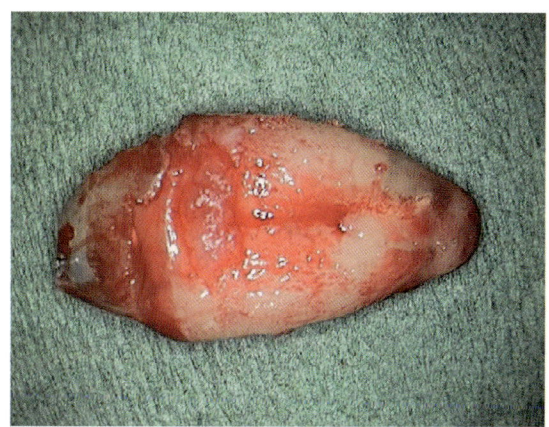

Extracted tooth 15

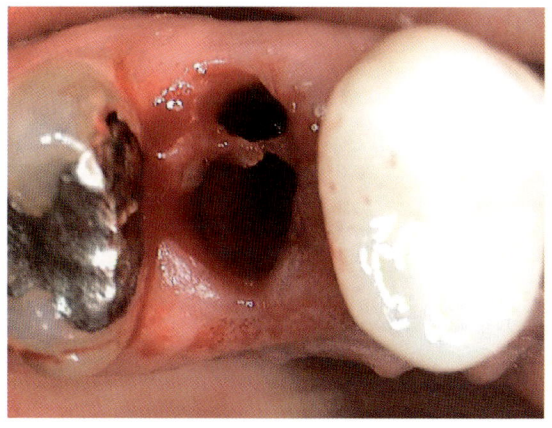

Alveolus after extraction, occlusal view

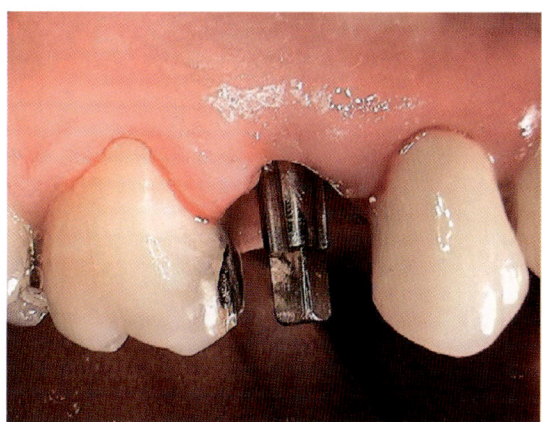

Implant in situ, vestibular view

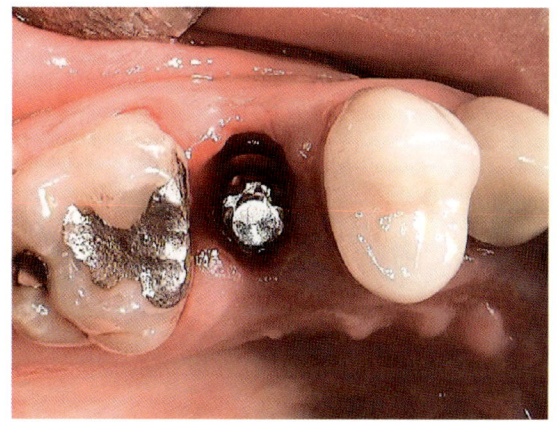

Implant, occlusal view

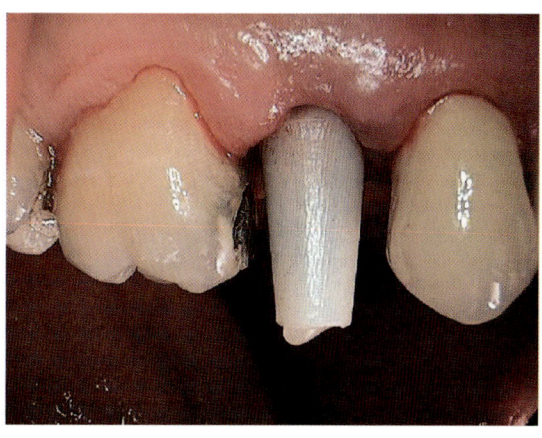

Cemented PC, vestibular view

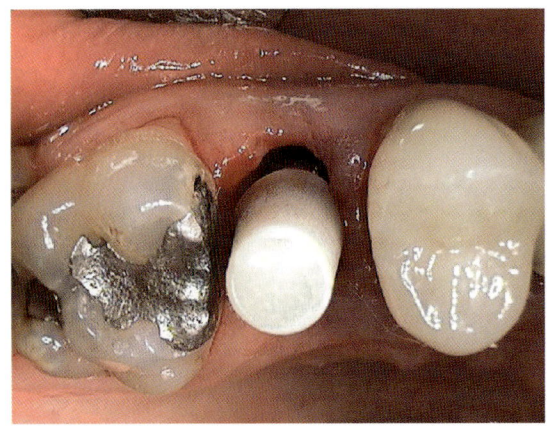

Cemented PC, occlusal view

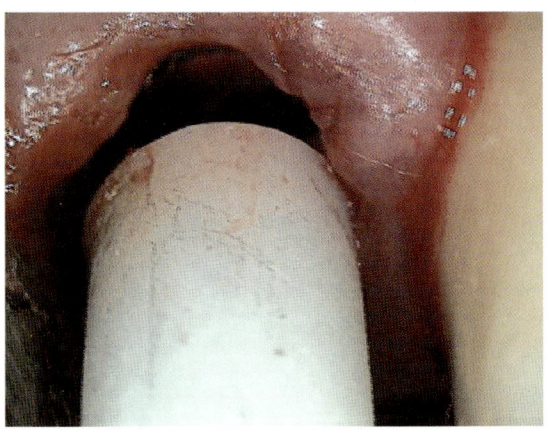

Cemented PC, macro image, vestibular view

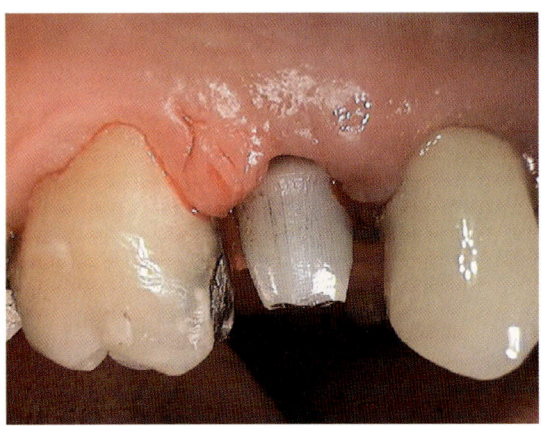

PC after preparation, vestibular view

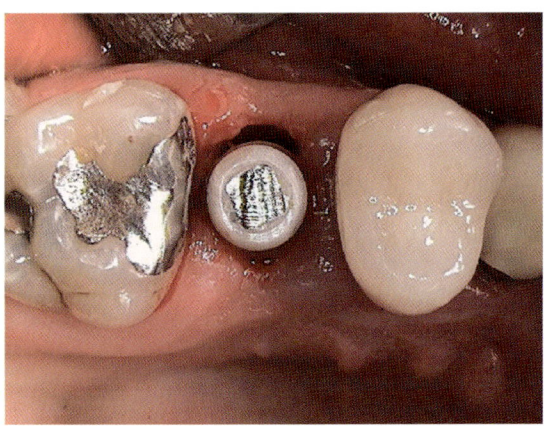

PC after preparation, occlusal view

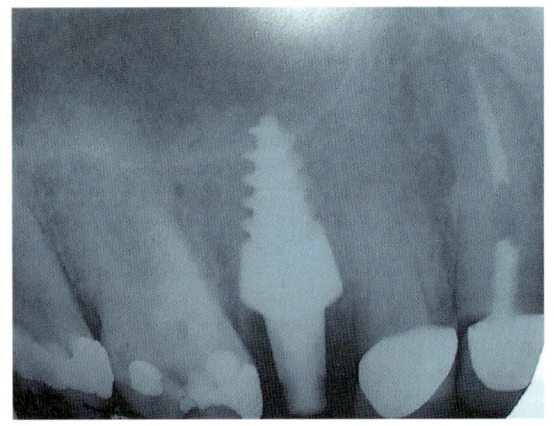

Radiographic control, panoramic radiograph

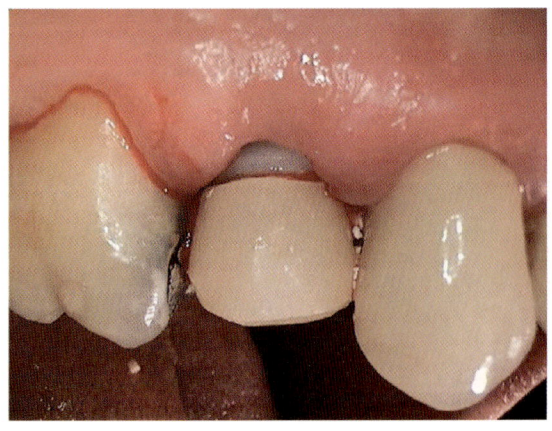

Dentist made temporary without ledge contact

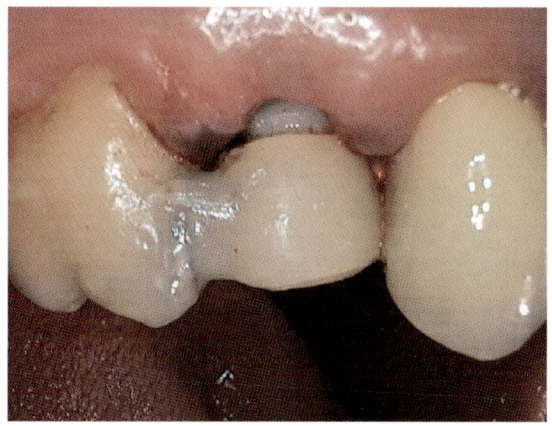

...with resin splinting

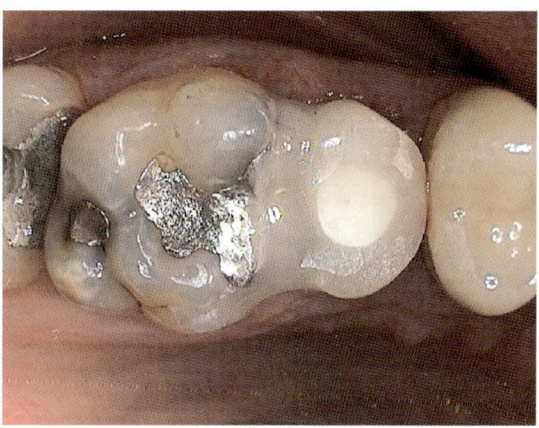

Splinted with neighbouring tooth, occlusal view

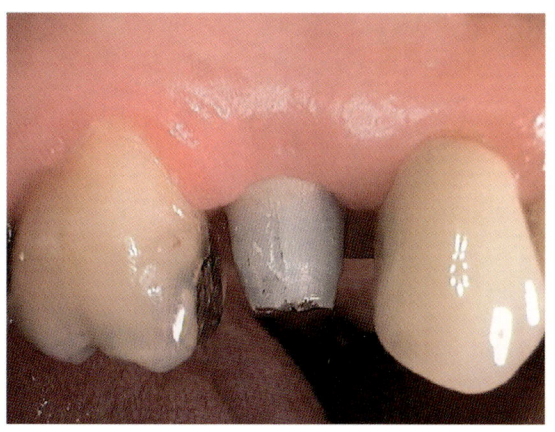

Situation before impression taking

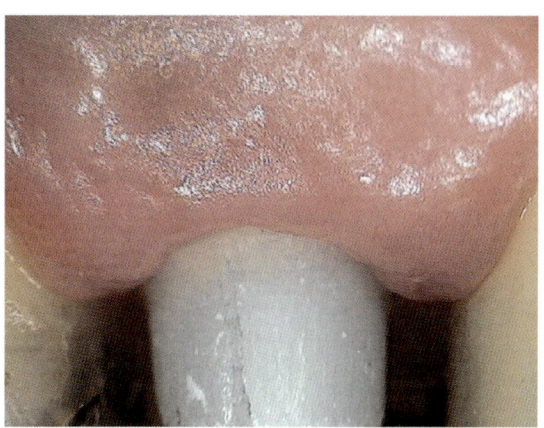

Before impression taking, macro image, gingiva free from inflammation

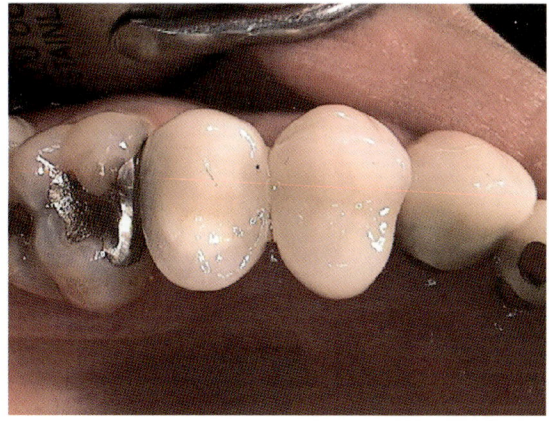

Final crown, occlusal view

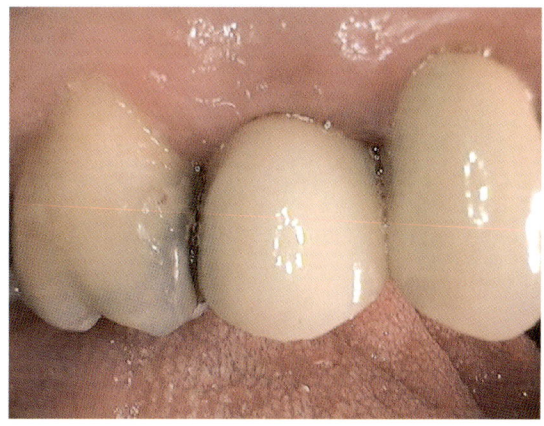

Final crown, vestibular view

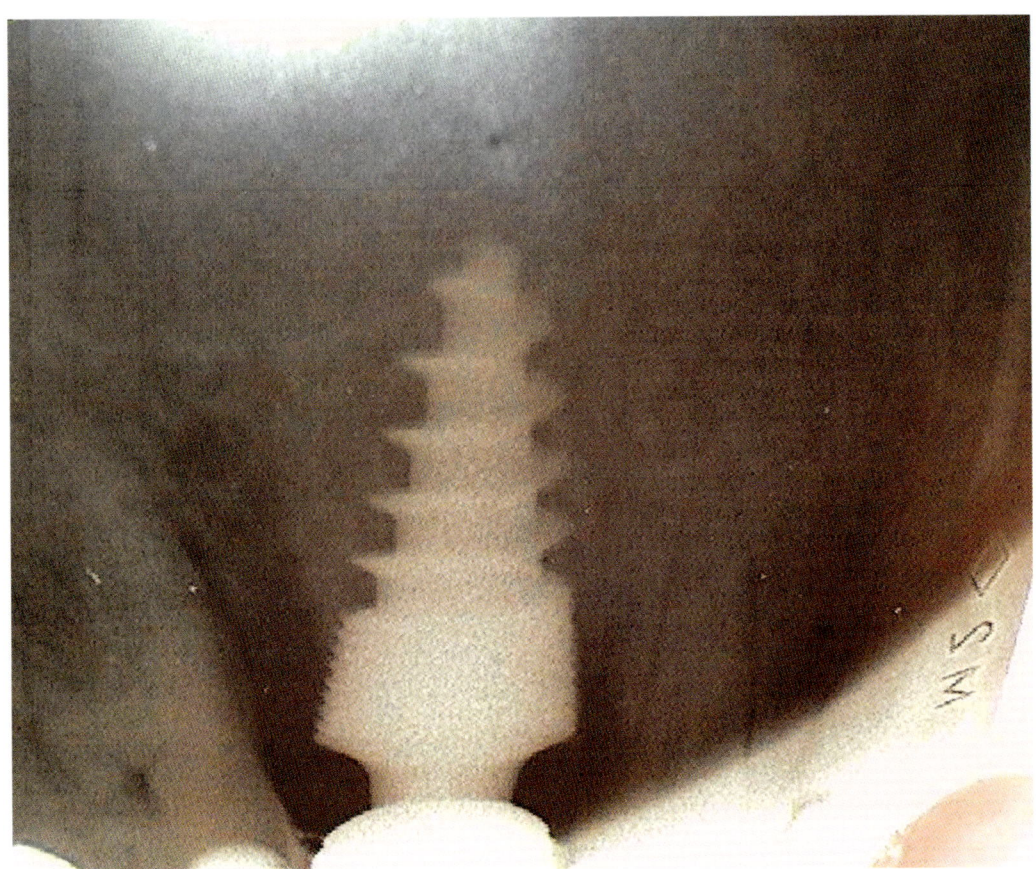

Final X-ray, zoomed picture

7.1.11/Case 11

Patient: female, 31 years old

25 immediate implant placement, zirconium dioxide crown

27/06/2011	25	extraction Champions® implant Ø 5.5 x 10 mm, >60 Ncm, Periotest 0 preparation dentist made temporary
28/06/2011		Wound control
14/08/2011	25	impression, Periotest 0
27/09/2011	25	cemented zirconium dioxide crown
Treatment period:		**3 months**
Remarks:		Implant placement into the scooped alveolus Late loading

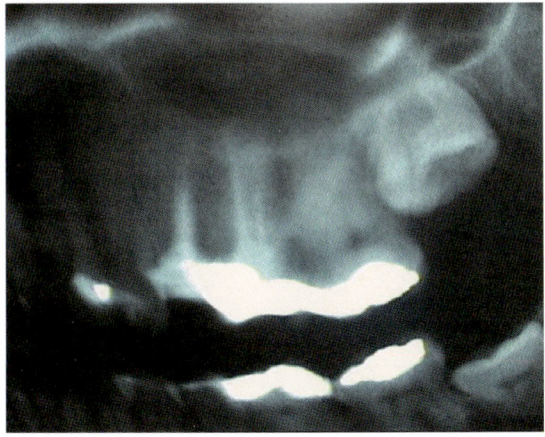

Initial panoramic radiograph

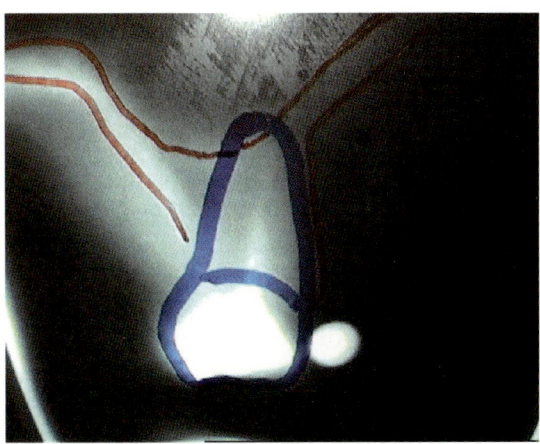

Cross-sectional image

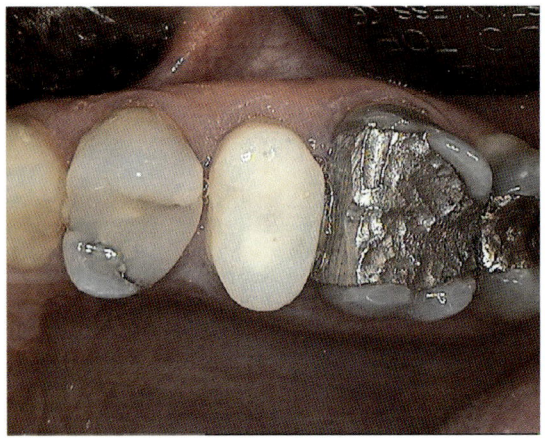

Before extraction of tooth 25

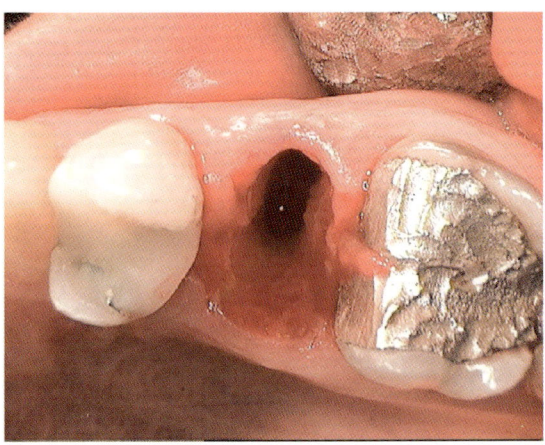

Alveolus after extraction of tooth 25

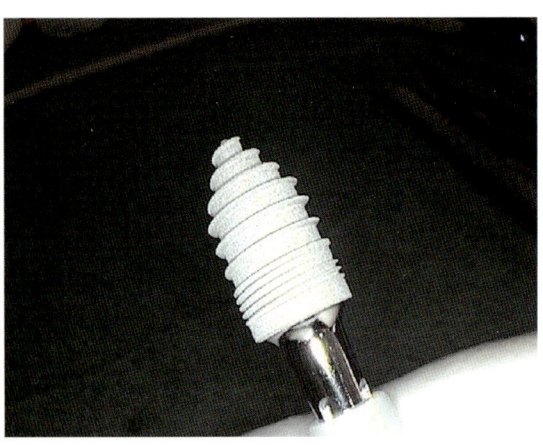

Implant ⌀ 5.5 x 10

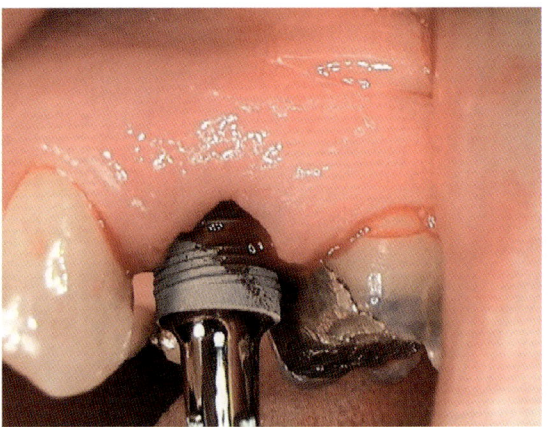

Implant placement at the beginning

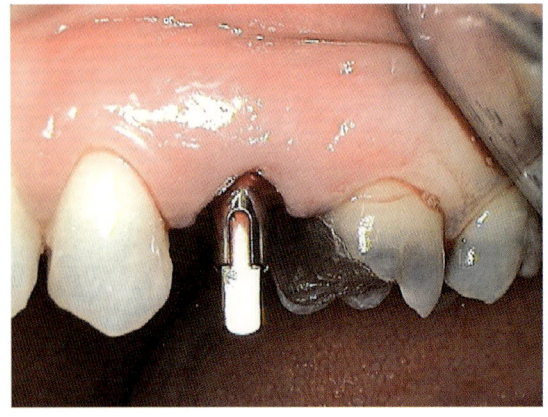

Completed implant placement, lateral view

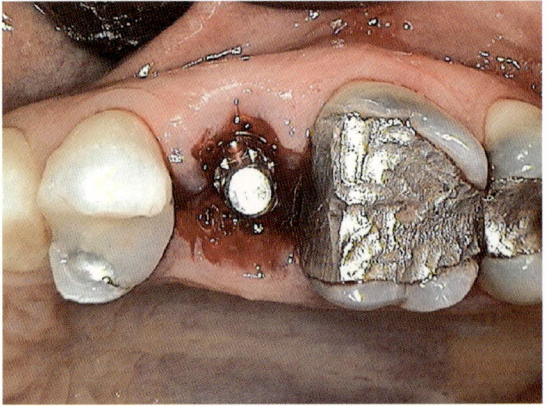

Completed implant placement, occlusal view

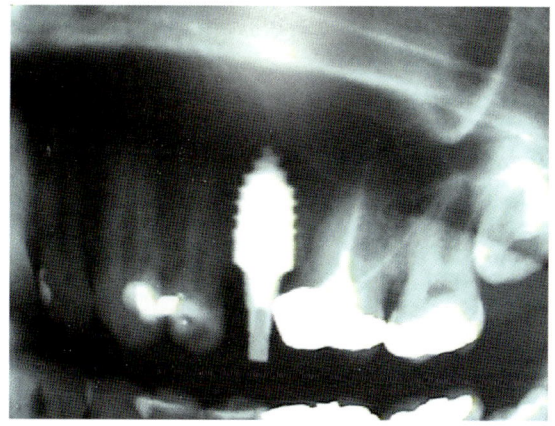

Panoramic radiographic control

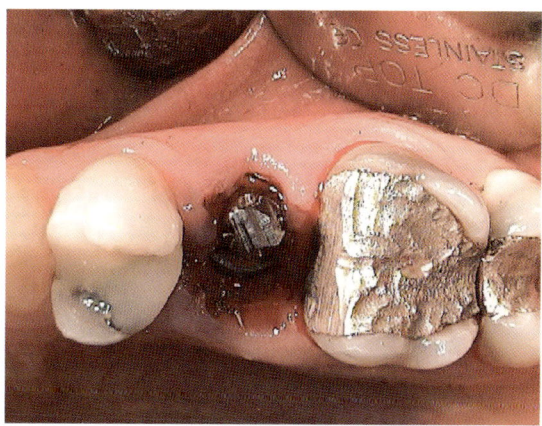

Prepared implant head, occlusal view

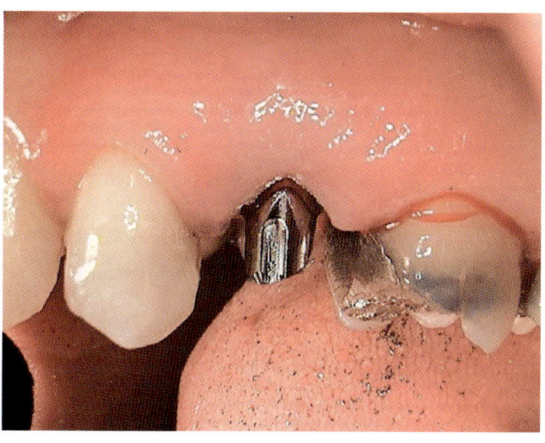

Prepared implant head, lateral view

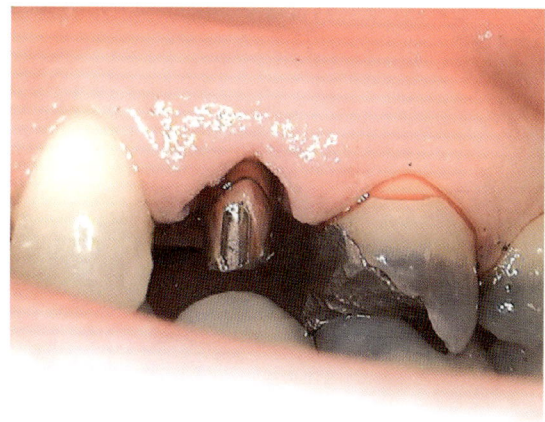

Prepared implant head in habitual occlusion

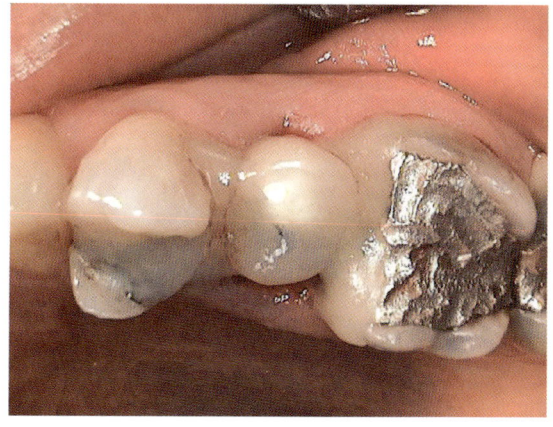

verblocktes ZA-Provisorium, Ansicht von okklusal

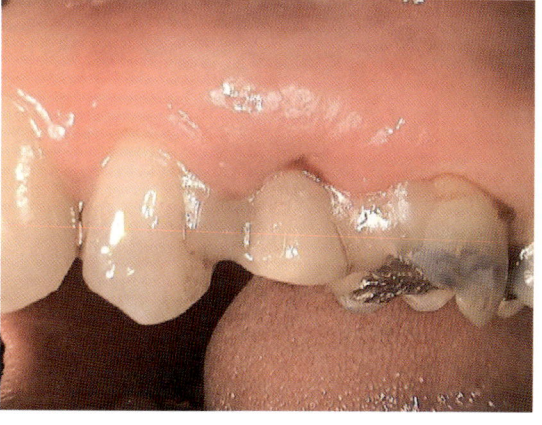

verblocktes ZA-Provisorium, Ansicht von lateral

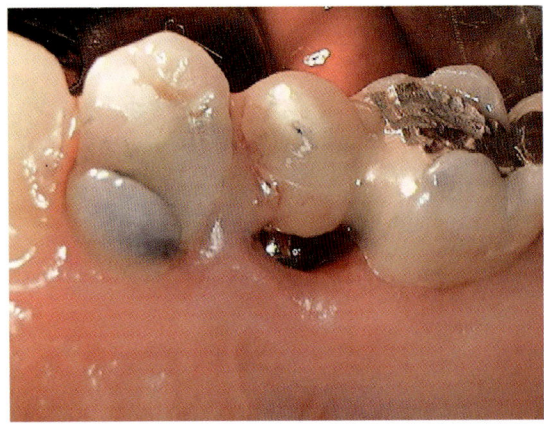

Splinted dentist made temporary, palatal view

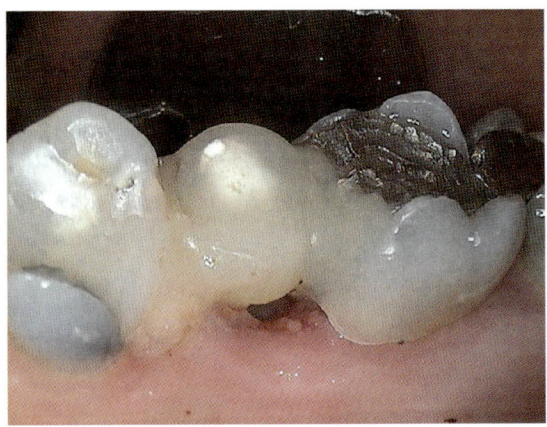

... and on the 1st postoperative day

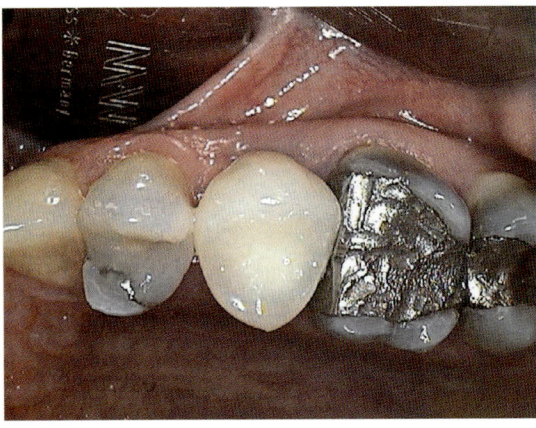

Final cemented crown, occlusal view

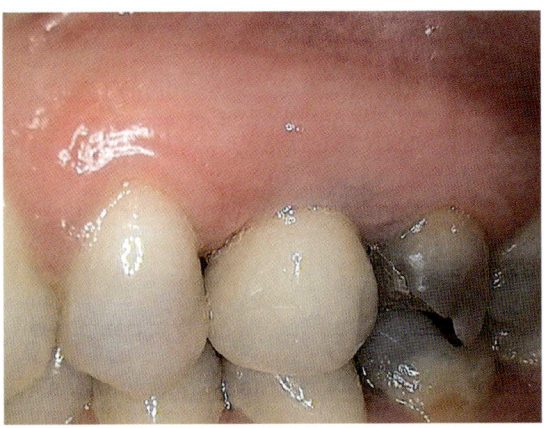

Final cemented crown, lateral view

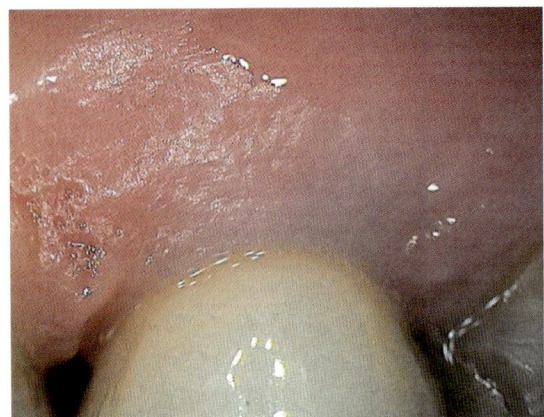

Final cemented crown, macro image

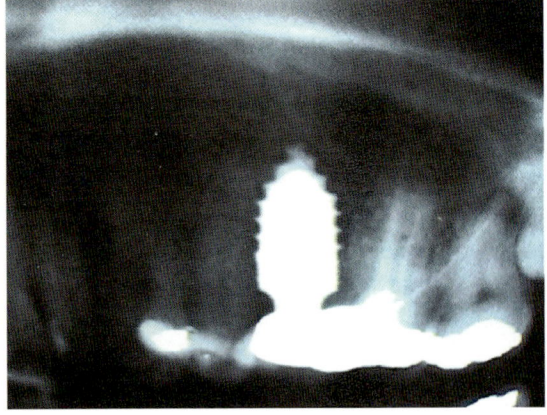

Radiograph final control, zoomed panoramic radiographic detail

7.1.12/Case 12

Patient: male, 66 years old

31,41 immediate implant placement, Prep-Caps zirconium dioxide crown

---

26/11/2009	31, 41, 42	extraction
	31, 42	Champions® implant Ø 3.0 x 16 mm, >40 Ncm
		zirconium Prep-Caps
		preparation
		splinted dentist made temporary
09/02/2010	31- 42	cemented zirconium dioxide crown

Treatment period: **2.5 months**

Remarks:
Immediate implant placement
Use of Prep-Caps
In case of incisor teeth in the lower jaw
an 1:1 implant placement can be abandoned.
Late loading

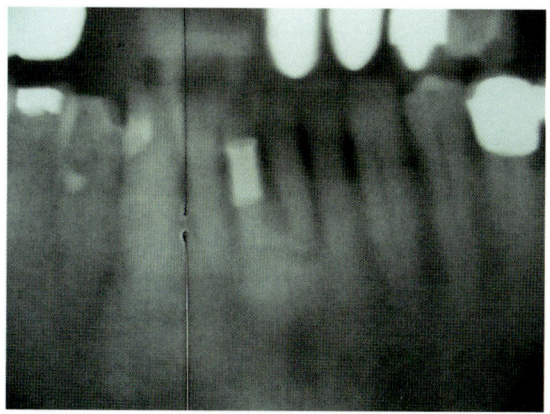

Panoramic radiograph with X-ray measuring device

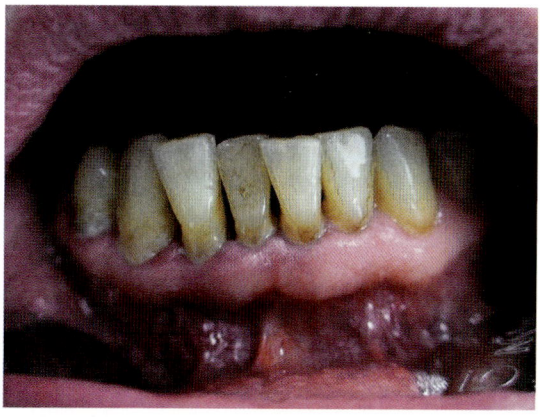

Clinical initial situation, anterior view

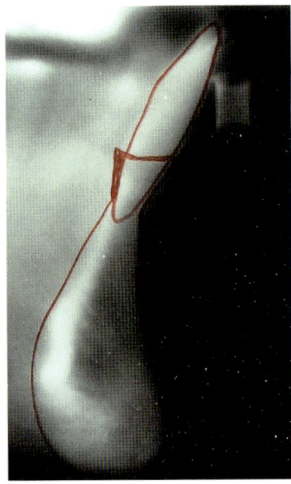

Cross-sectional radiography

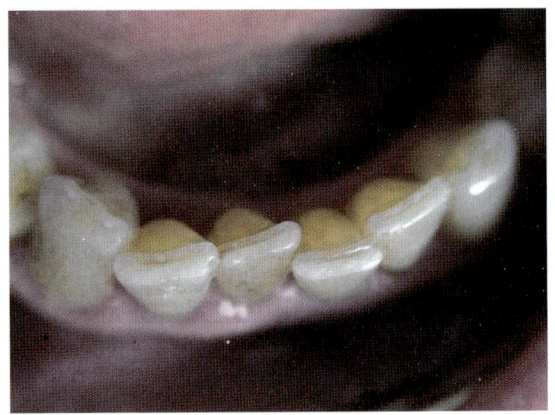

Clinical initial situation, occlusal view

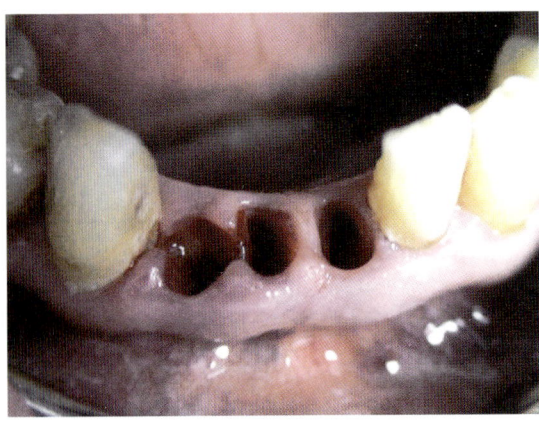

...and alveoli after extraction

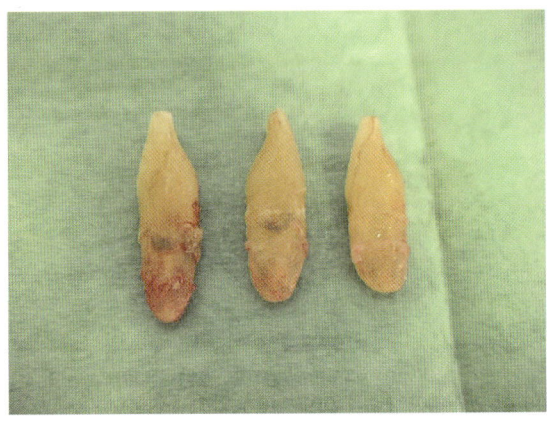

Extracted teeth

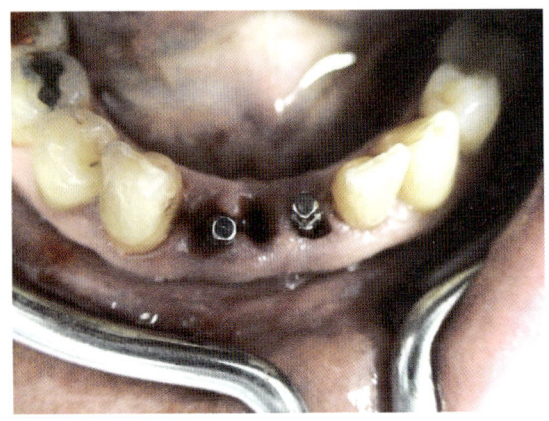

31, 42 implant placement

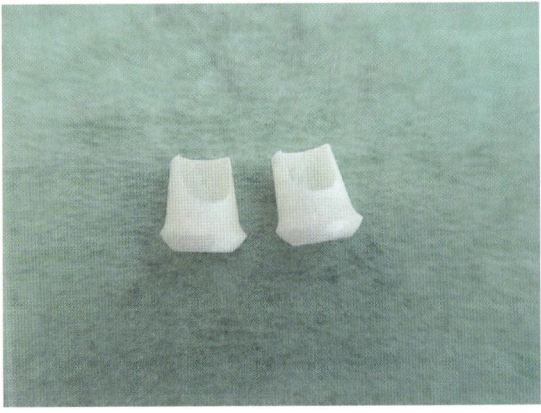

selected PCs...

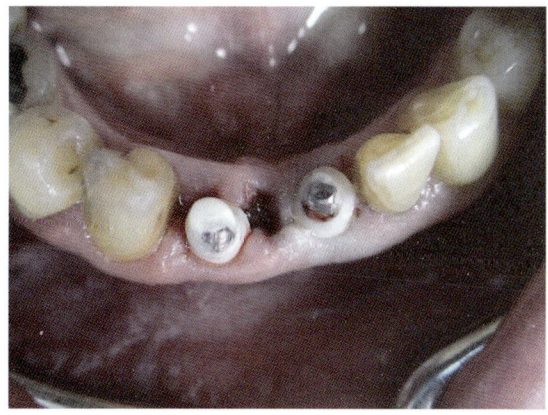

...cemented and prepared

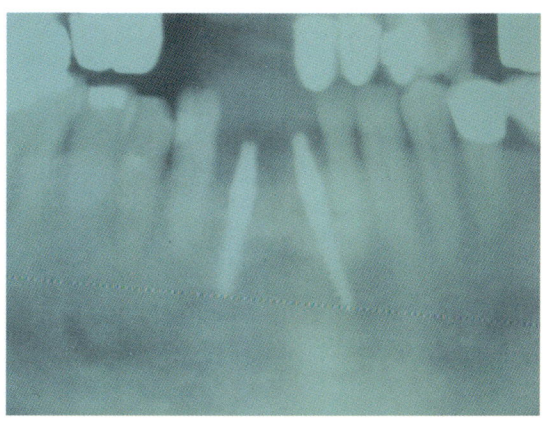

Panoramic radiographic control of the implants

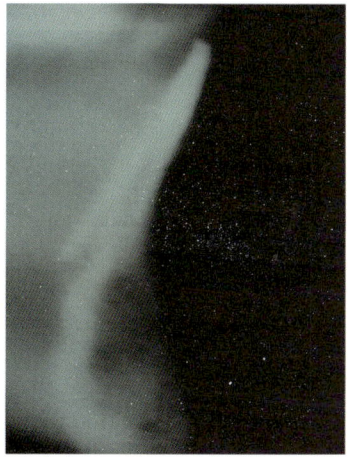

Radiographic control, cross-sectional image

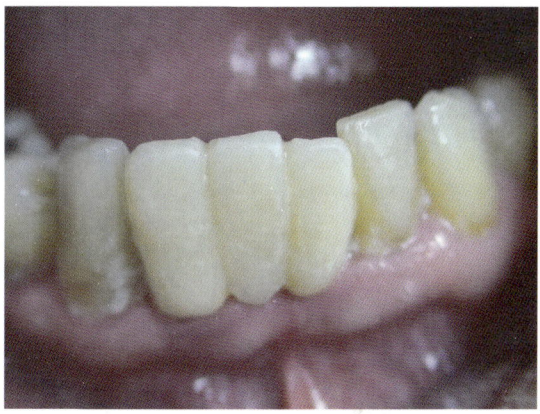

Cemented dentist made temporary

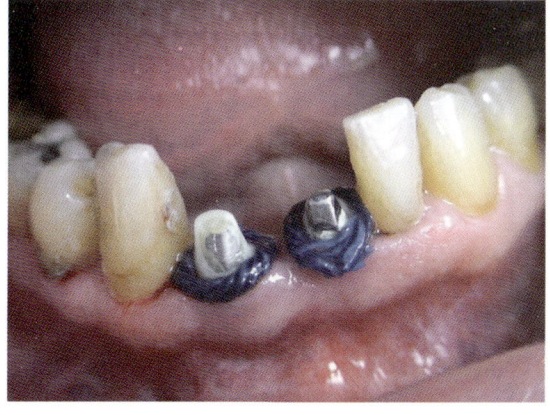

Retraction sutures before impression taking

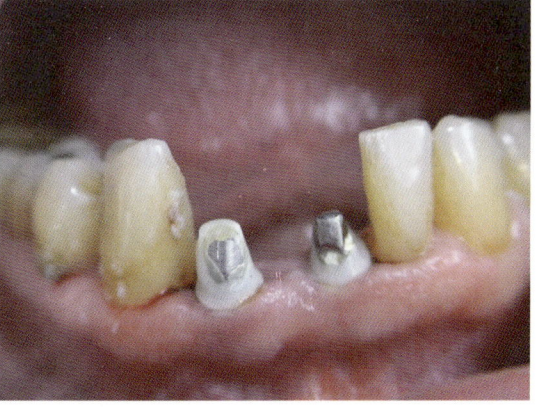

Prepared implant heads with PC before impression taking

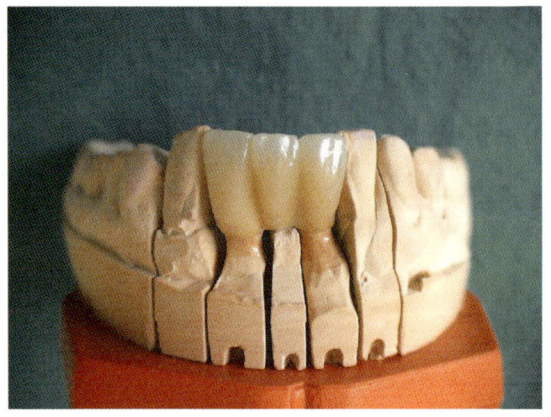

Bridge onto the cast, anterior view

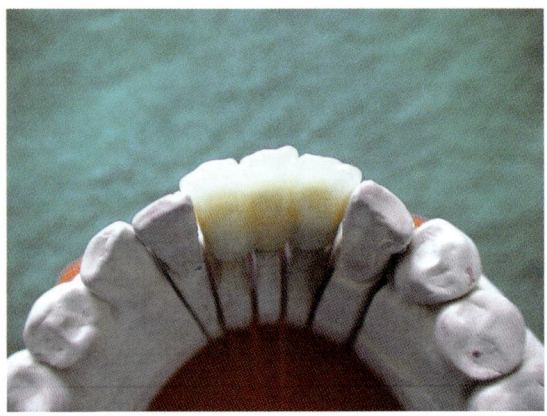

Bridge onto the cast, occlusal view

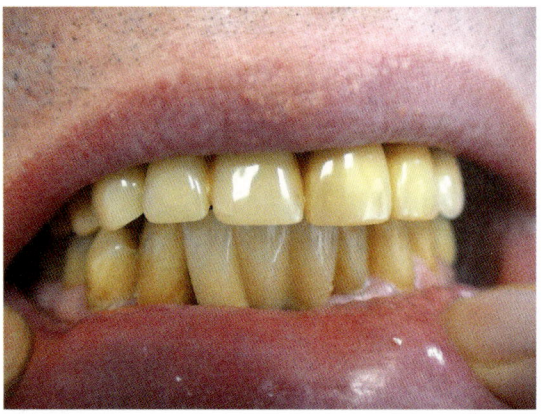

Cemented bridge in labial view

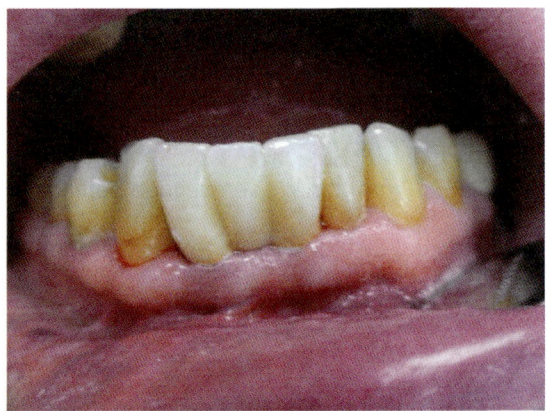

Cemented bridge, anterior view

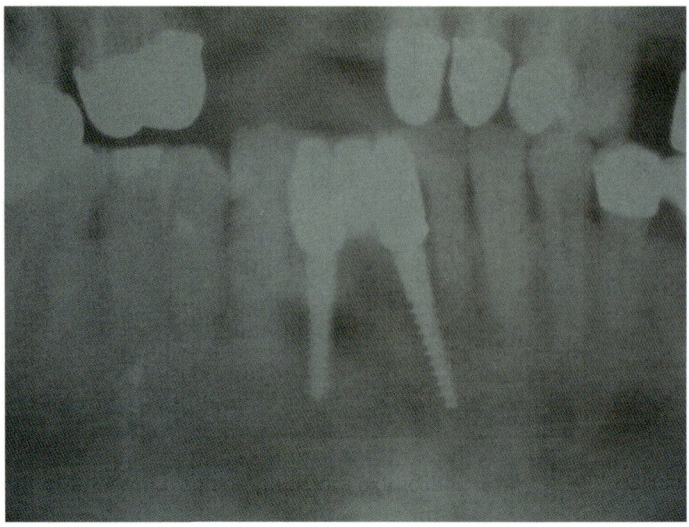

Cemented bridge,
panoramic radiographic control,
detail

7.1.13/Case 13

Patient: female, 52 years old

36, 2 implants, zirconium dioxide crown

21/06/2011	36	extraction
29/09/2011	36m	Champions® implant Ø 3.5 x 10 mm, >50 Ncm, Periotest -5
	36d	Champions® implant Ø 3.5 x 10 mm, >50 Ncm, Periotest -4 impression cemented dentist made temporary
10/10/2011	36	cemented zirconium dioxide crown
Treatment period:		**1.5 weeks**
Remarks:		For single lower molar teeth always 2 implants are inserted to achieve a better static and anti-rotation protection. Early loading

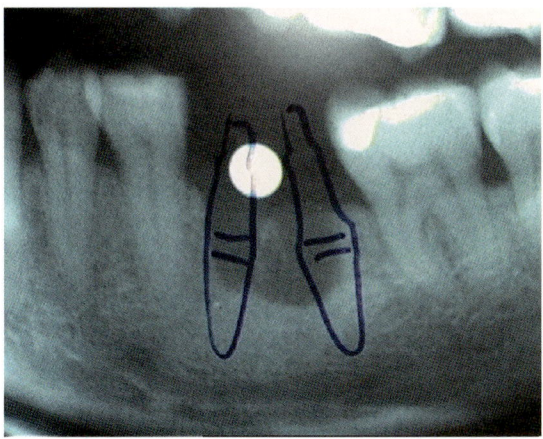

Planned treatment, zoomed radiographic detail

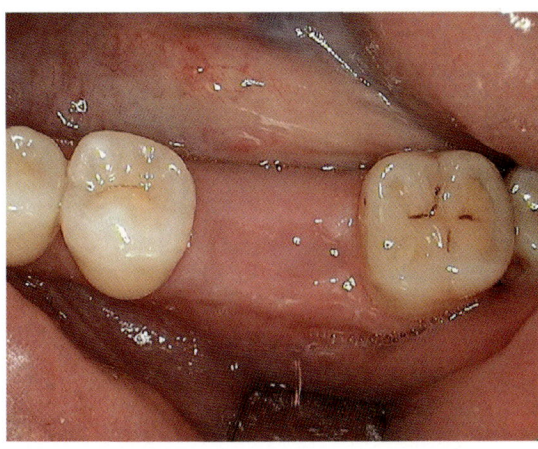

Clinical situation, occlusal view

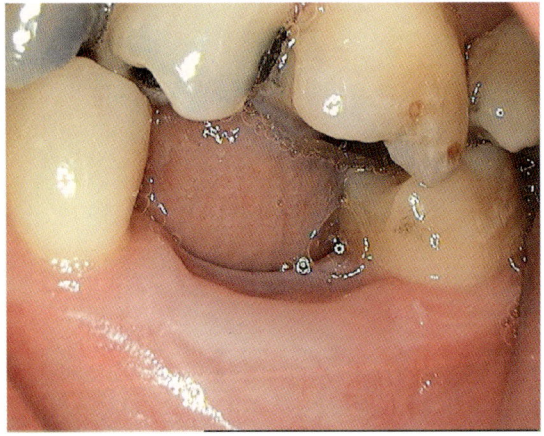

Clinical initial situation, lateral view

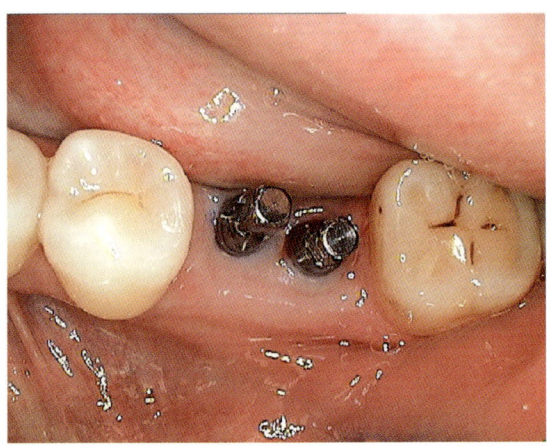

After implant placement, occlusal view

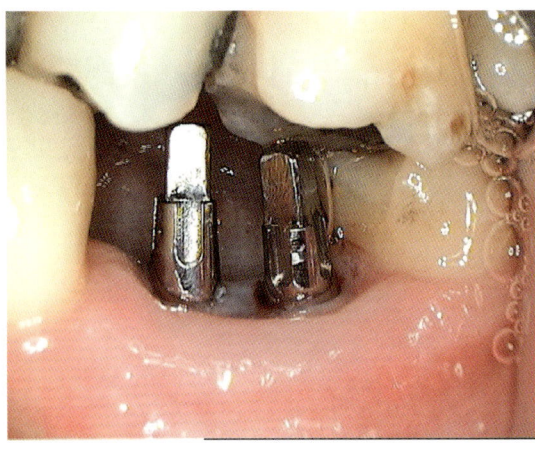

After implant placement, lateral view

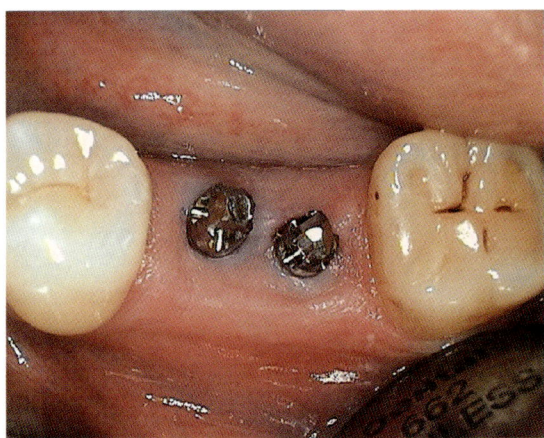

After preparation of implant heads, occlusal view

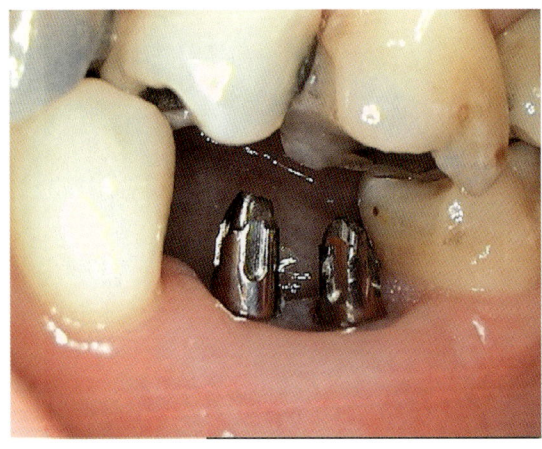

After preparation of implant heads, lateral view

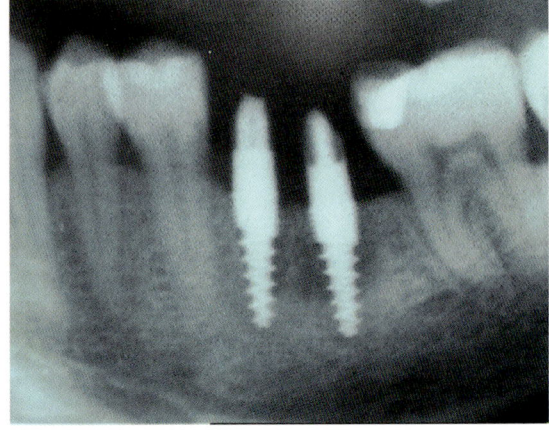

Radiographic control

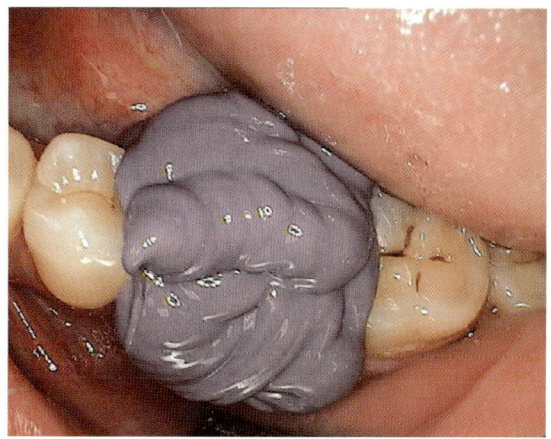

Impression taking at the beginning

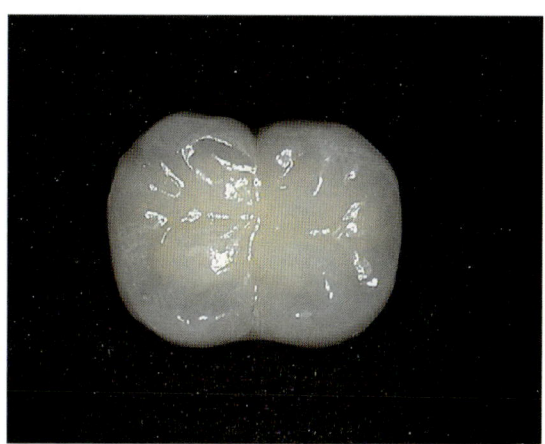

Final crown, occlusal view

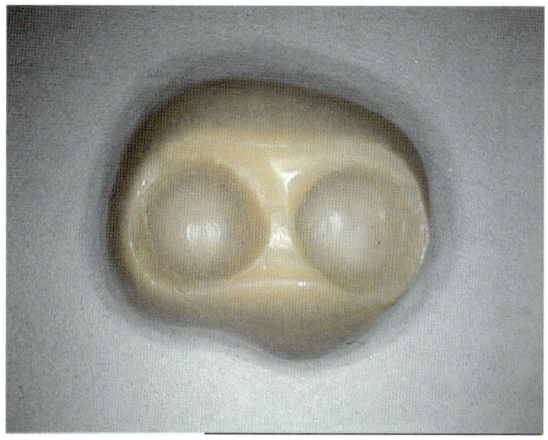

Final crown, basal view

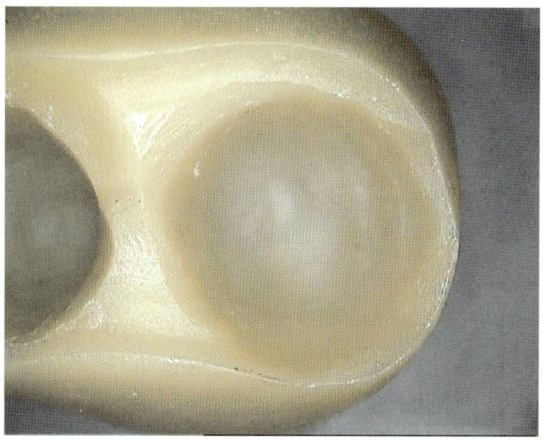

Final crown, detailed image, basal view

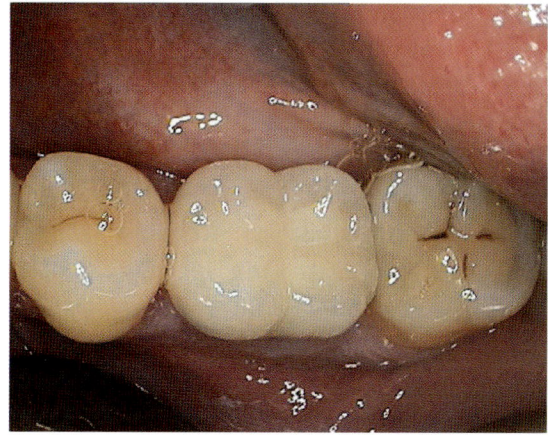

Cemented crown, occlusal view

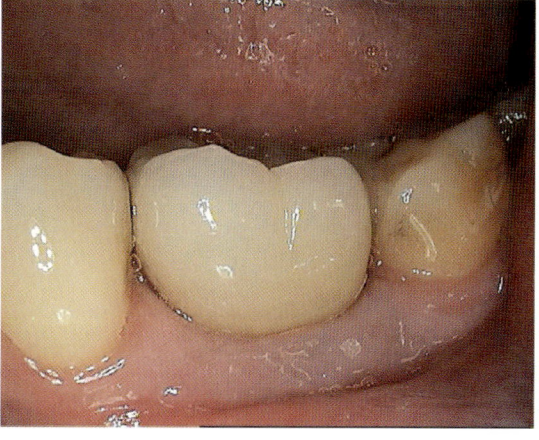

Cemented crown, lateral view

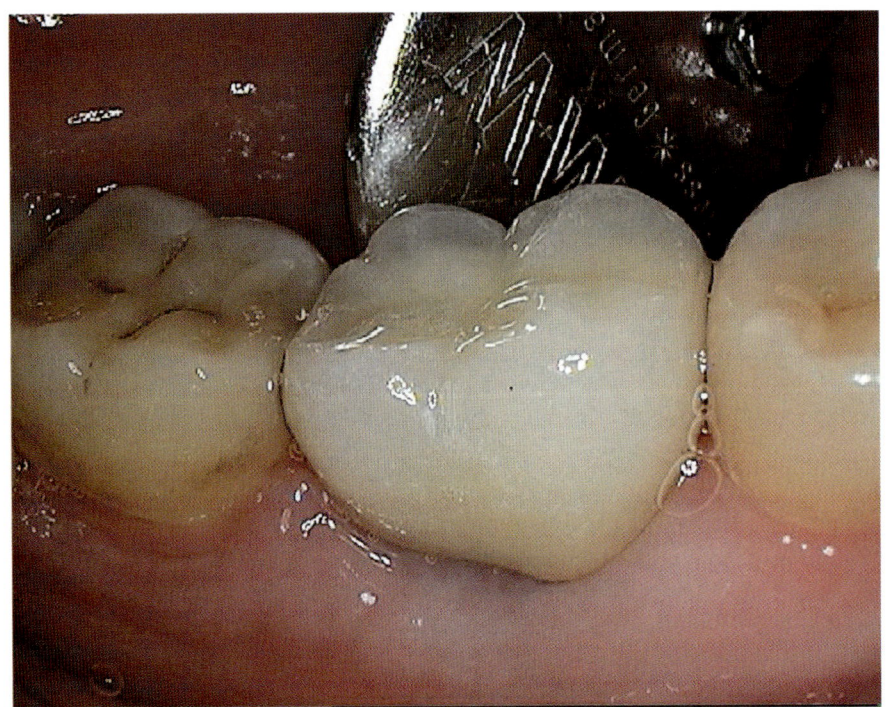

Cemented crown, lingual view

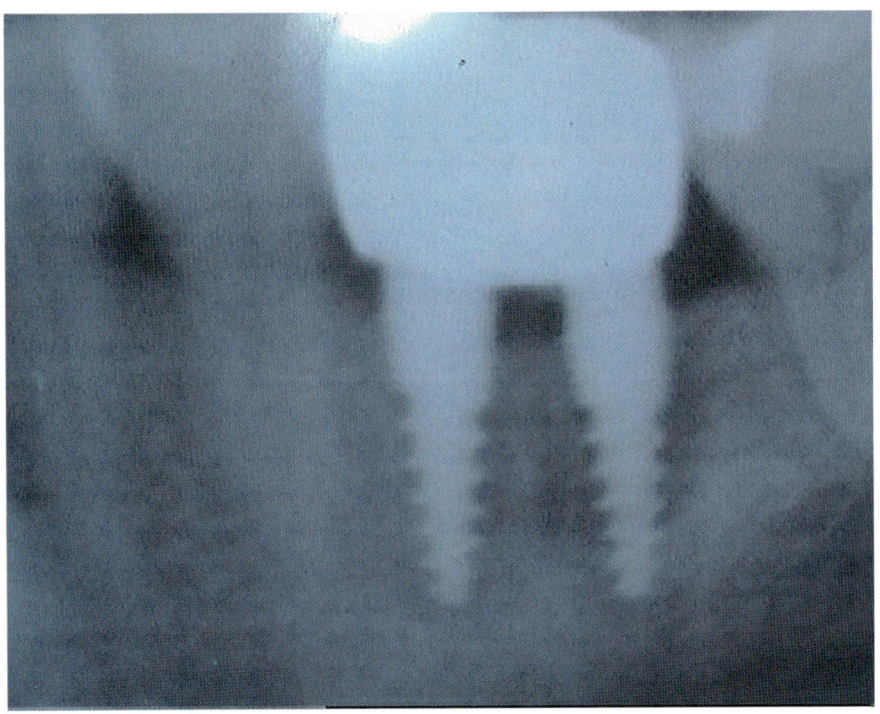

Final radiographic control

7.1.14/Case 14

Patient: female, 75 years old

11,21 immediate implant placement, Prep-Caps, splinted crown

06/12/2010	11,21	extraction Champions® implant Ø 4.5 x 14 mm, >40 Ncm, zirconium Prep-Caps, preparation cemented dentist made temporary
07/12/2010	11,21	cemented laboratory made temporary
14/02/2011	11,21	impression
01/03/2011		Cemented double crown
Treatment period:		**3 months**
Remarks:		Extremely protruded upper jaw The family dentist said: "An implant placement is out of question in this case!"

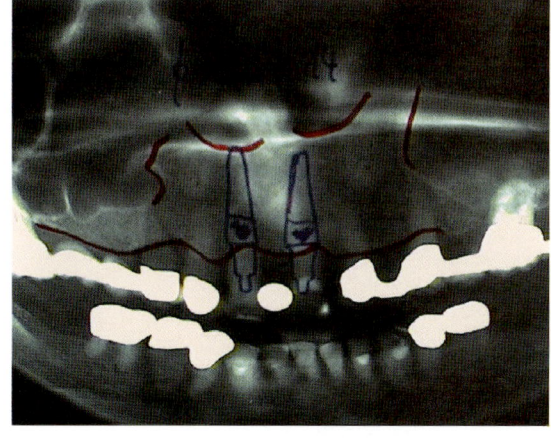

Planned treatment, initial panoramic radiograph

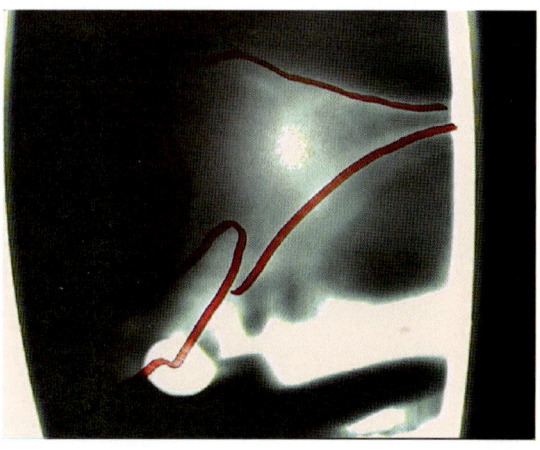

Cross-sectional image

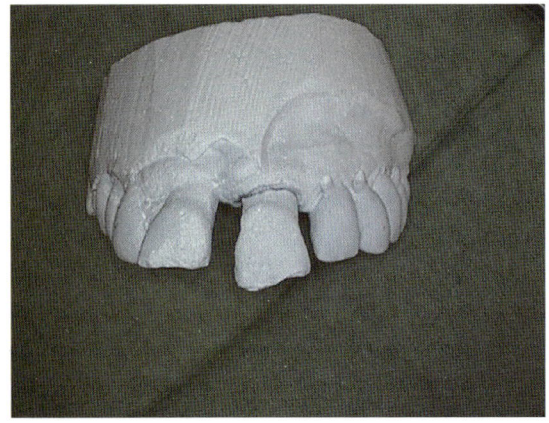

Situation model

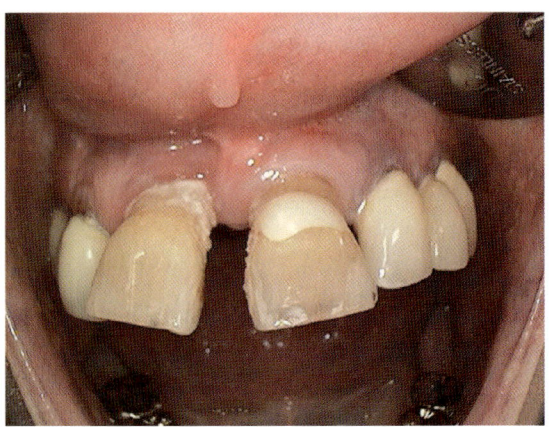

Clinical initial situation, anterior view

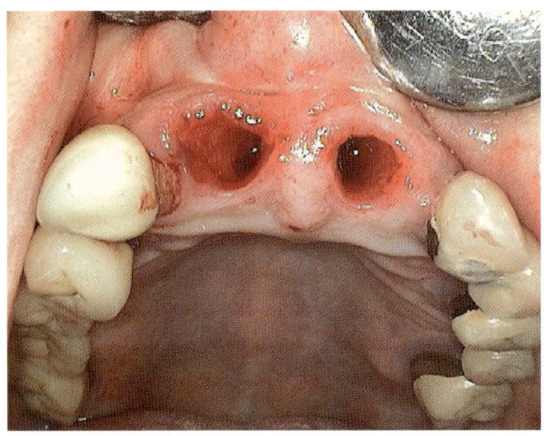

Alveoli 11, 21, situation after extraction

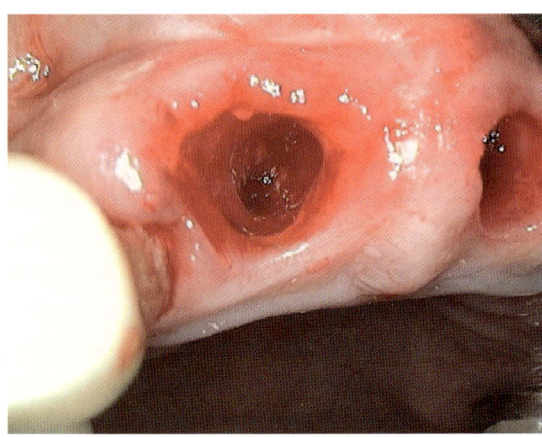

11 palatal pilot hole preparation

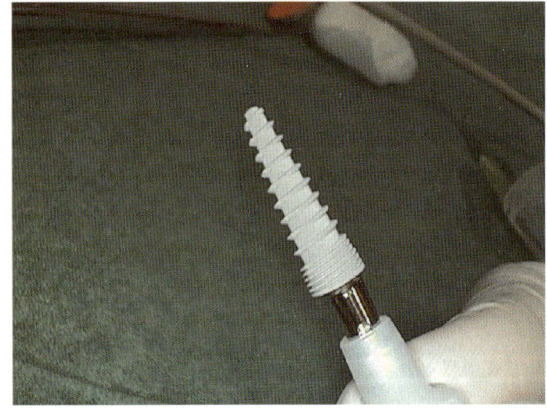

Champions® implant

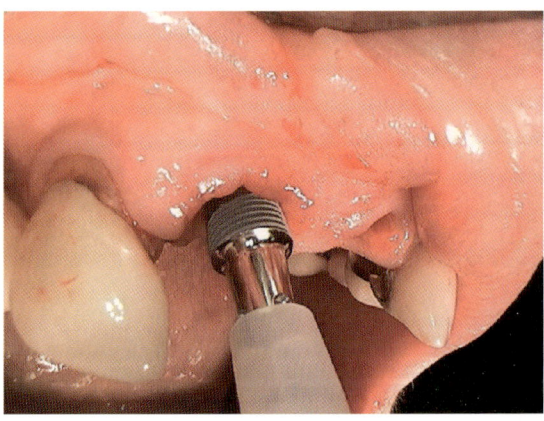

Insertion at the beginning

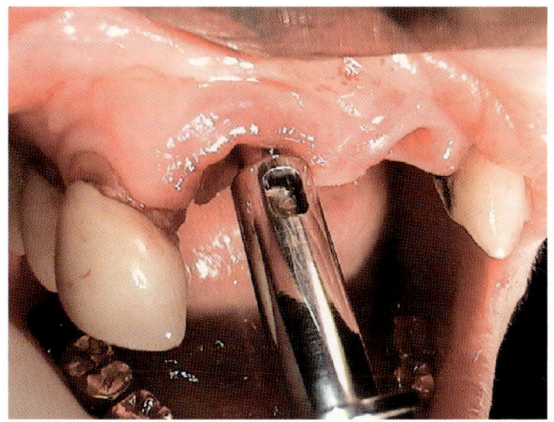

Attached carrier at the end of the insertion

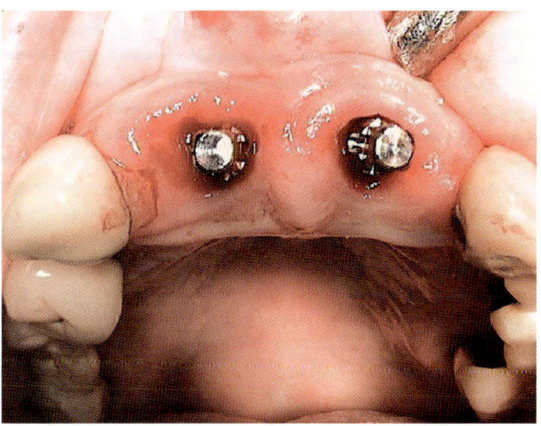

Completed implant placements, occlusal view

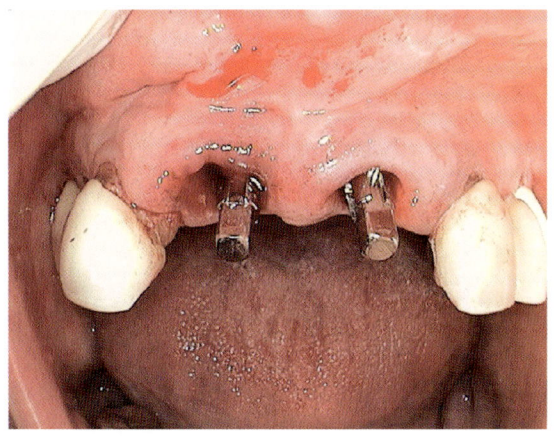

Completed implant placement, anterior view

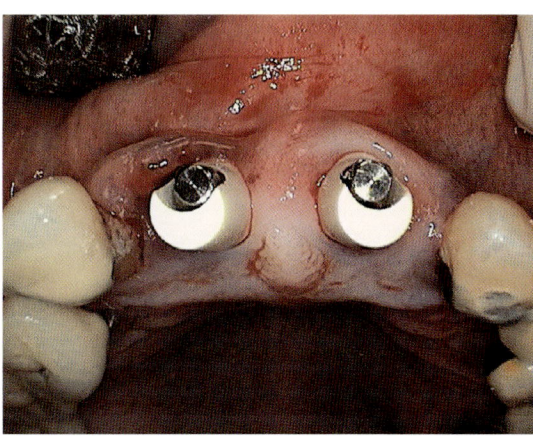

PC try-in

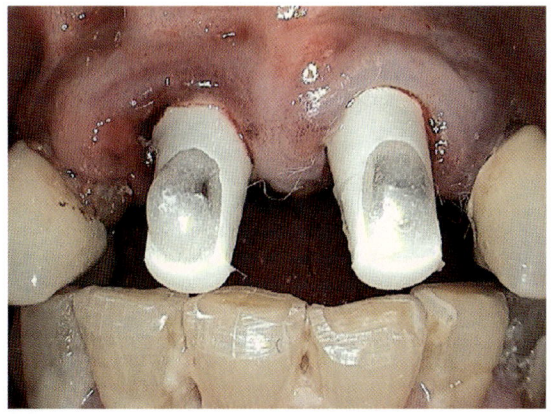

Cemented PC, anterior view

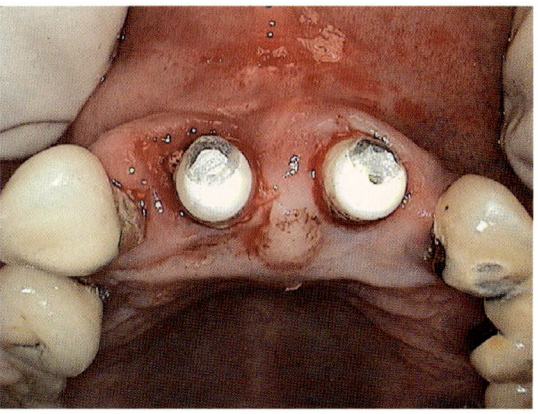

Prepared PC, occlusal view

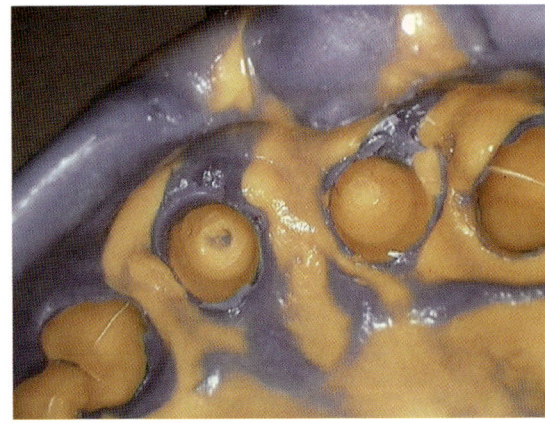

Impression taking of the prepared PC

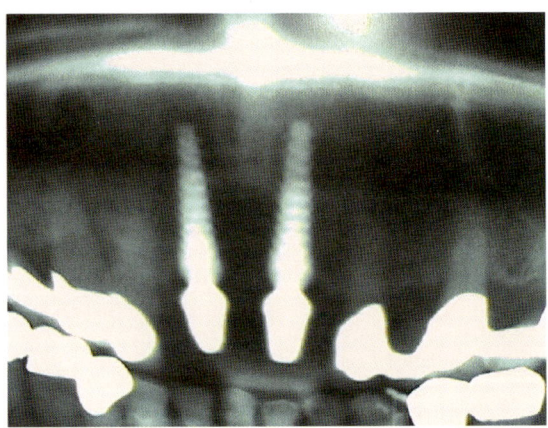

Panoramic radiographic control

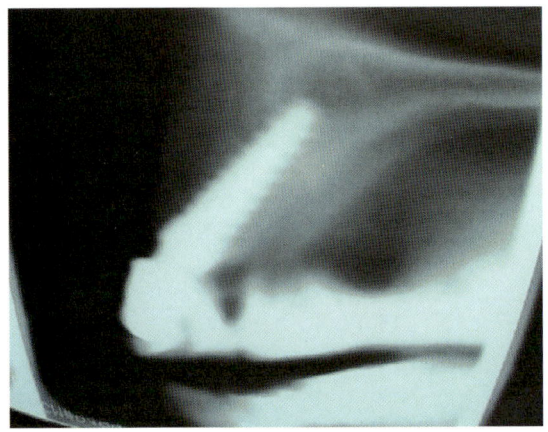

Cross-sectional image

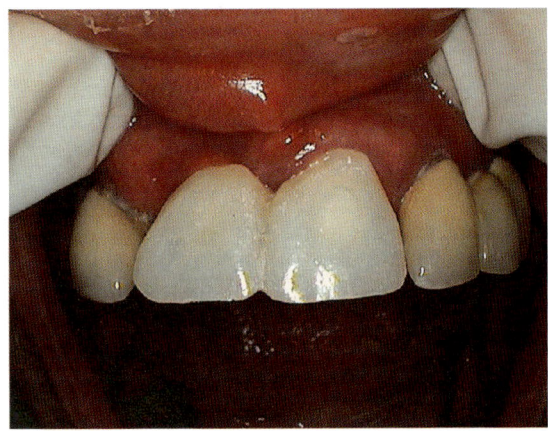

Cemented dentist made temporary

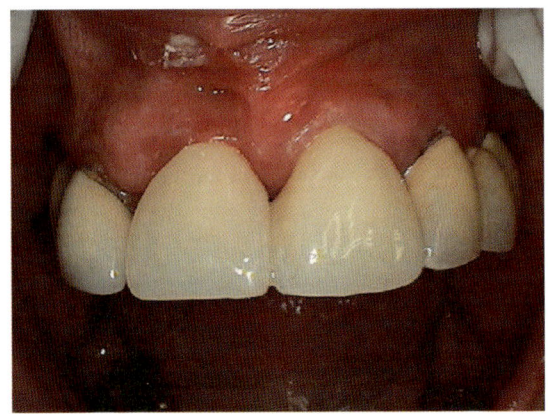

Cemented laboratory made temporary, anterior view

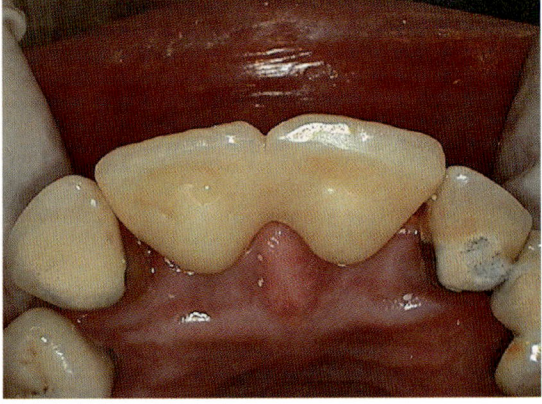

Cemented laboratory made temporary, palatal view

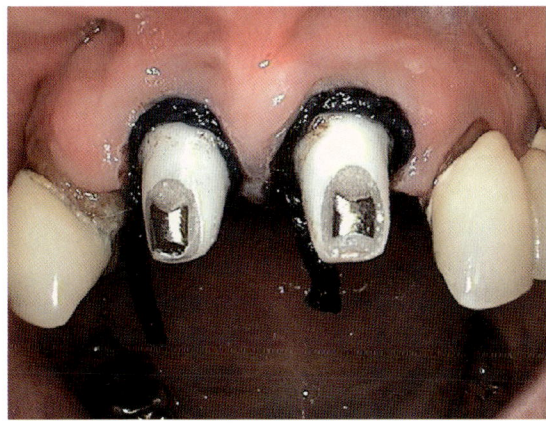

11, 12 with retraction sutures, before impression taking

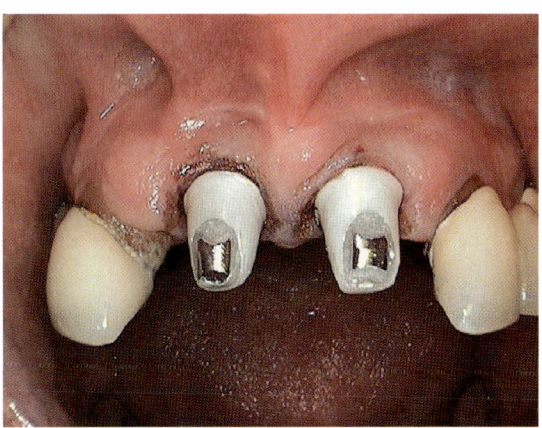

Ledge illustration after gingival retraction

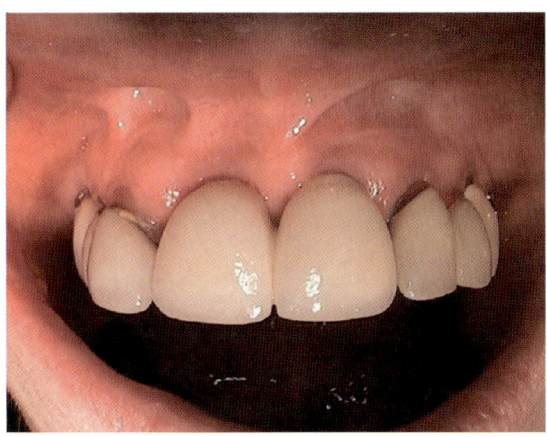

Final cemented splinted crown, anterior view

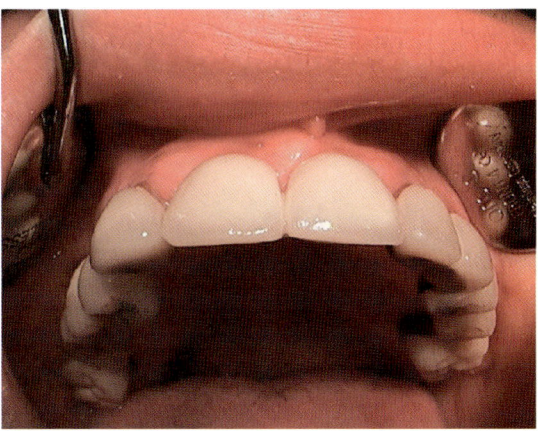

Final cemented splinted crown, incisal view

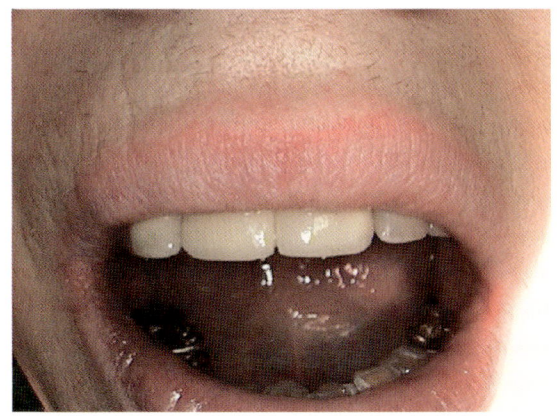

Smile line

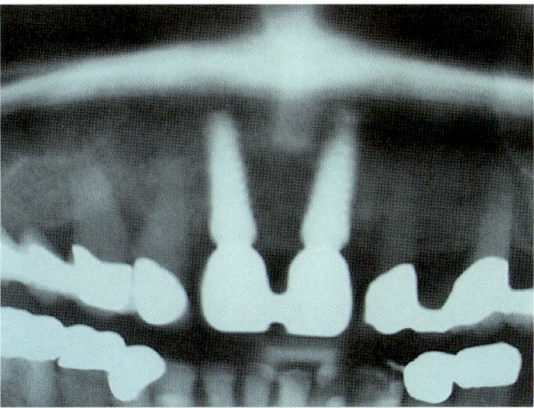

Final panoramic radiographic control

3 - 4 implants

7.2.1/Case 15

Patient: female, 58 years old

35,36, 3 implants, paranerval implant placement, splinted crown

---

15/02/2010	35	Champions® implant Ø 3.5 x 12 mm, 60 Ncm, PT -5
	36m	Champions® implant Ø 3.5 x 12 mm, 70 Ncm, PT -7
	36d	Champions® implant Ø 3.5 x 14 mm, 70 Ncm, PT -7 impression cemented dentist made temporary
22/02/2010	35-36	cemented zirconium dioxide splinted crown
10/10/2011		Radiographic control and control images
Treatment period:		**1 week**
Remarks:		Paranerval late implant placement, early loading 20 months after implant placement the gingiva is completely free from irritation. The splinted crownhas loosened and has been cemented once again.

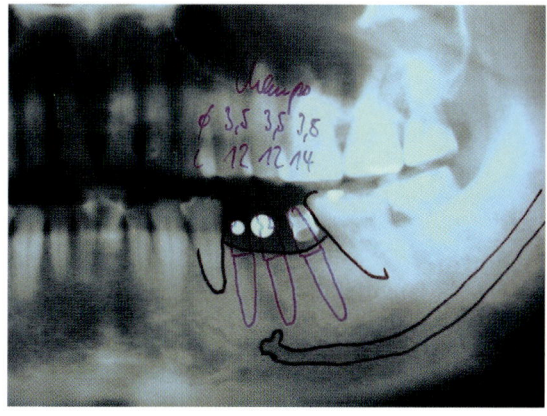

Panoramic radiograph for planned treatment

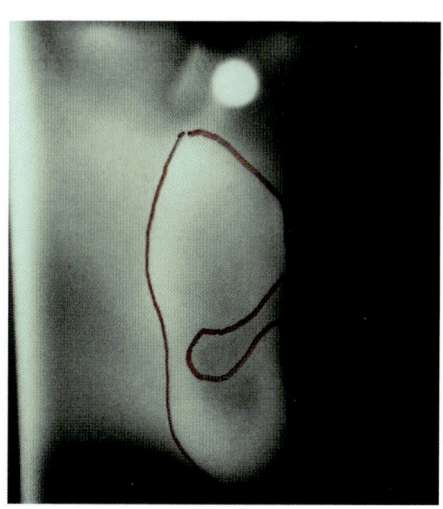

Cross-sectional image

91

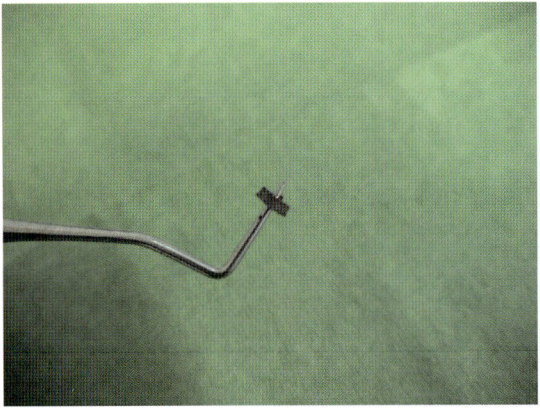

Probe and rubber ring for the measurement of the gingival thickness

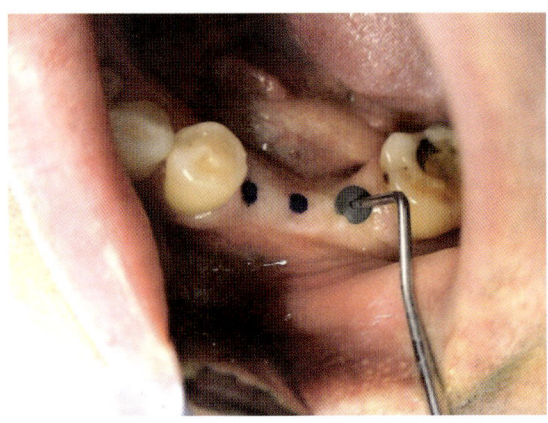

Measurement of gingival thickness

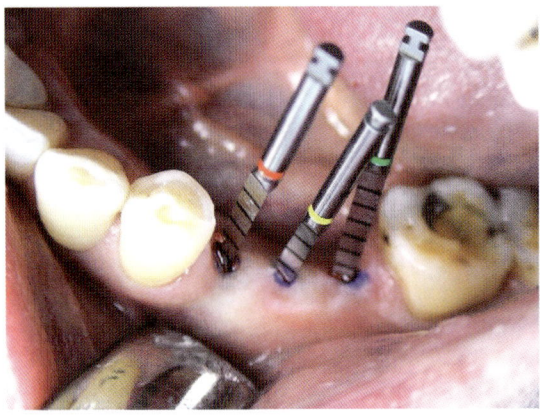

Pilot hole preparation

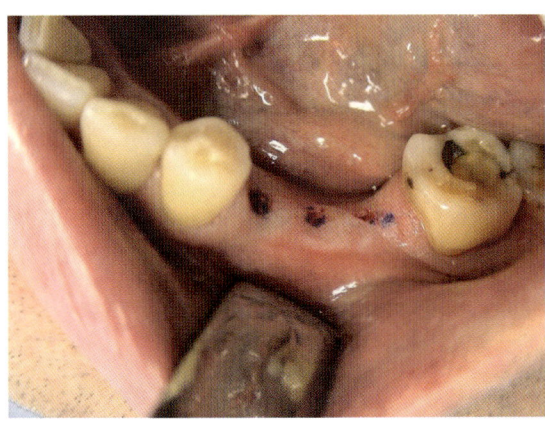

Clinical situation after pilot hole preparation

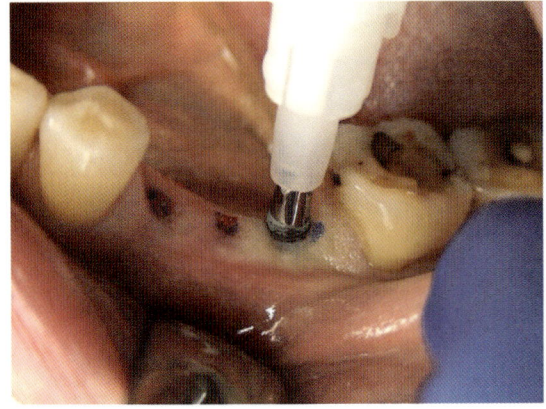

Clinical situation, implant placement at the beginning

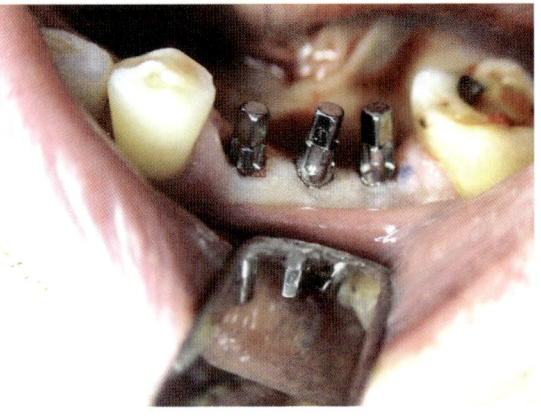

Completed insertion

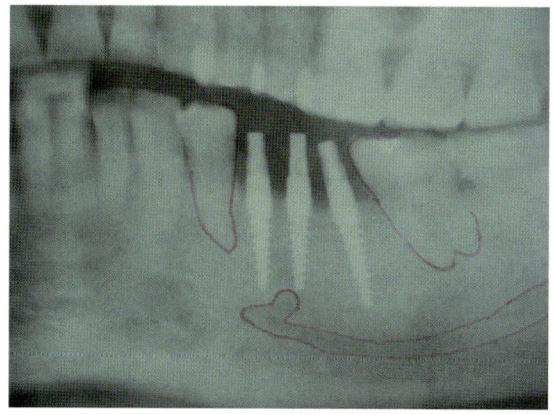

Panoramic radiographic control

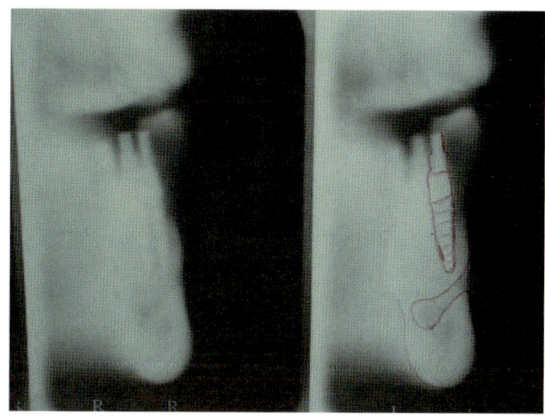

Radiographic control, cross-sectional images

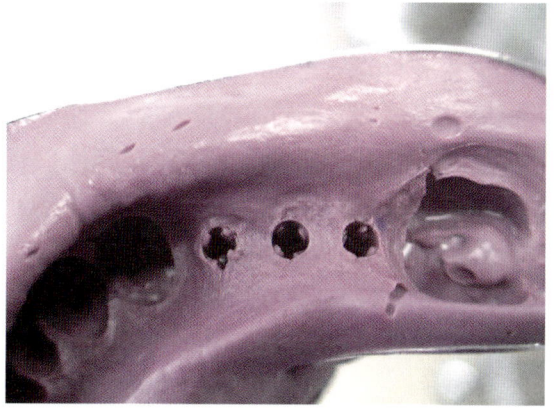

Impression

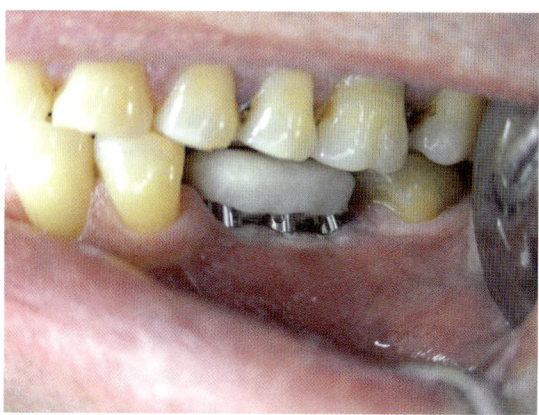

Dentist made temporary

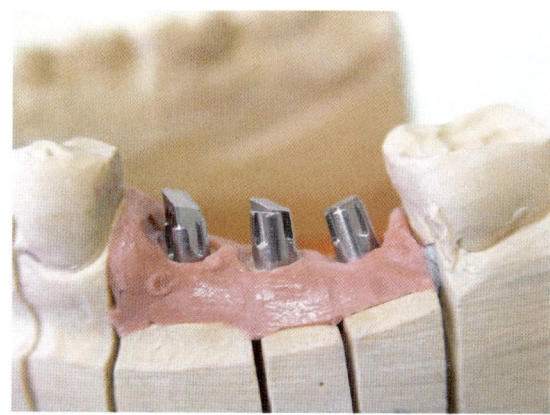

Implant head preparation on cast

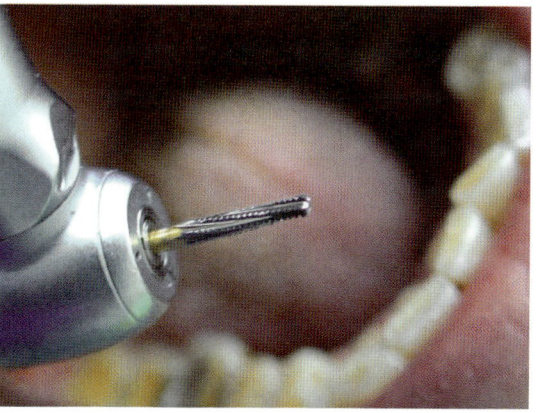

Bone mill for implant head preparation in mouth

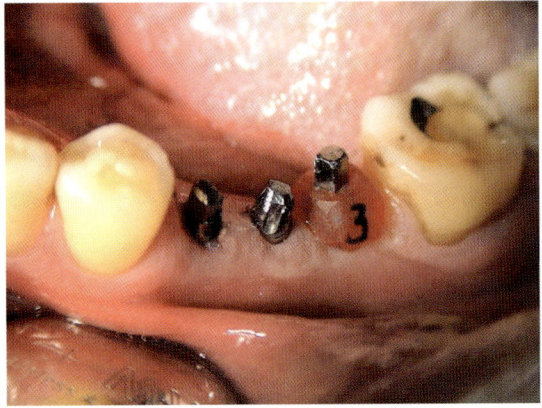

Attached plastic cap before implant head preparation

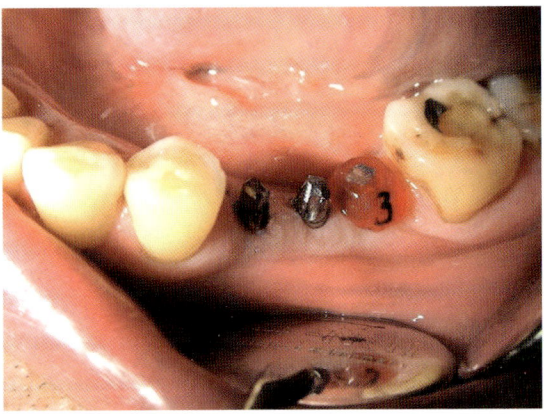

Attached plastic cap after implant head preparation

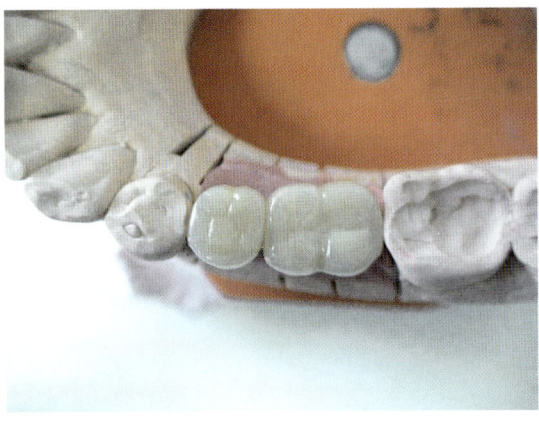

Final splinted crown, occlusal view

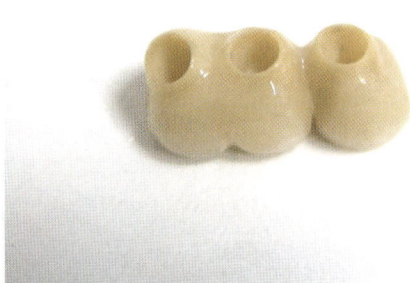

Final splinted crown, basal view

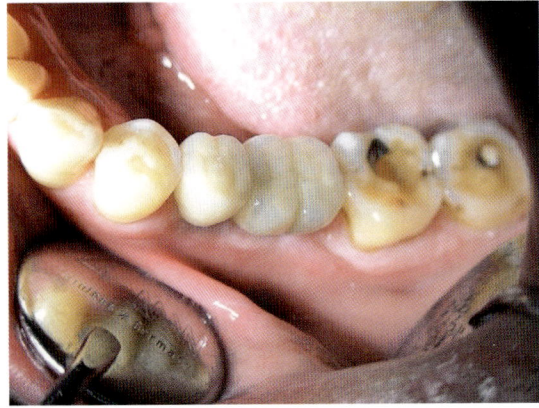

Final splinted crown, occlusal view

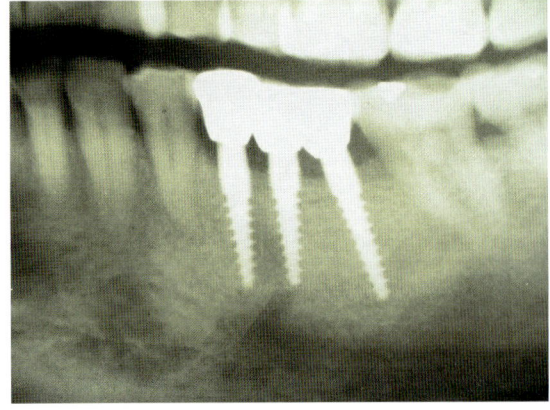

Panoramic radiographic control

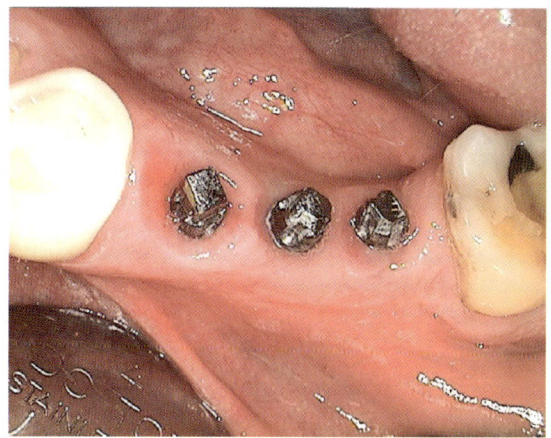

Clinical situation after 20 months...

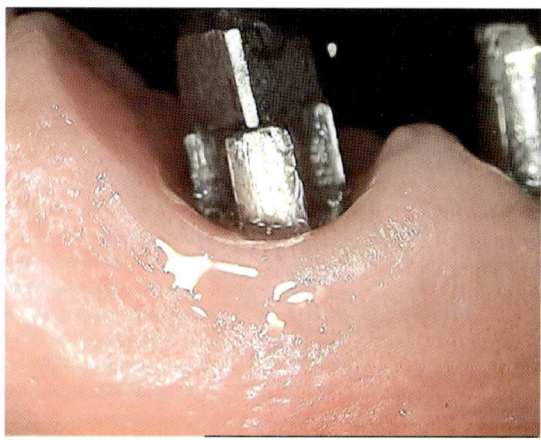

...macro image...

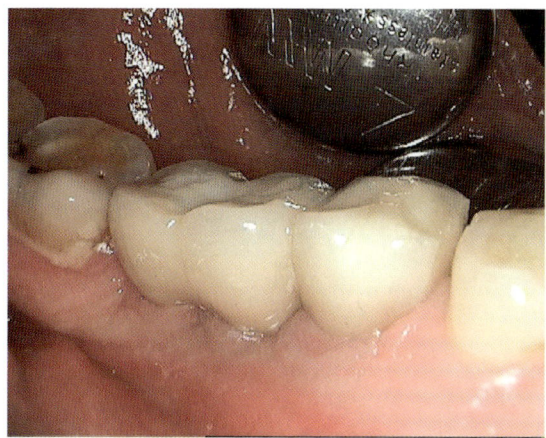

...in situ...

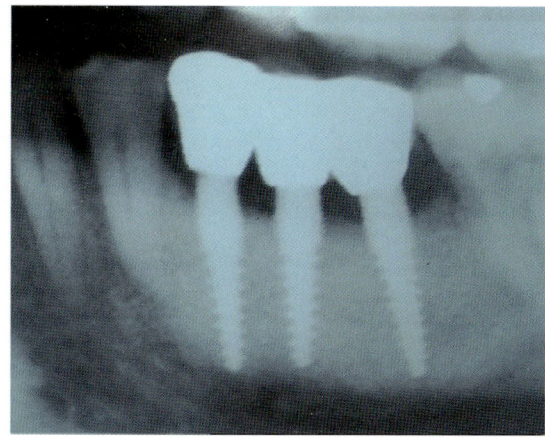

...detail of the panoramic radiograph, zoomed

7.2.2/Case 16

Patient: male, 51 years old

35,36 implant placements, splinted crowns

10/05/2011	36	extraction
28/06/2011	35	Champions® implant Ø 3.0 x 10 mm, >50 Ncm, Periotest - 3
	36m	Champions® implant Ø 3.0 x 10 mm, >60 Ncm, Periotest - 4
	36d	Champions® implant Ø 3.5 x 8 mm, >60 Ncm, Periotest - 3 preparation of implant heads splinted dentist made temporary
02/09/2011		Impression, Periotest: equal values
09/09/2011	35-36	cemented zirconium dioxide splinted crown
Treatment period:		**2.5 months**
Remarks:	36	curved implant! late loading

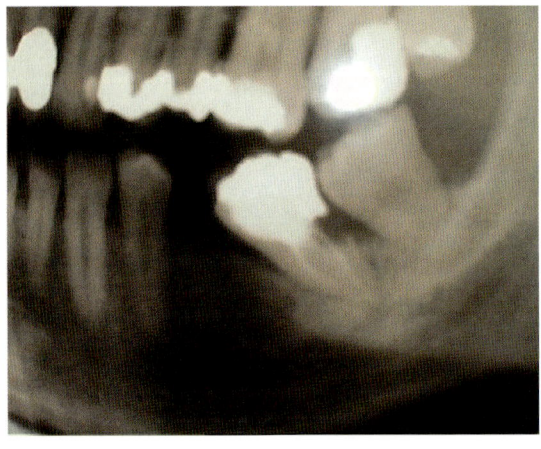

Panoramic radiograph before extraction

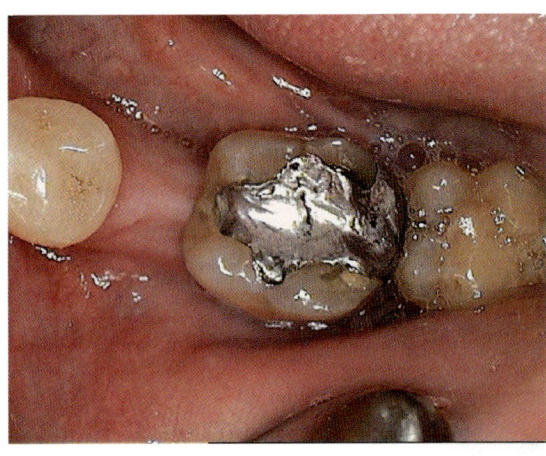

Clinical situation before extraction, occlusal view

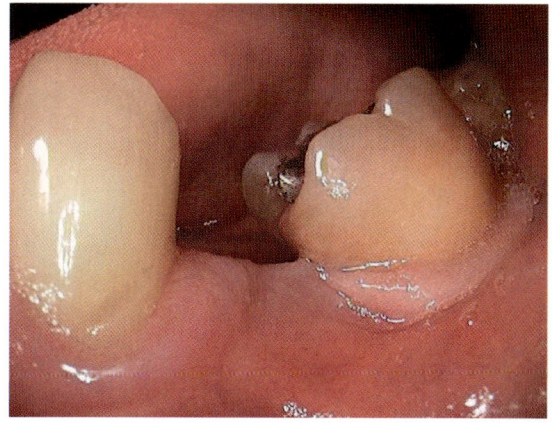

Clinical situation before extraction, lateral view

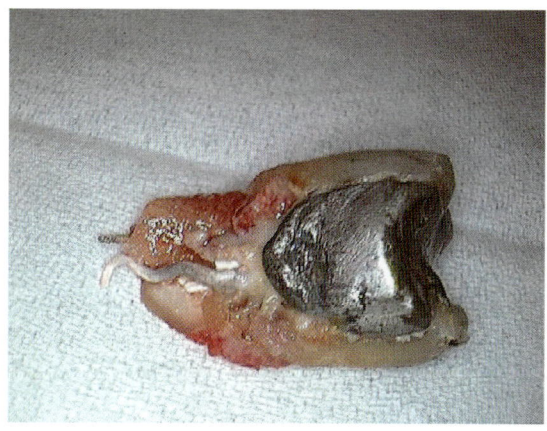

36 extracted mesial root

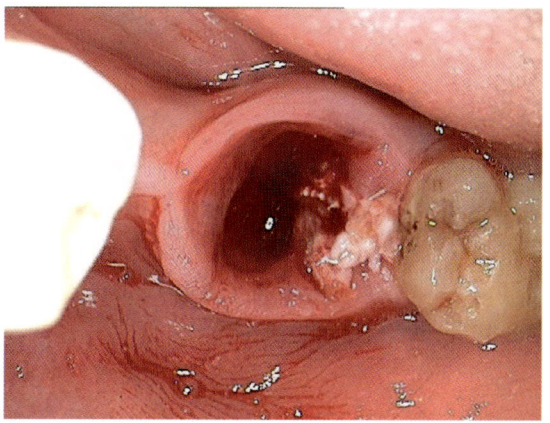

Distal root after fracture

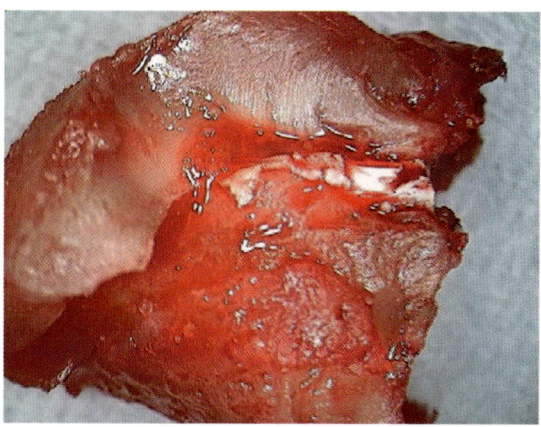

Macro image after extraction

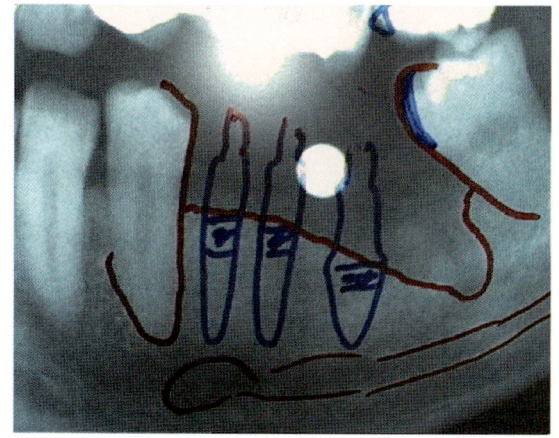

Planned implant placement, panoramic radiograph

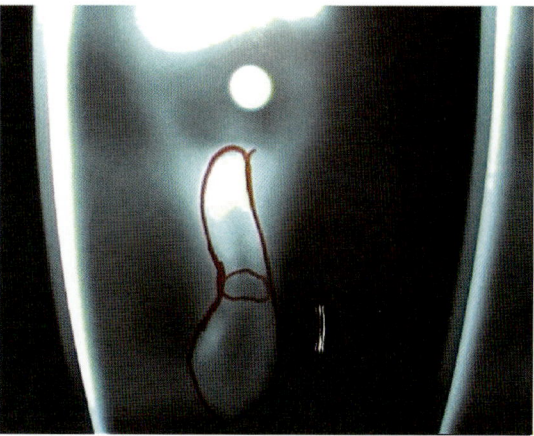

Cross-sectional image

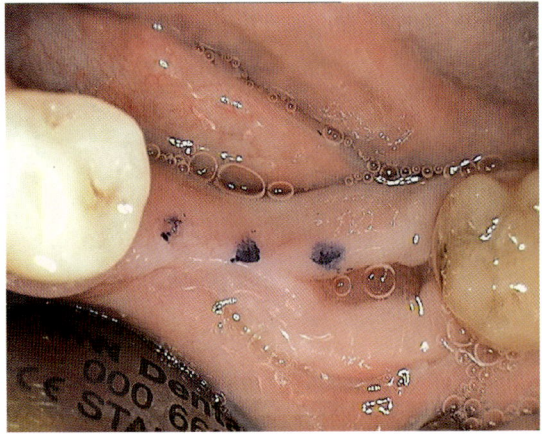

Clinical situation before implant placement

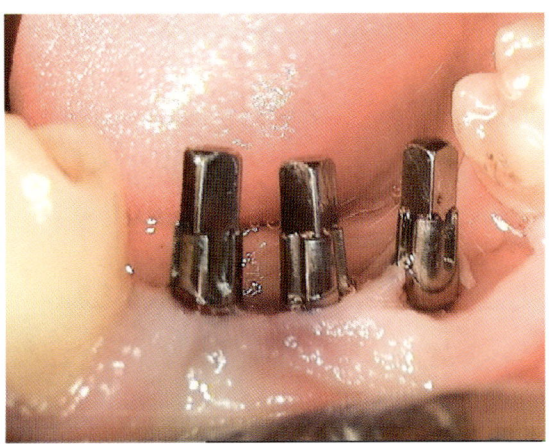

Implant placement, lateral view

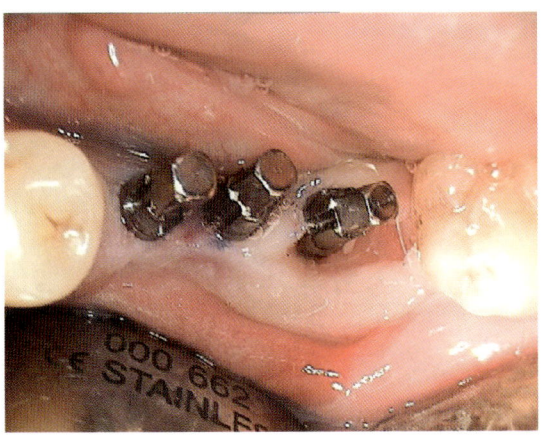

Implant placement, occlusal view

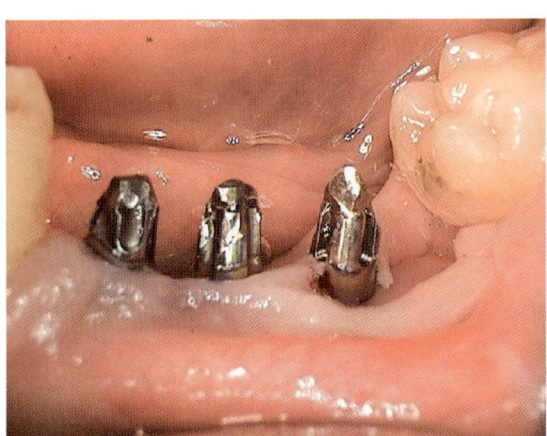

Preparation of implant heads, lateral view

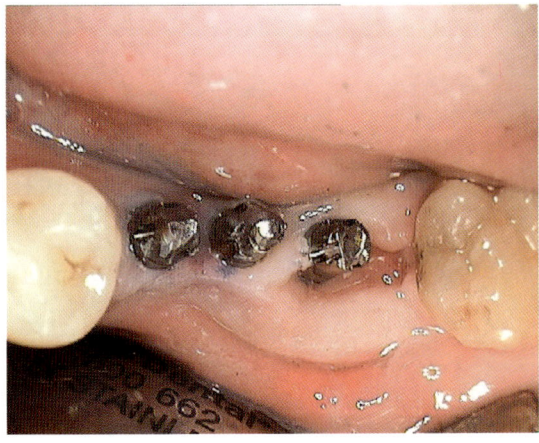

Prepared implant heads, occlusal view

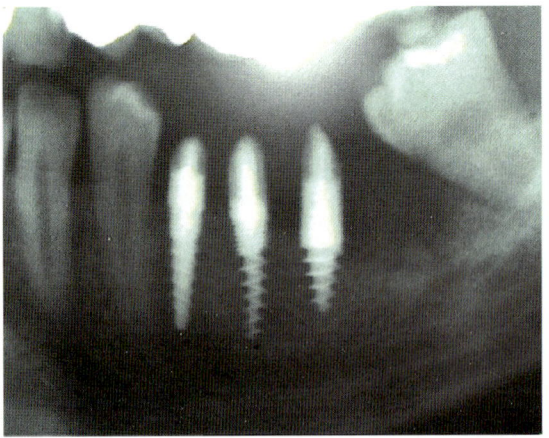

Panoramic radiographic control

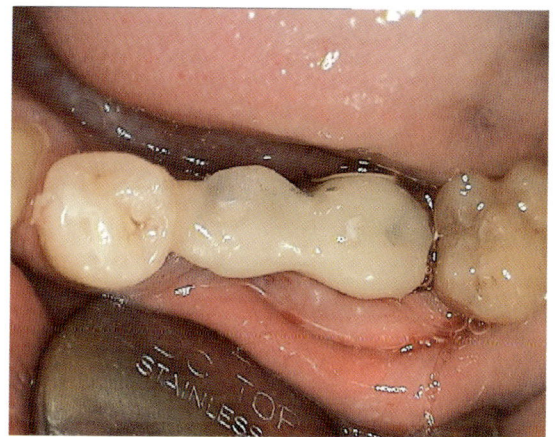

Dentist made temporary

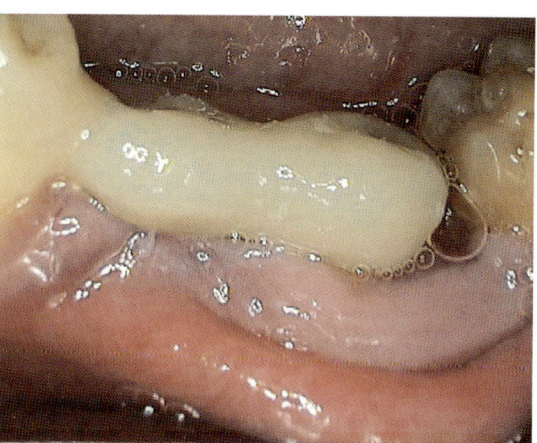

Splinted dentist made temporary

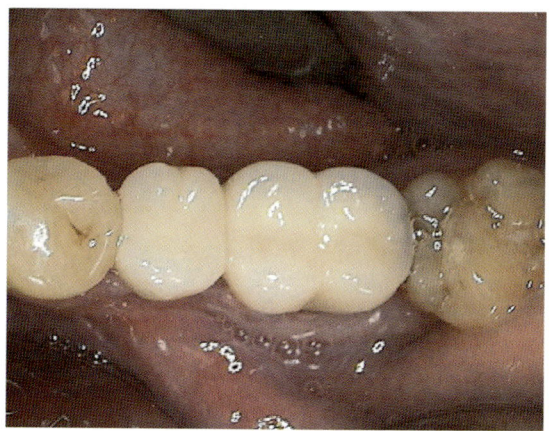

Final cemented splinted crown, occlusal view

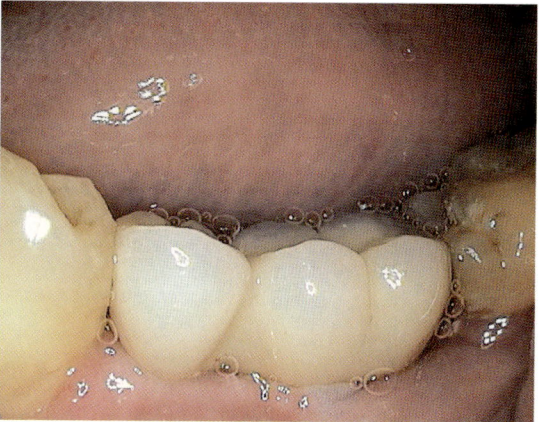

Final cemented splinted crown, lateral view

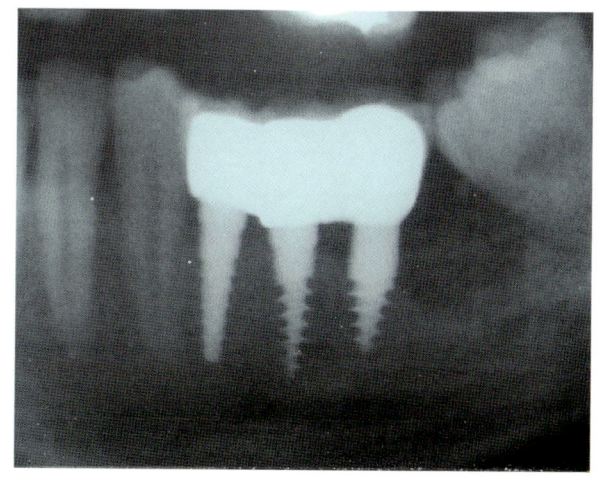

Final X-ray, zoomed panoramic radiograph

7.2.3/Case 17

Patient: female, 44 years old

44,-47 implants
plastic caps, splinted crown

06/10/2009	44	Champions® implant Ø 3.0 x 14 mm, >60 Ncm
	45, 46, 47	Champions® implant Ø 3.5 x 8 mm, >60 Ncm, Periotest -4 bone spreading impression cemented dentist made temporary
08/10/2009	44-47	preparation of the abutments cemented zirconium dioxide splinted crown

Treatment period: **2 days**

Remarks: Paranerval late implant placement, immediate loading
Grinding caps made in the laboratory have been attached onto the implants in mouth and all overhanging sections of the implant heads removed.

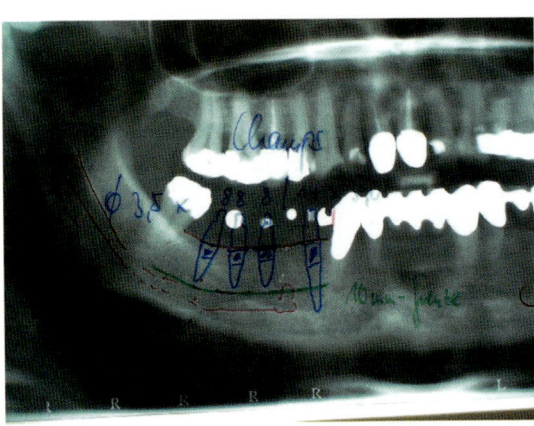

Panoramic radiograph for planned treatment

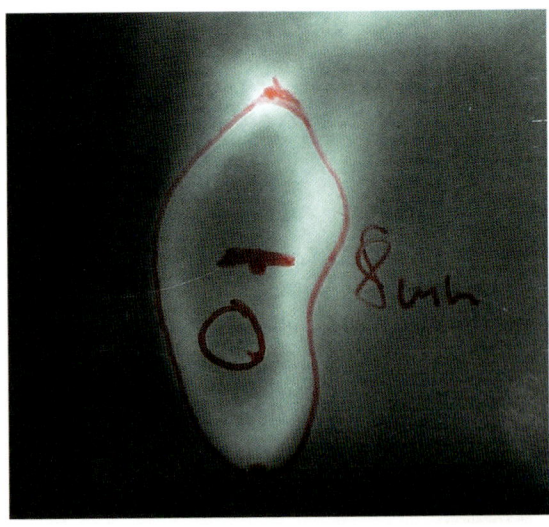

X-ray planning, cross-sectional image

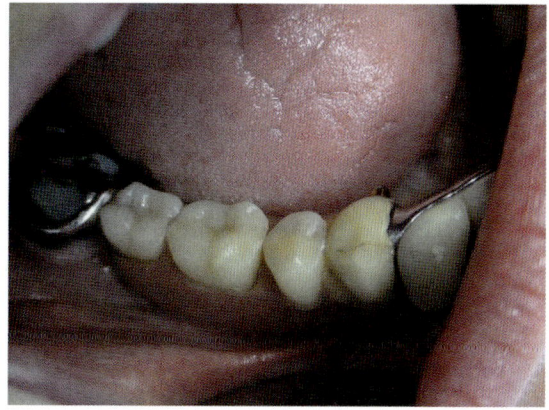

Clinical initial situation with integrated prosthesis

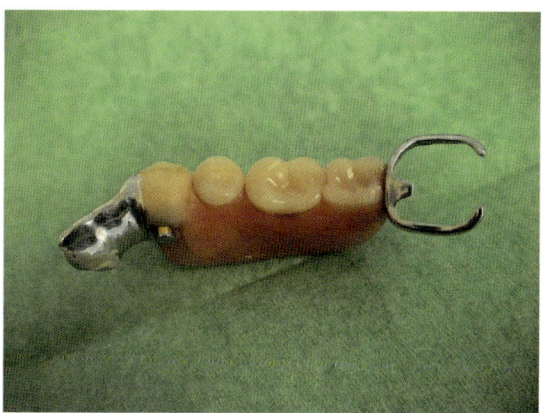

Former prosthesis

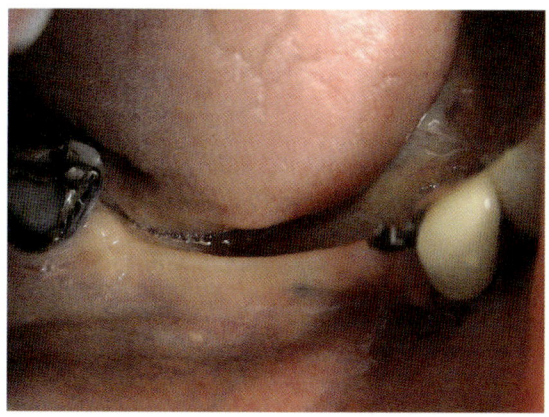

Clinical initial situation without prosthesis

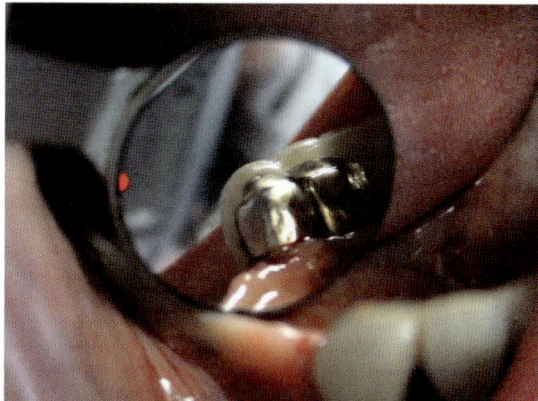

Detached attachment element 43

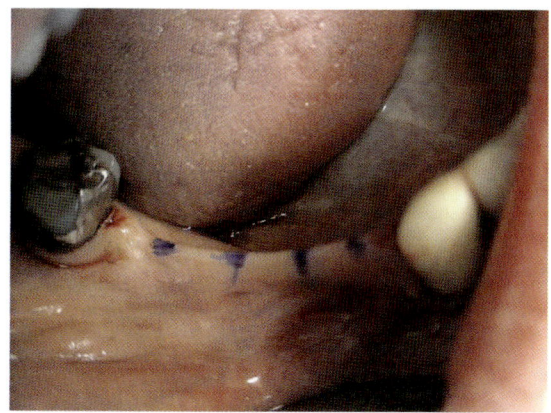

Marked positions for planned implants

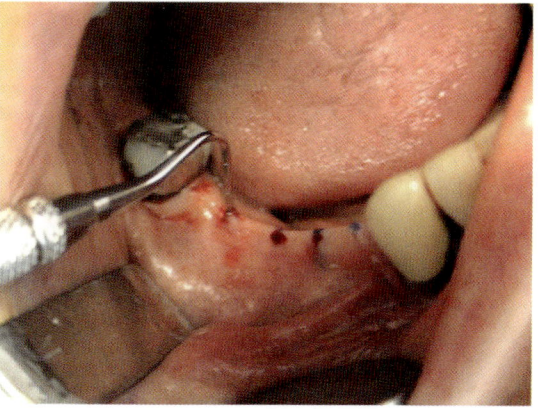

Pilot hole preparation

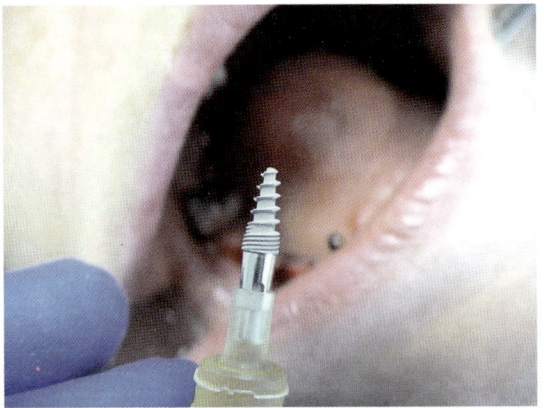

Implant placement at the beginning

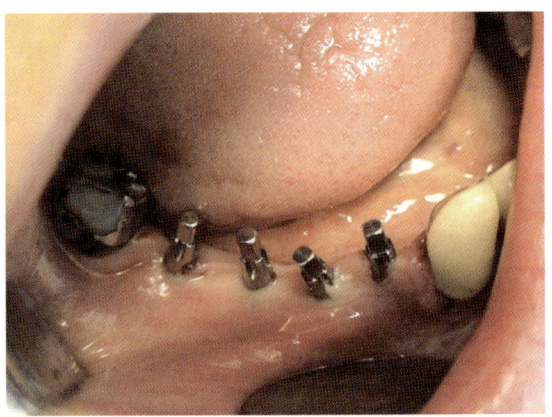

Completed implant placement

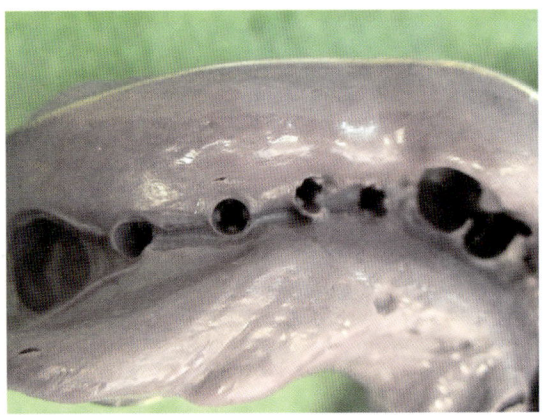

Impression for final dental prosthesis

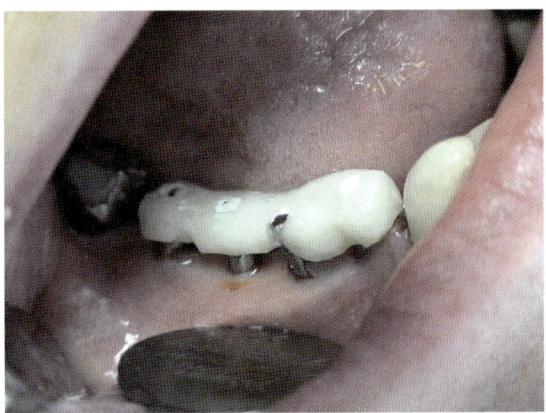

Cemented dentist made temporary

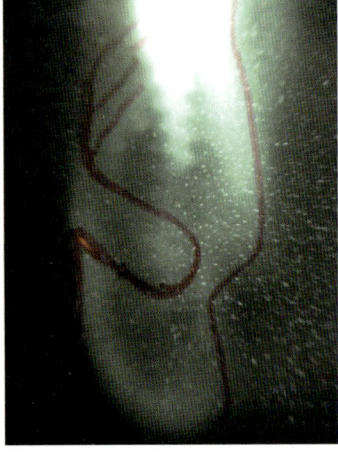

Radiograph control, cross-sectional image after implant placement; paranerval implant placement

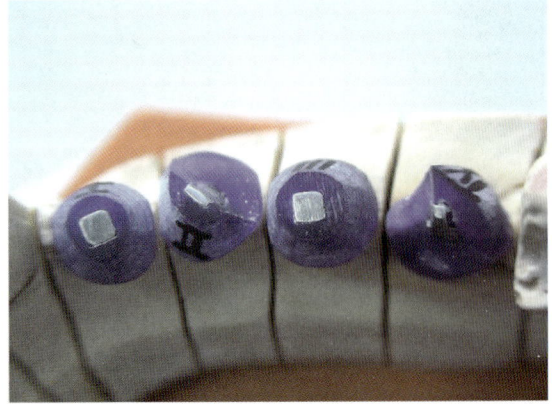

Plastic caps for the preparation of implant heads

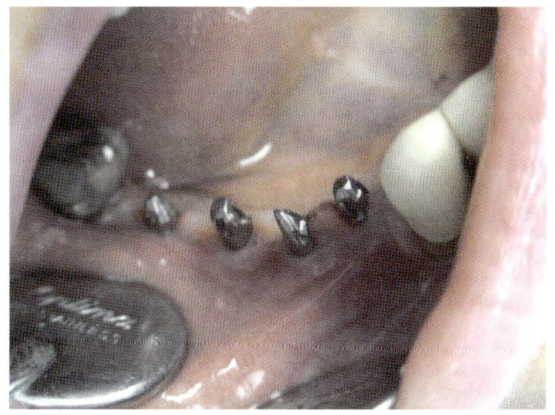

Clinical situation before dental prosthesis integration

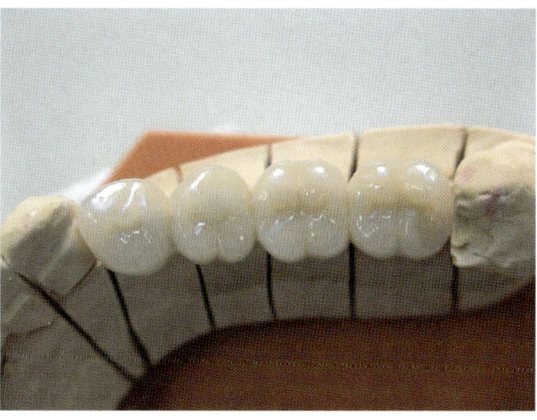

splinted crown on cast

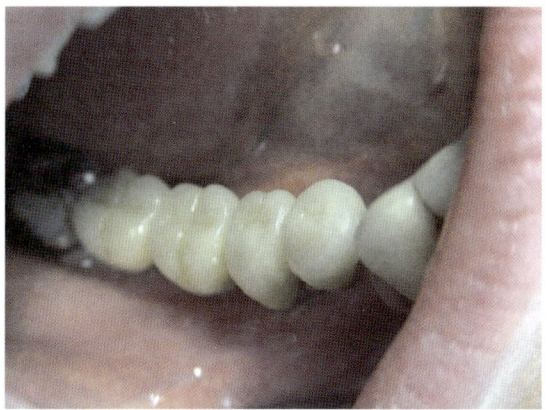

splinted crown in mouth

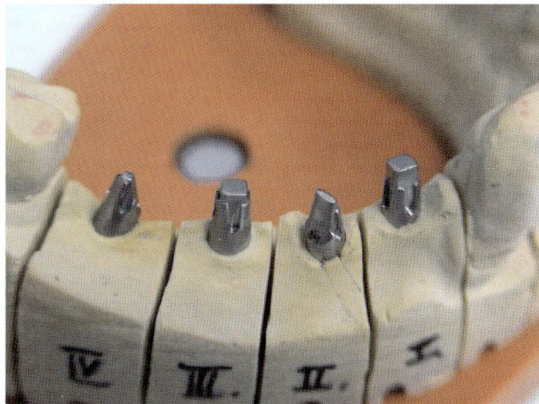

Simulated preparation of implant heads onto the cast made in the laboratory

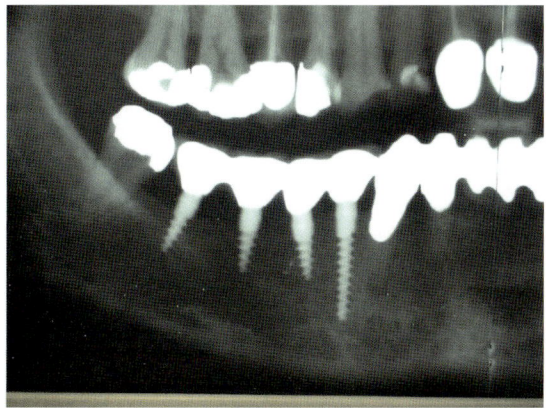

Radiograph control, panoramic radiograph

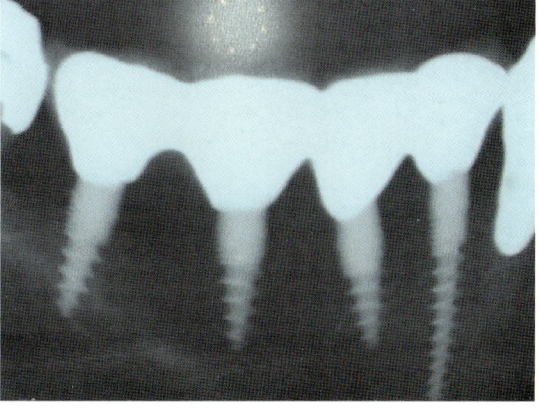

Radiograph control, panoramic radiograph, zoomed detail

7.2.4/Case 18

Patient: female, 55 years old

35, 36, 37 implant placement, splinted crown

May 2011	35	extraction performed by the family dentist
07/07/2011	35	Champions® implant Ø 4.5 x 10 mm, 20 Ncm, Periotest -4
	36m	Champions® implant Ø 3.5 x 10 mm, 40 Ncm, Periotest -4
	36d	Champions® implant Ø 3.5 x 10 mm, 60 Ncm, Periotest -6
	37	Champions® implant Ø 3.5 x 8 mm, >20 Ncm, Periotest -4 cemented dentist made temporary
16/09/2011		Impression Periotest: 35 -5, 36m -5, 36d -6, 37 -4
26/09/2011	35-37	cemented zirconium dioxide splinted crown
Treatment period:		**2.5 months**
Remarks:		Between the implants no cleaning gaps are required!

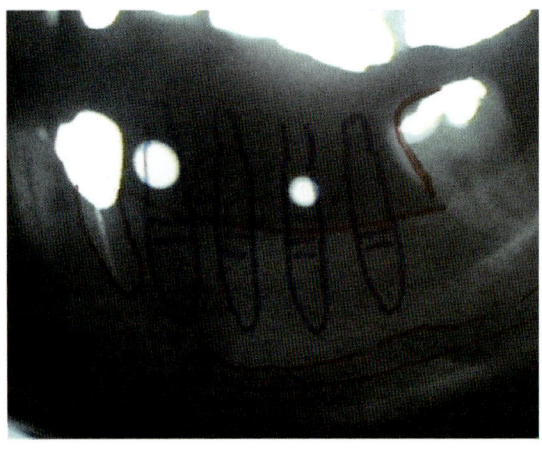

Panoramic radiograph for planned treatment

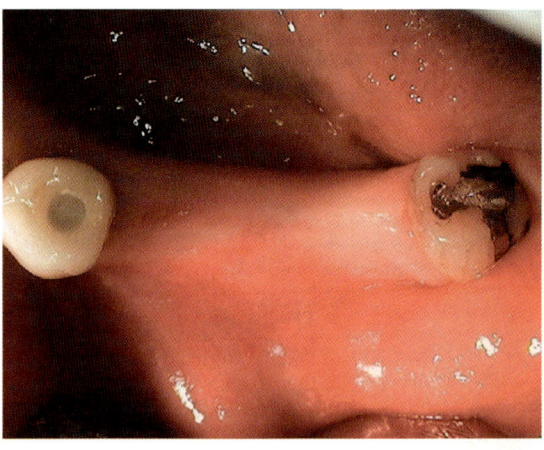

Clinical initial situation, occlusal view

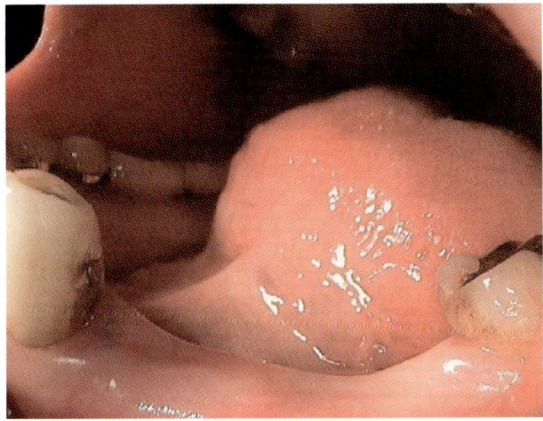

Clinical initial situation, lateral view

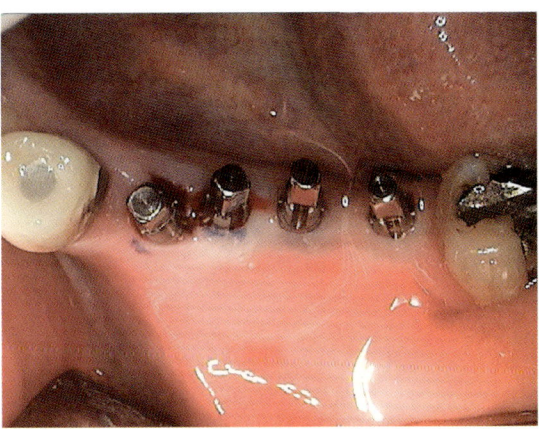

Completed implant placement, occlusal view

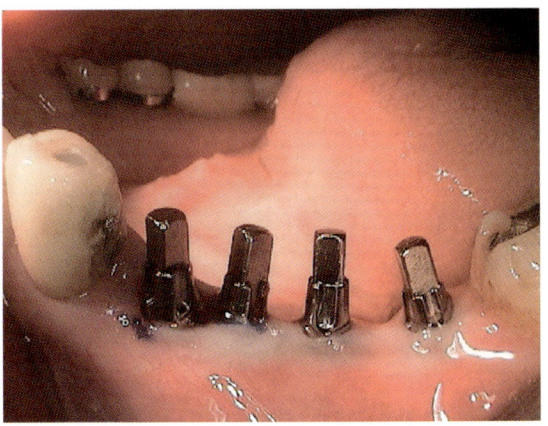

Completed implant placement, lateral view

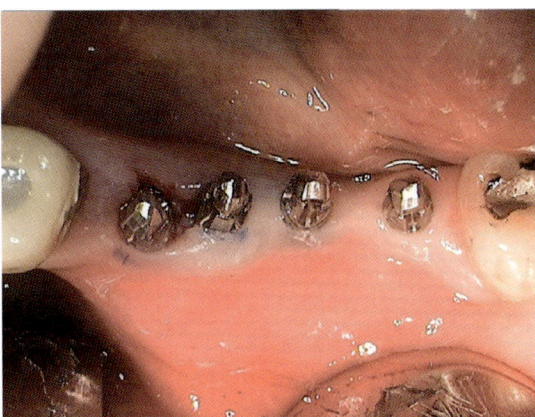

Prepared implant heads, occlusal view

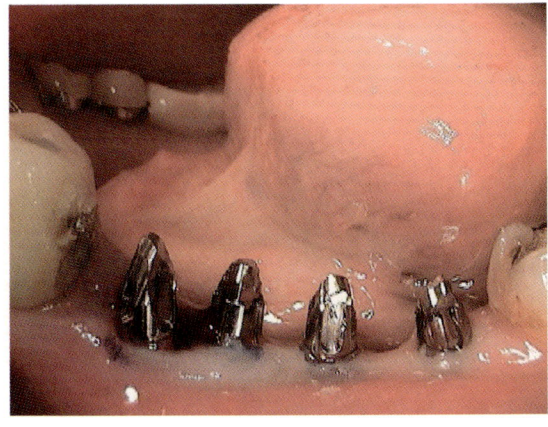

Prepared implant heads, lateral view

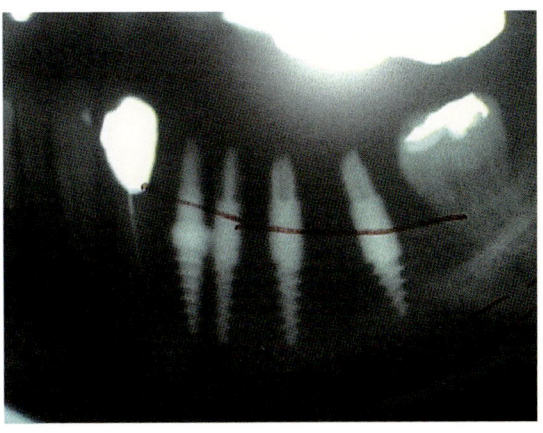

Panoramic radiographic control

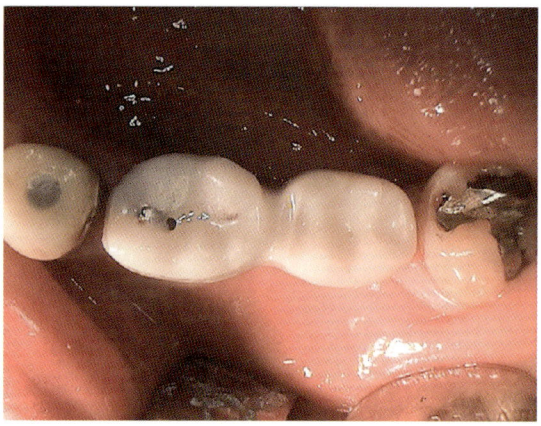

Dentist made temporary, occlusal view

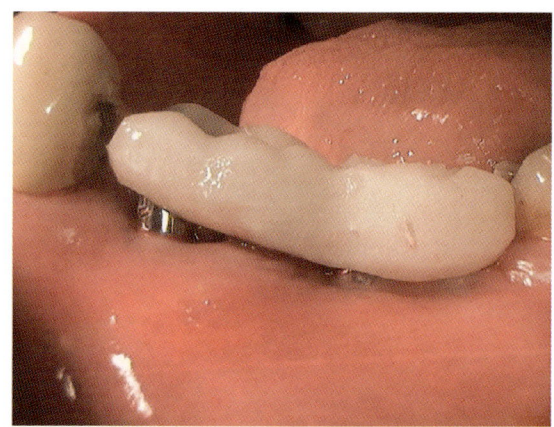

Dentist made temporary, lateral view

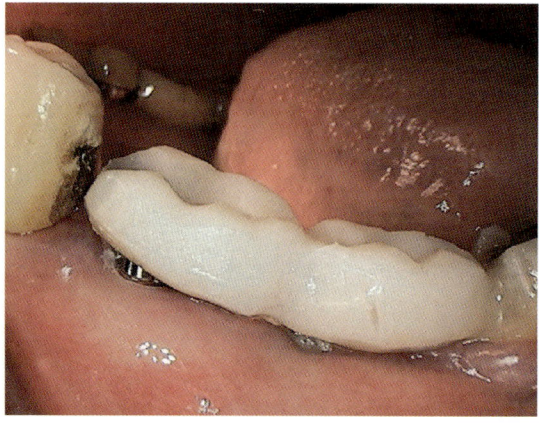

Dentist made temporary before impression taking

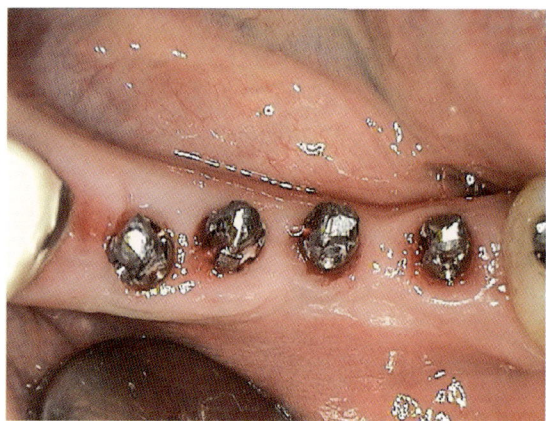

Clinical situation before impression taking

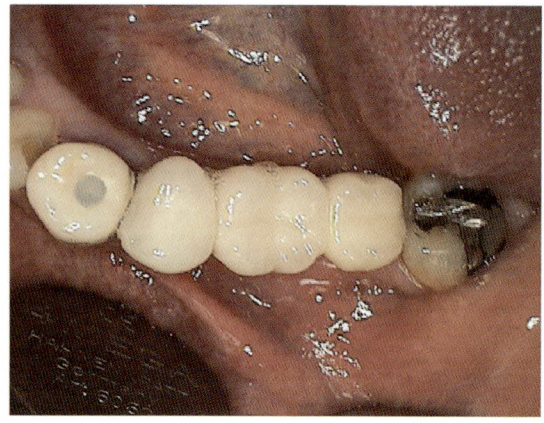

Cemented splinted crown, occlusal view

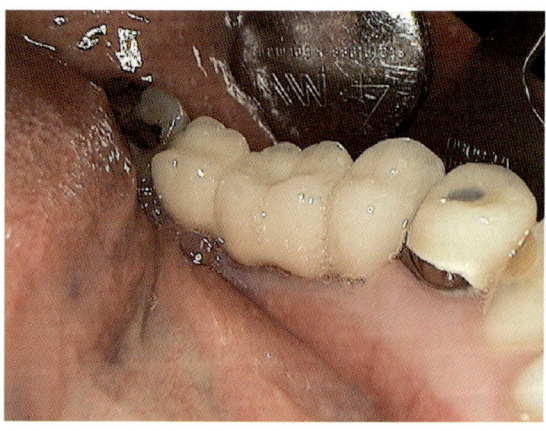

Cemented splinted crown, lingual view

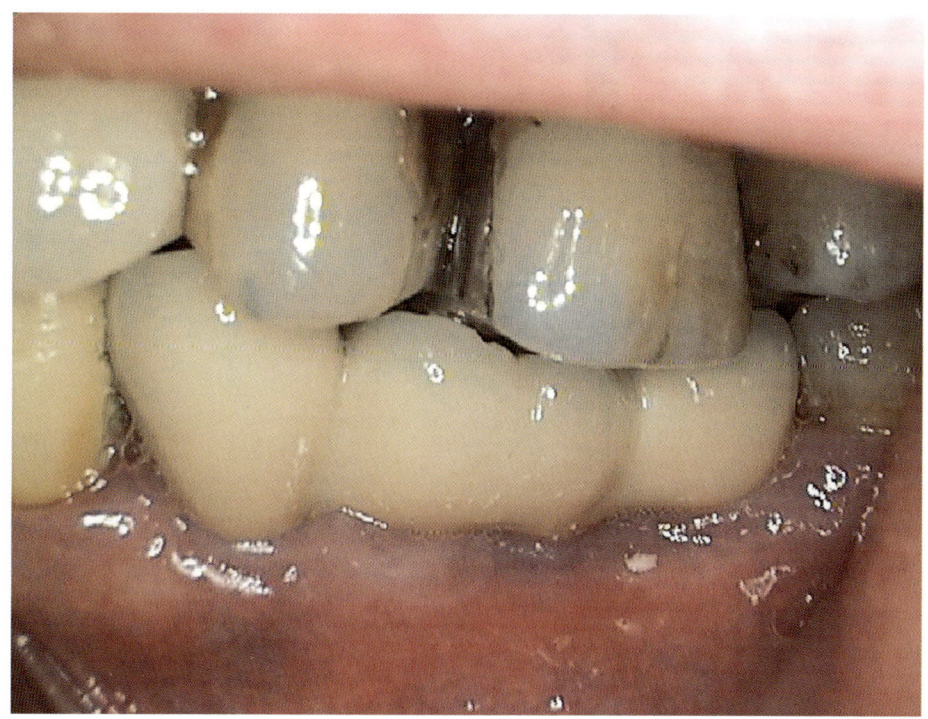

Cemented splinted crown, lateral view

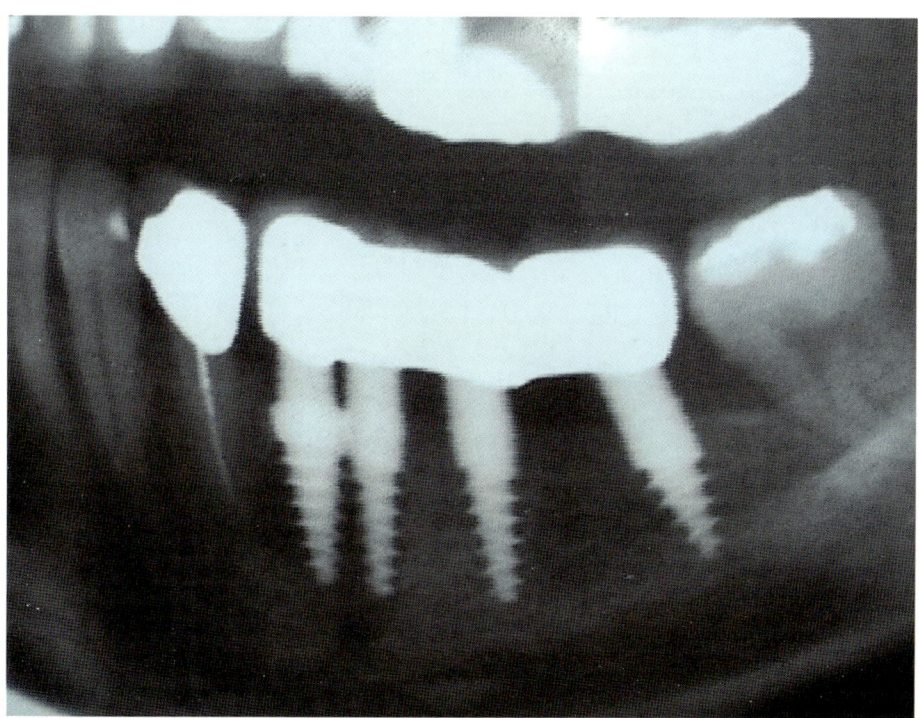

Cemented splinted crown; panoramic radiographic control; zoomed detail

7.2.5/Case 19

Patient: male, 30 years old

24-26 4 implants, splinted crown

14/02/2011	24	Champions® implant Ø 3.5 x 12 mm, >30 Ncm
	25	Champions® implant Ø 4.5 x 12 mm, 30 Ncm
	26m	Champions® implant Ø 4.5 x 12 mm, >40 Ncm
	26d	Champions® implant Ø 4.5 x 10 mm, 20 Ncm indirect sinus lift stump preparation dentist made temporary
15/02/2011		Cemented laboratory made temporary
16/05/2011		Impression, cemented dentist made temporary
30/05/2011	24-26	cemented zirconium dioxide splinted crown
21/09/2011		Panoramic radiograph required for an additional implant placement

Treatment period:

Remarks:

3.5 months

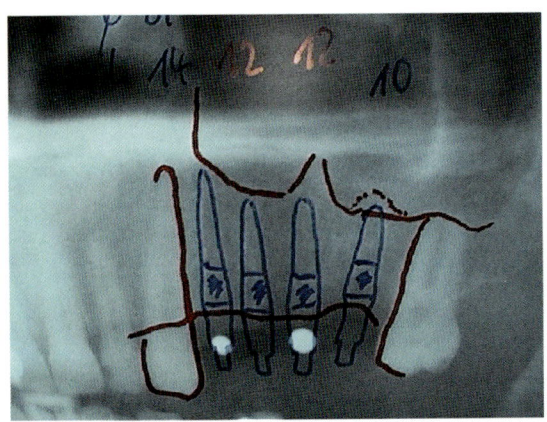

Panoramic radiograph for planned treatment

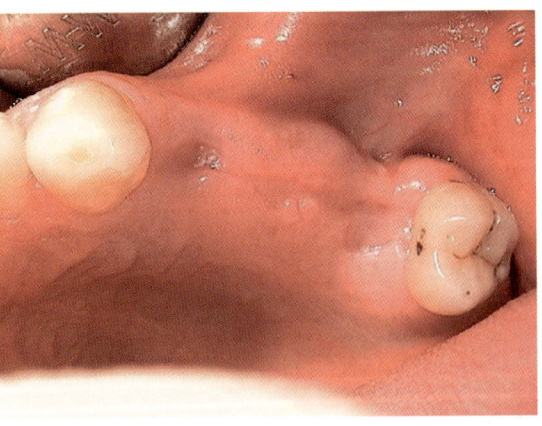

Clinical initial situation

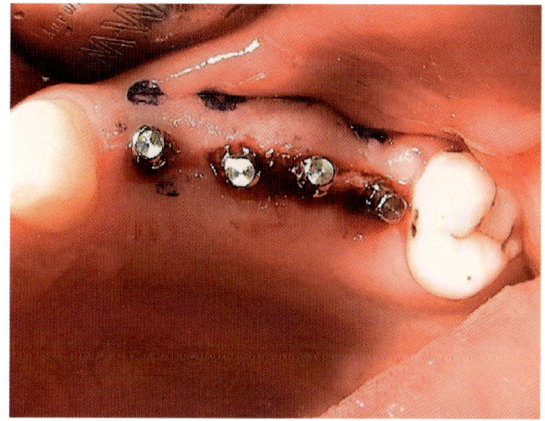

Situation after implant placement, occlusal view

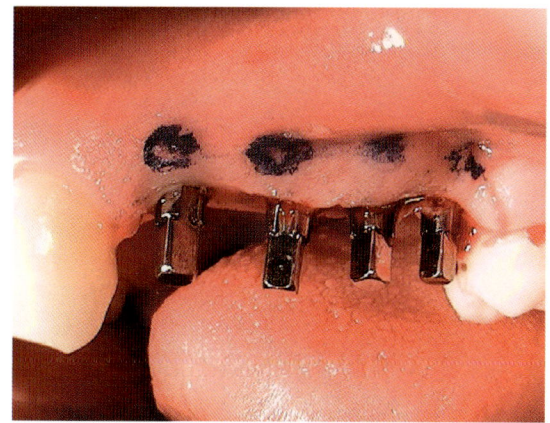

Situation after implant placement, lateral view

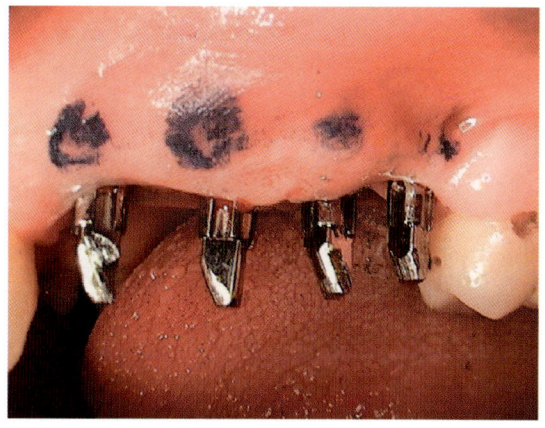

After implant head preparation, lateral view

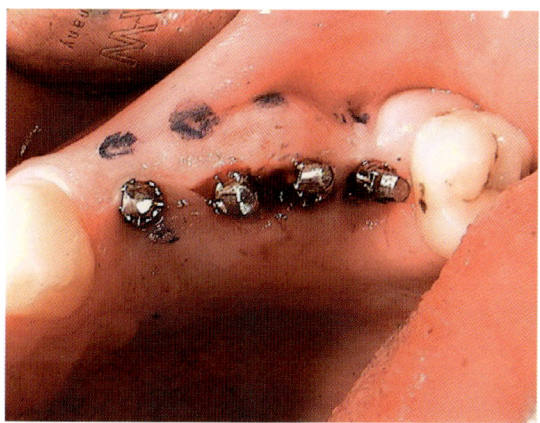

After implant head preparation, occlusal view

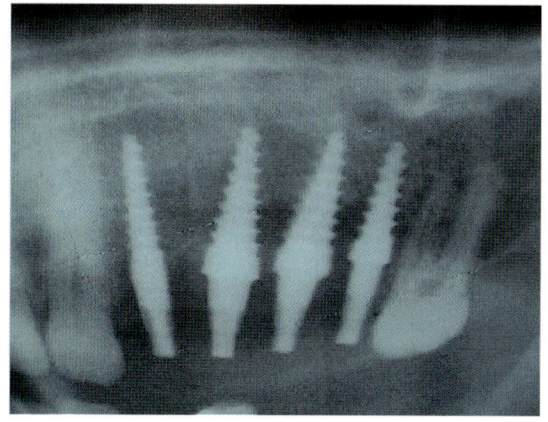

Panoramic radiographic control

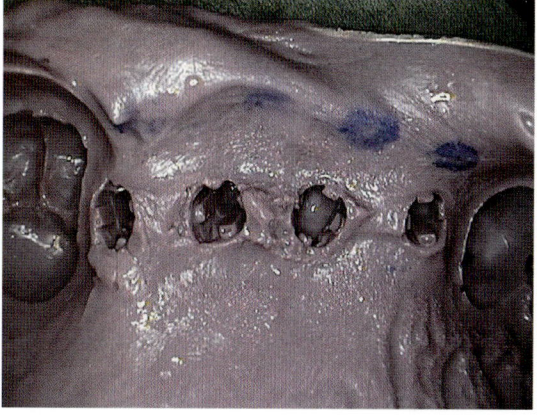

Impression taking for the laboratory made

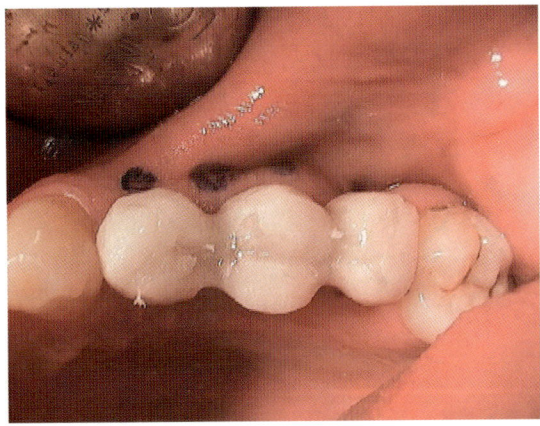

Dentist made temporary, occlusal view

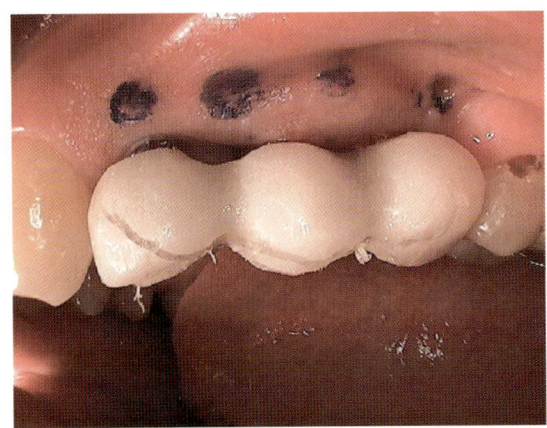

Dentist made temporary, lateral view

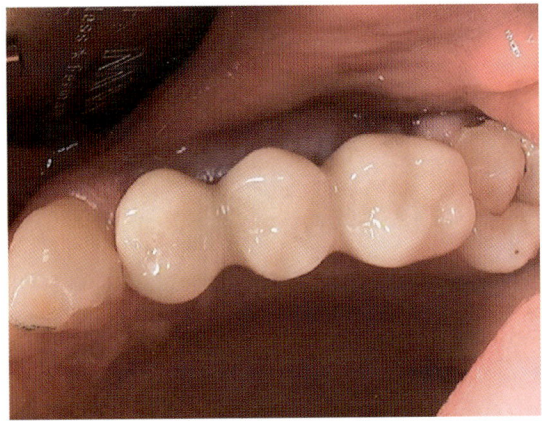

Laboratory made temporary 1st postoperative day, occlusal view

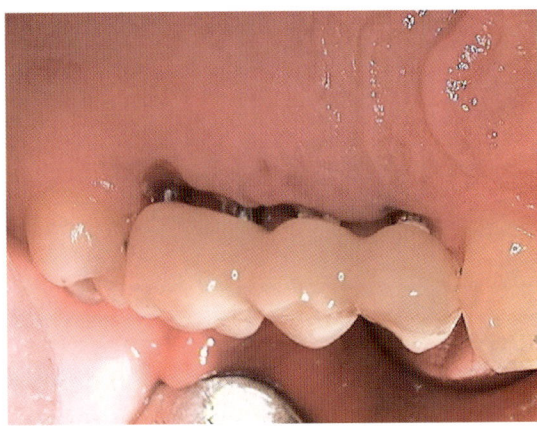

Laboratory made temporary 1st postoperative day, palatal view

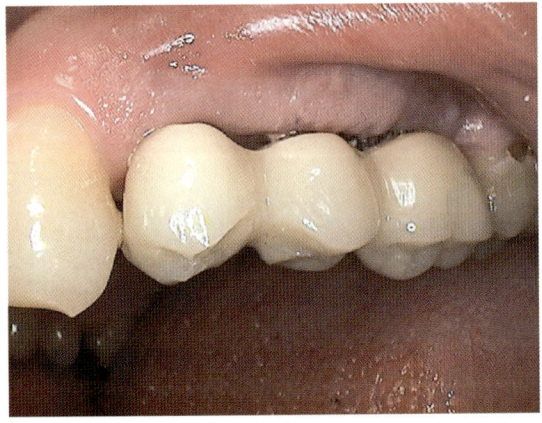

Laboratory made temporary, 1st postoperative day, lateral view

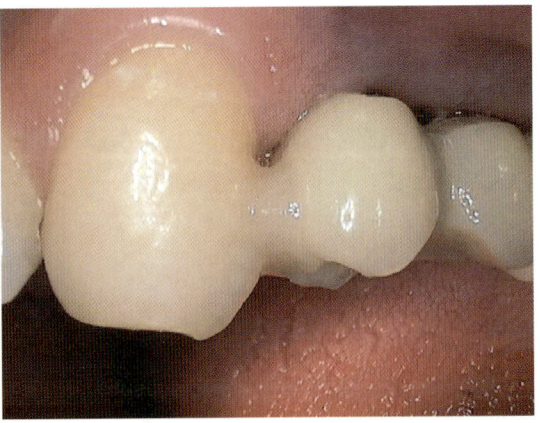

Laboratory made temporary with splinting, lateral view

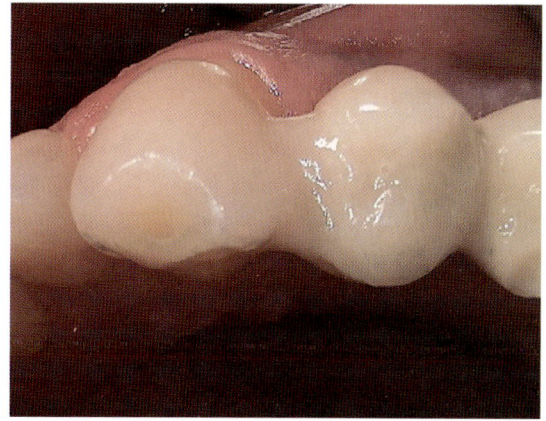

Laboratory made temporary with splinting, occlusal view

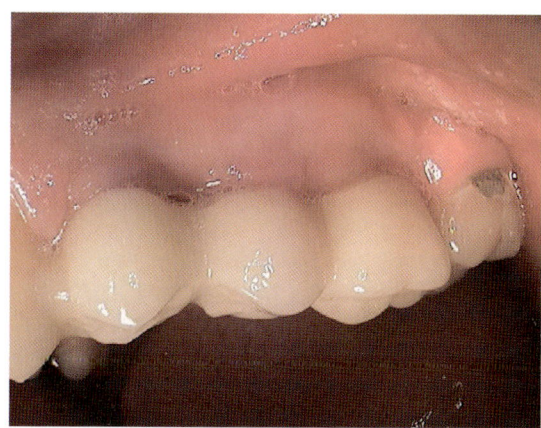

Clinical situation before impression taking

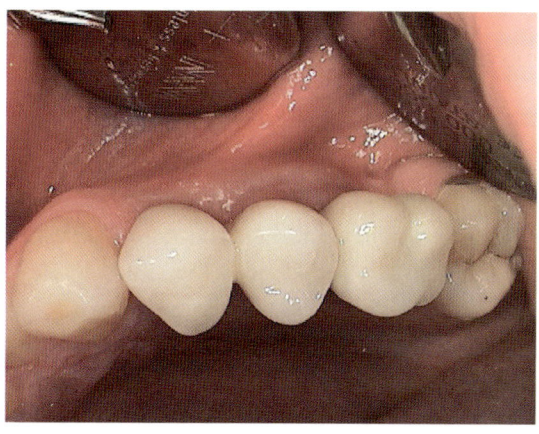

Final cemented splinted crown, occlusal view

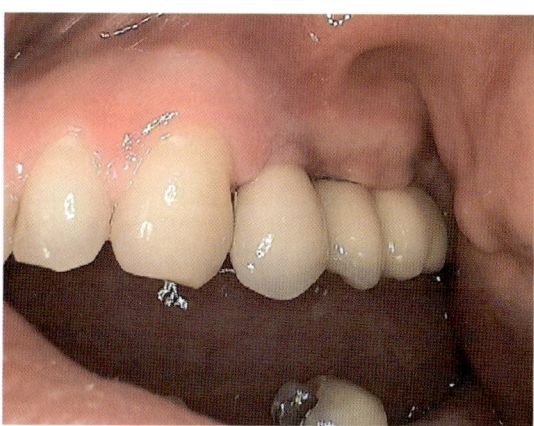

Final cemented splinted crown, lateral view

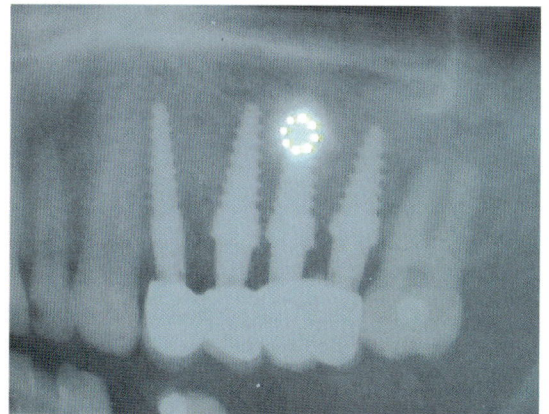

Final panoramic radiographic control

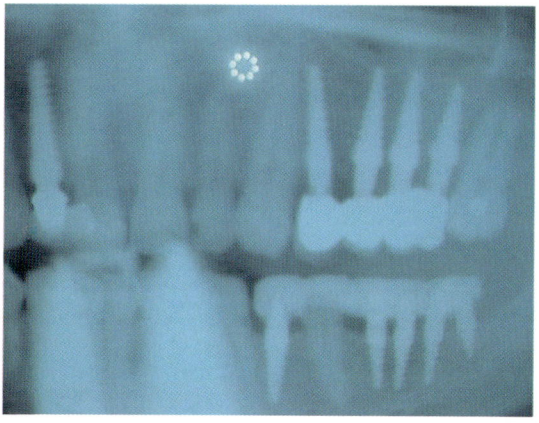

Panoramic radiographic control after 4 months due to additional implant placement

7.2.6/Case 20

Patient: male, 68 years old

24-26 4 implants,
zirconium dioxide splinted crown

02/05/2011	27 24-26	extraction 4 Champions® Implants Ø 3.5 x 6, 8, 10, 12mm indirect sinus lift preparation cemented dentist made temporary
27/06/2011		Impression
11/07/2011	24-26	cemented zirconium dioxide splinted crown
Treatment period:		**2.5 months**
Remarks:		Avoiding a direct sinus lift by using several short implants Late loading

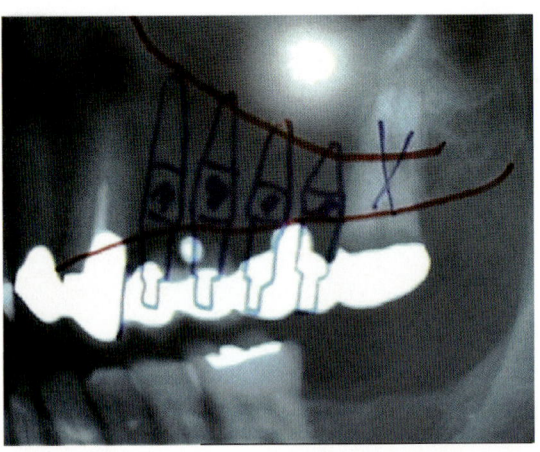

Panoramic radiograph for planned treatment

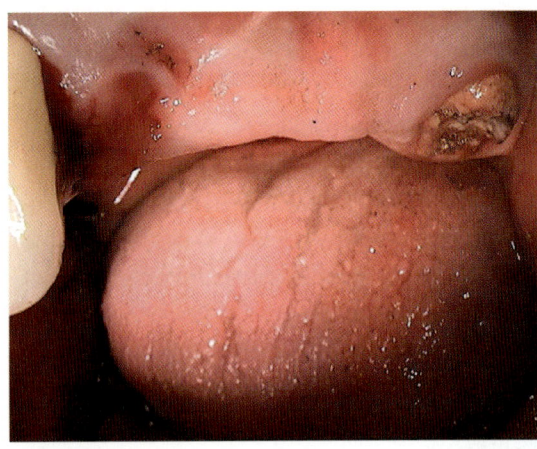

Clinical situation after bridge removal

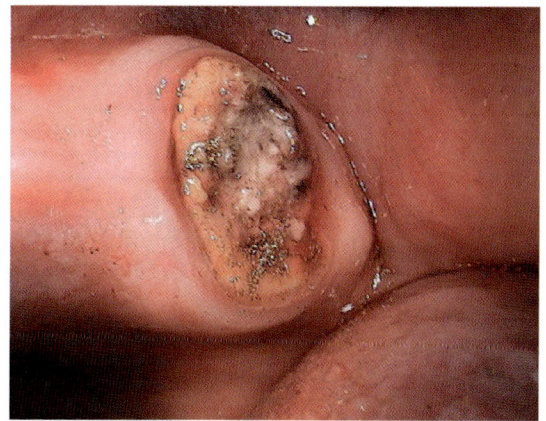

...and macro image

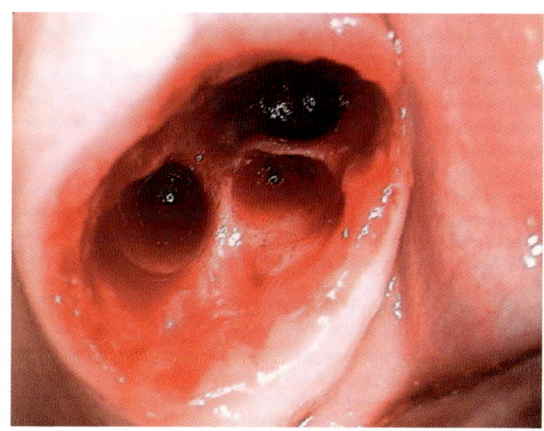

Alveolus 27 after extraction

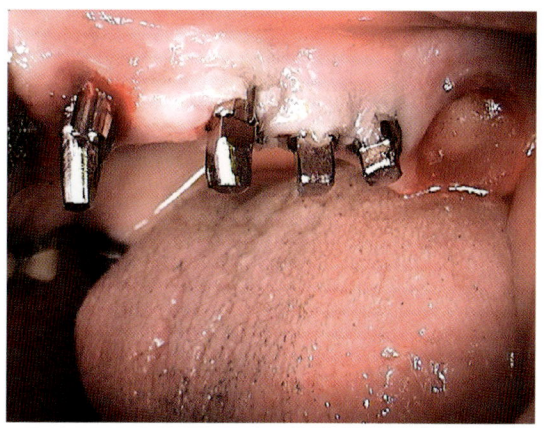

24-26 implant placement, lateral view

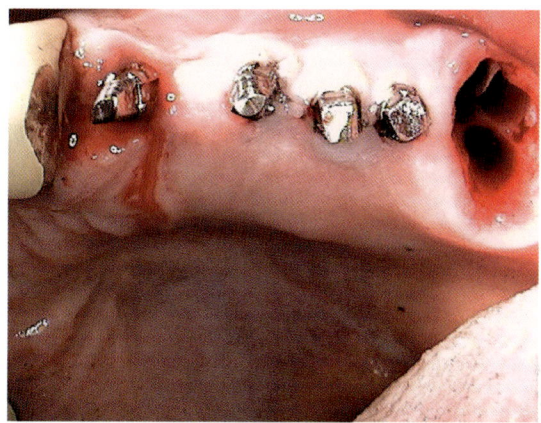

24-26 implant placement, occlusal view

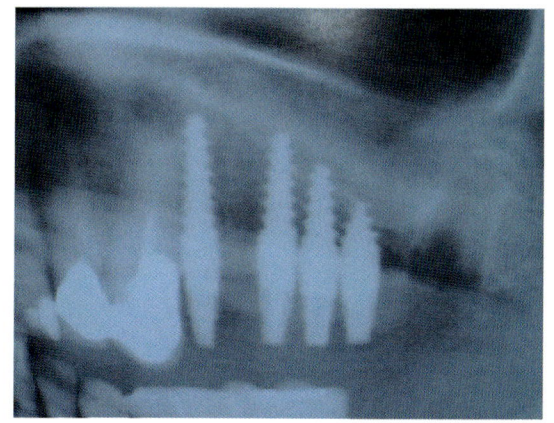

Panoramic radiographic control

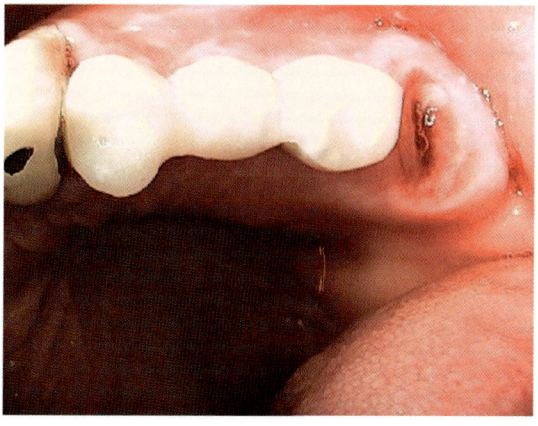

Cemented dentist made temporary, occlusal view

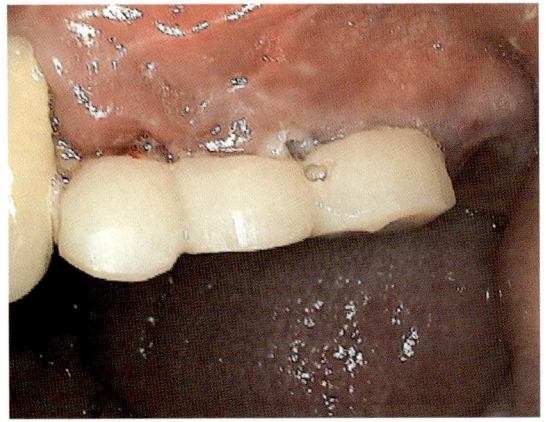

Cemented dentist made temporary, lateral view

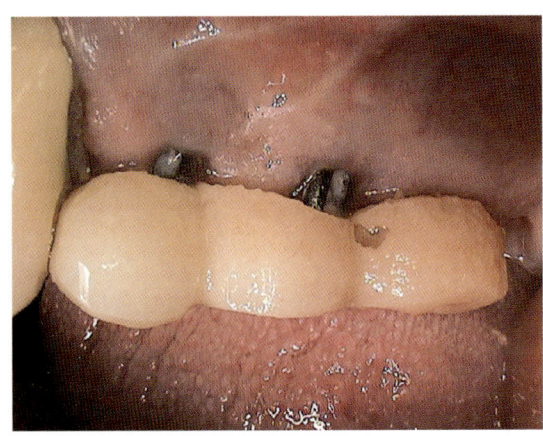

Cemented dentist made temporary, before impression taking

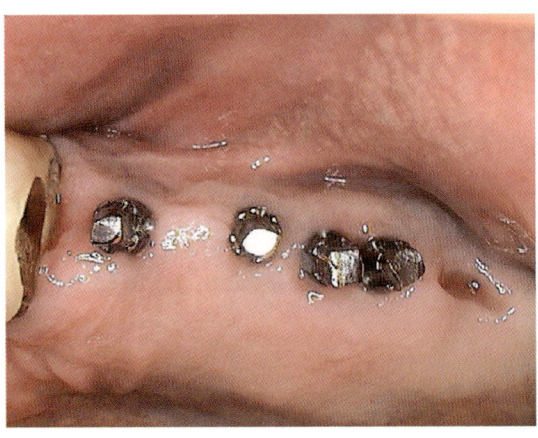

Clinical situation before impression taking...

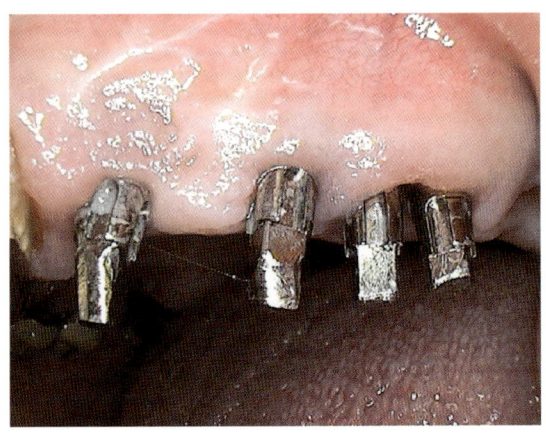

...detailed image...

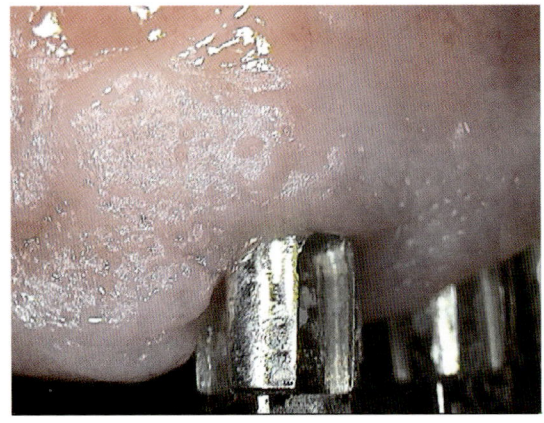

...macro image...

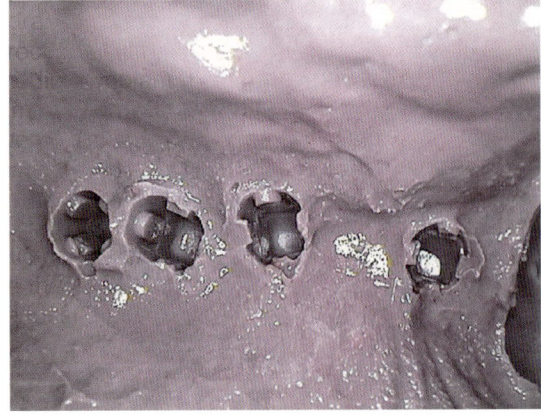

Impression

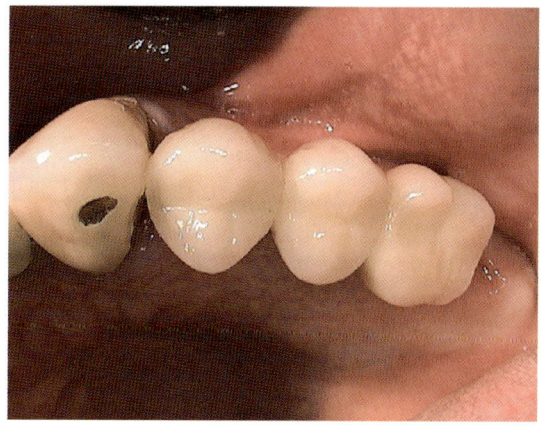

Final cemented splinted crown, occlusal view

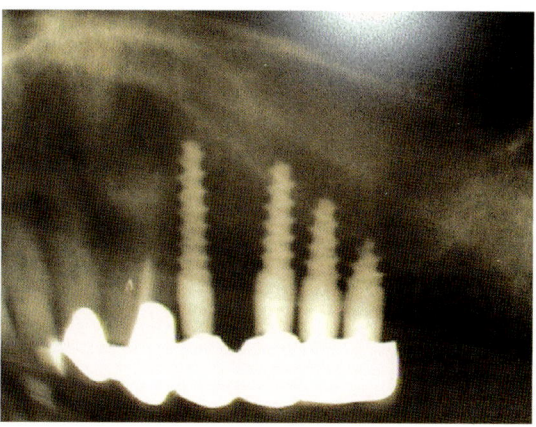

Final cemented splinted crown, panoramic radiographic control, detail

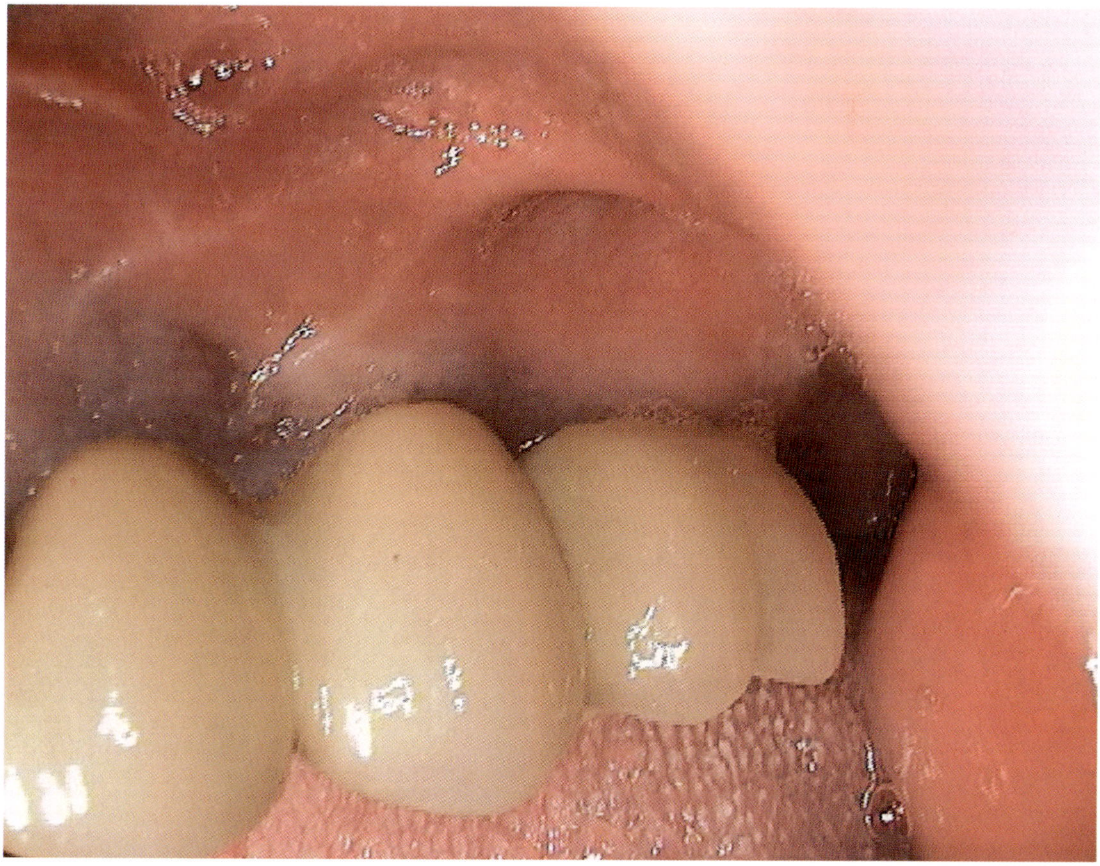

Final cemented splinted crown, lateral view

7.2.7/Case 21

Patient: male, 55 years old

14,16, 17 4 implants, laboratory made temporary
14-17 splinted crown

09/11/2010	13,15	crown lengthening, preparation
	14	Champions® implant Ø 3.0 x 14 mm, 30 Ncm
	16m	Champions® implant Ø 3.5 x 8 mm, >40 Ncm
	16d	Champions® implant Ø 4.5 x 8 mm, >60 Ncm
	17	Champions® implant Ø 4.5 x 8 mm, 25 Ncm
	13-17	cemented dentist made temporary
10/11/2011		Cemented laboratory made temporary
15/01/2011		Impression
02/02/2011	13-17	cemented zirconium dioxide splinted crown
Treatment period:		**3 months**
Remarks:		Avoiding a sinus lift Late implant placement, late loading

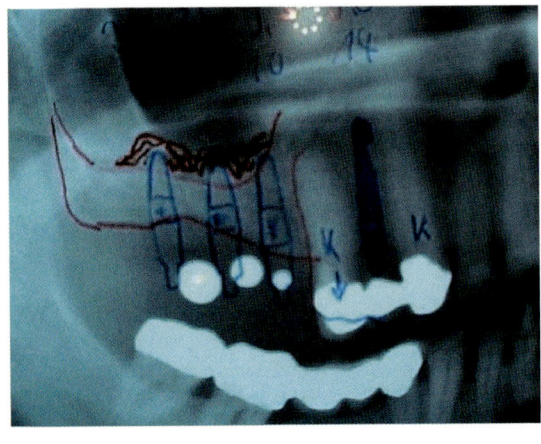

Panoramic radiograph for planned treatment

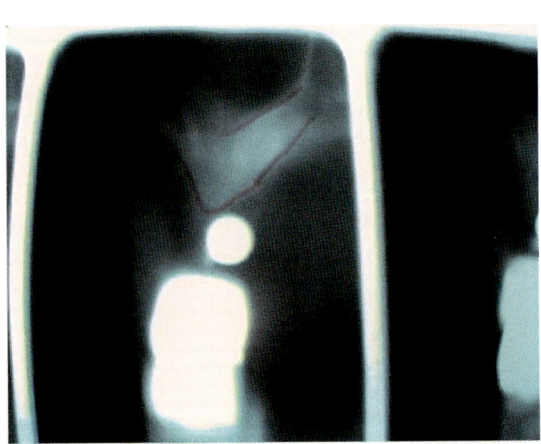

Cross-sectional image

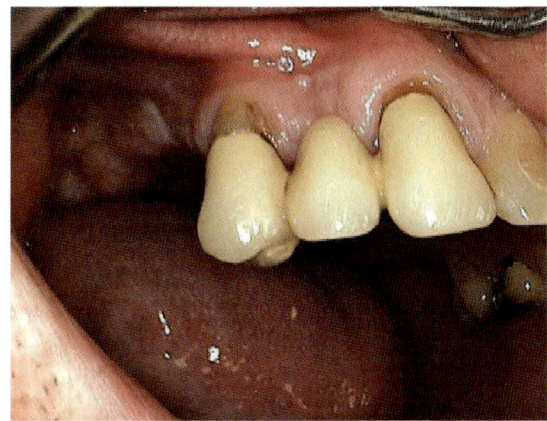

Clinical initial situation...

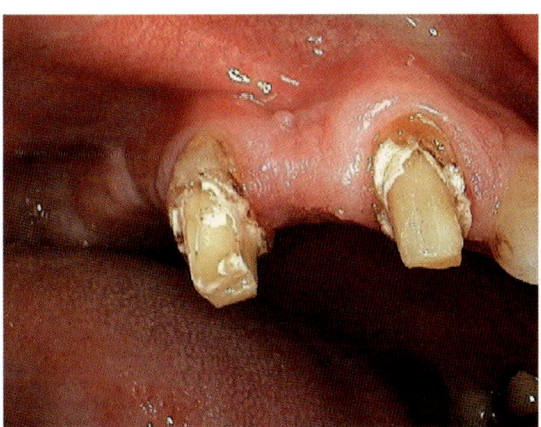

...after bridge removal...

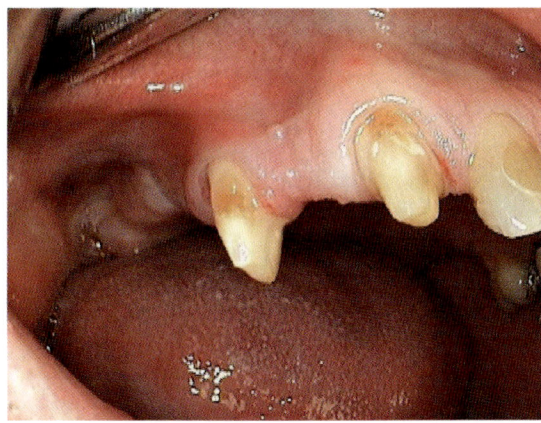

...and teeth preparation

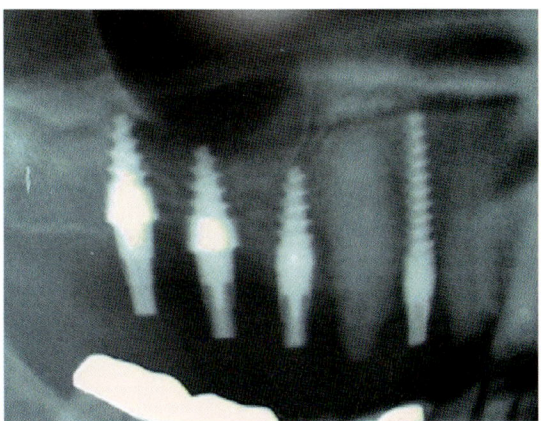

Panoramic radiographic control

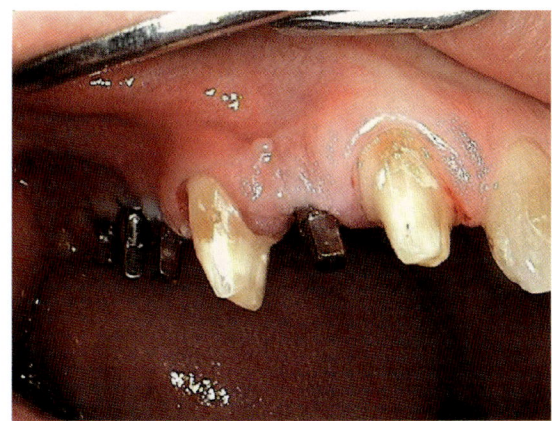

Clinical situation after implant placement...

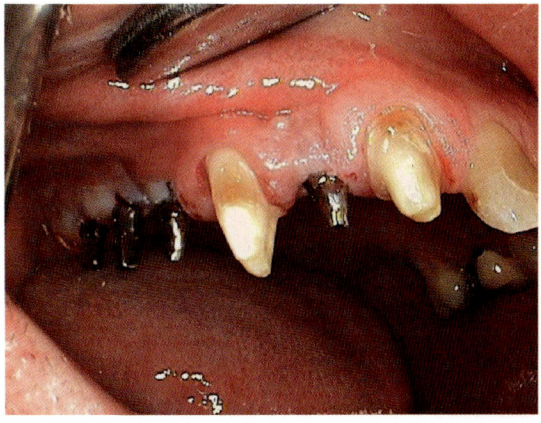

...and implant head preparation

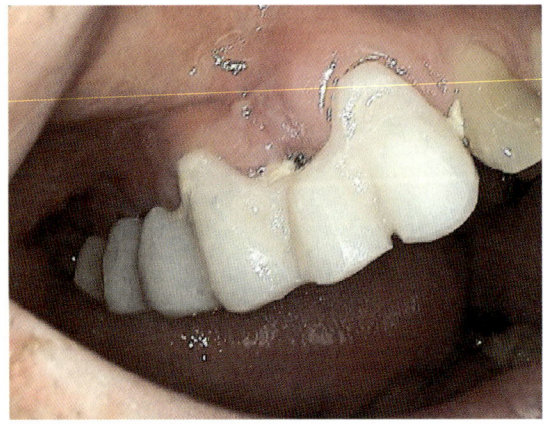

Cemented dentist made temporary

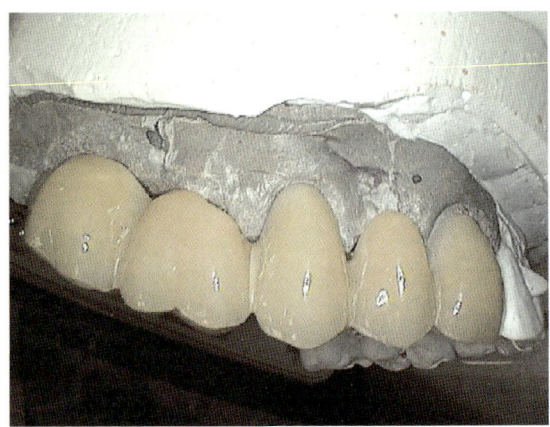

Laboratory made temporary onto the cast

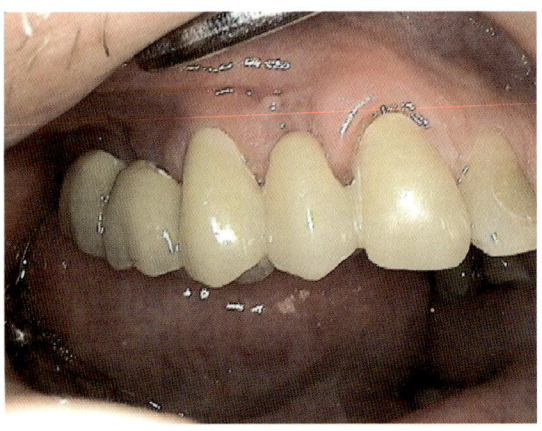

Laboratory made temporary, lateral view

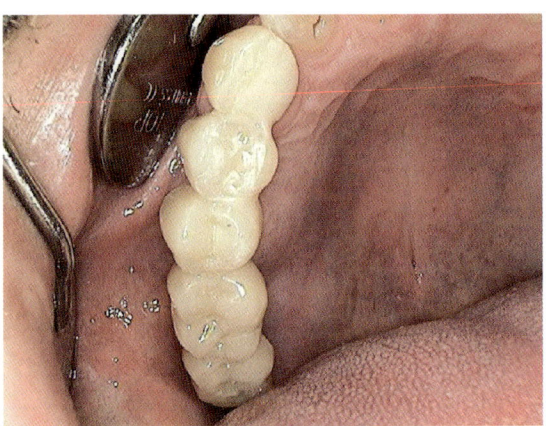

Laboratory made temporary, occlusal view

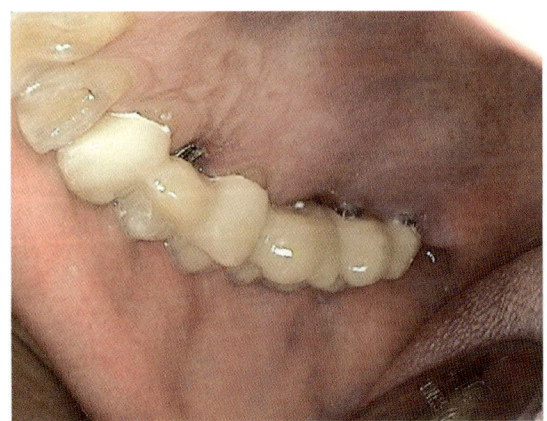

Laboratory made temporary, palatal view

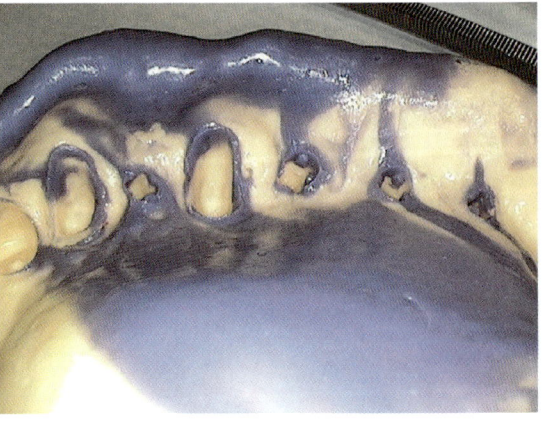

Impression taking for the final splinted crown

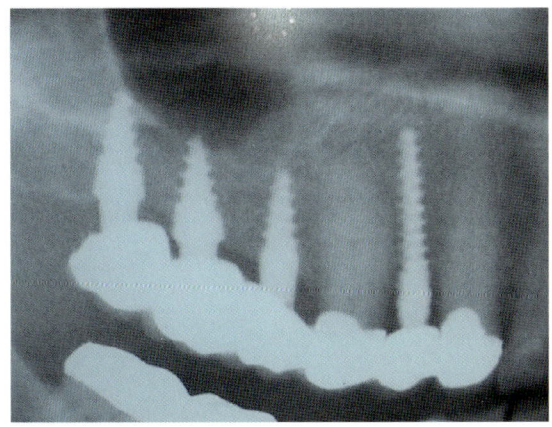

Cemented splinted crown, panoramic radiographic control

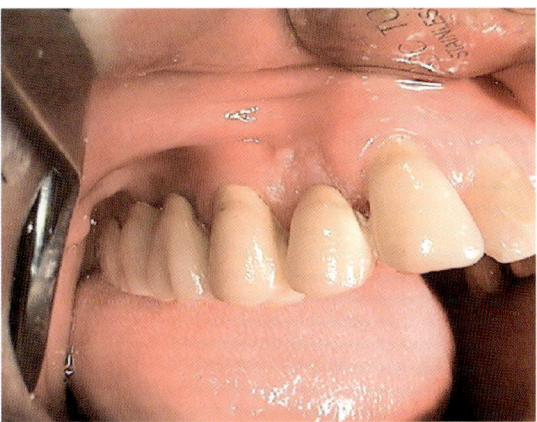

Cemented splinted crown, lateral view

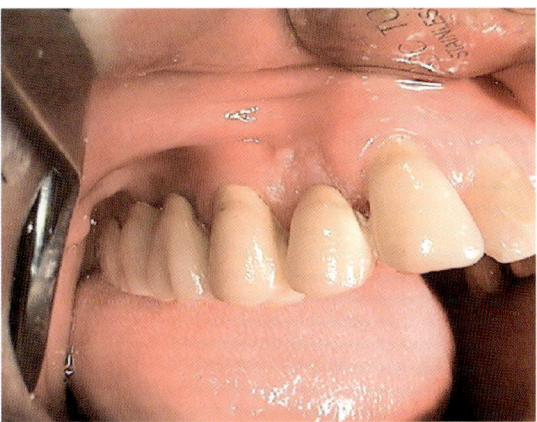

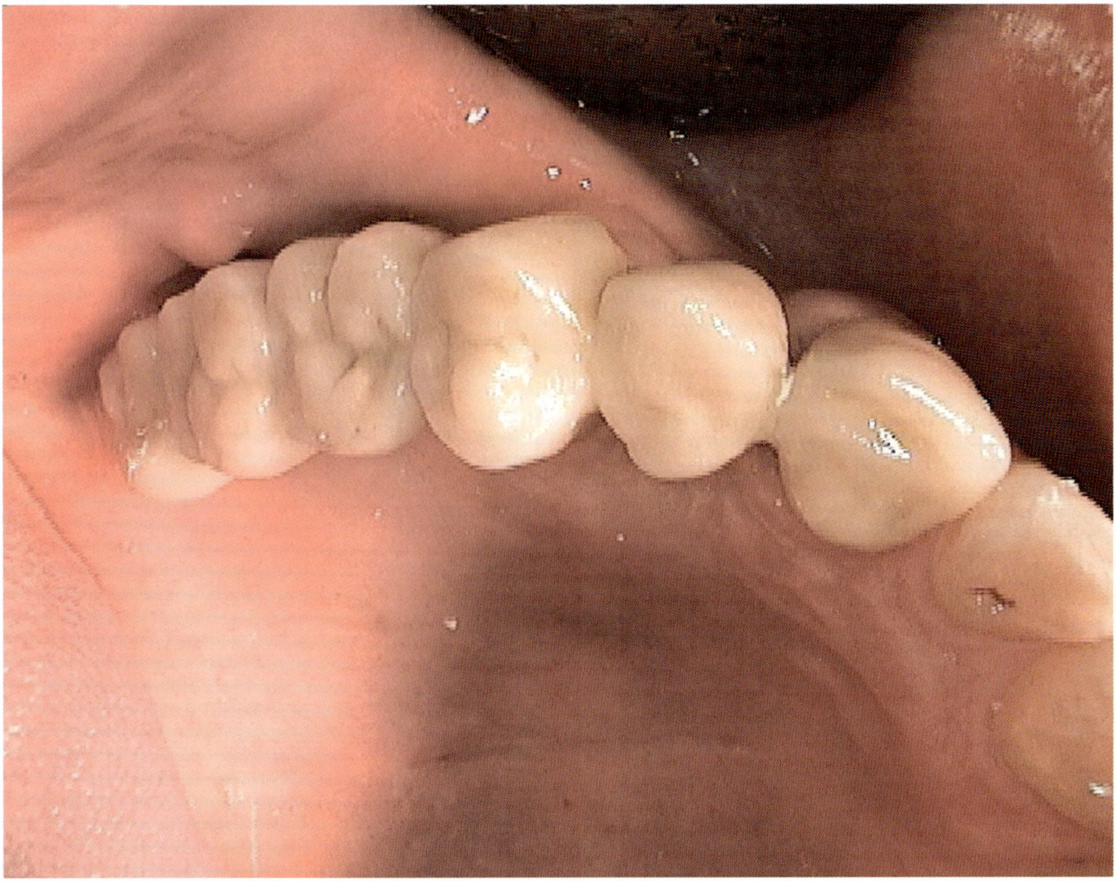

Cemented splinted crown, occlusal view

Patient: female, 61 years old

34, 35, 36 implant placement, splinted crown

17/02/2011	34	Champions® implant Ø 3.0 x 14 mm, >60 Ncm, Periotest - 3
	35	Champions® implant Ø 3.5 x 6 mm, >50 Ncm, Periotest - 2
	36m	Champions® implant Ø 3.5 x 6 mm, >60 Ncm, Periotest 0
	36d	Champions® implant Ø 3.5 x 6 mm, >60 Ncm, Periotest 4 impression cemented dentist made temporary
25/02/2011	34-36	cemented zirconium dioxide splinted crown

Treatment period: **1 week**

Remarks: Lower jaw, right side: Implant placement 15 months ago
Here also: Early loading
No bone loss after 15 months!

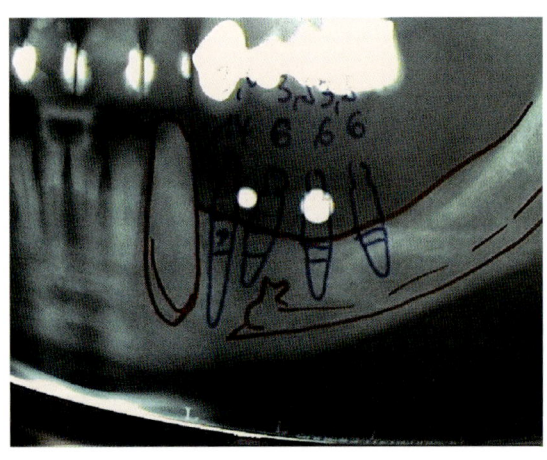

Planned treatment, initial panoramic radiograph

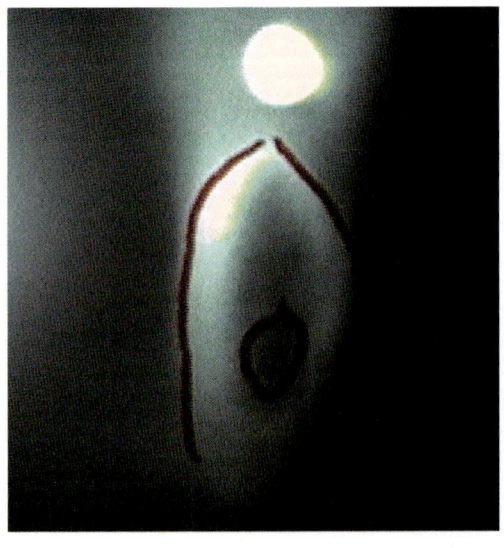

X-ray, cross-sectional image

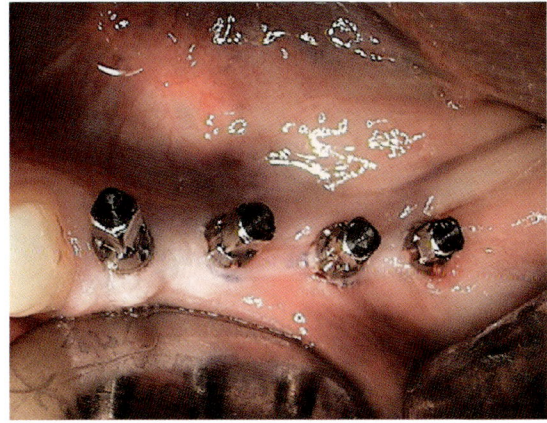

After implant placement, occlusal view

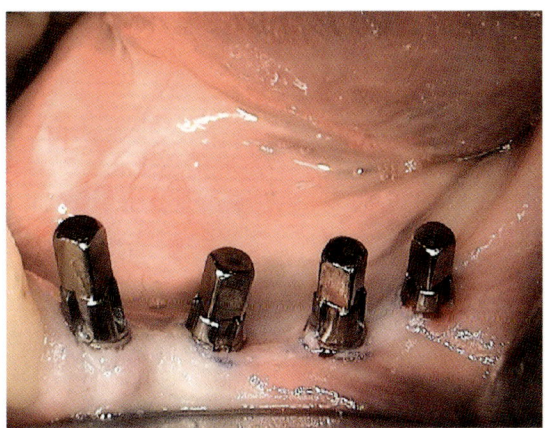

After implant placement, lateral view

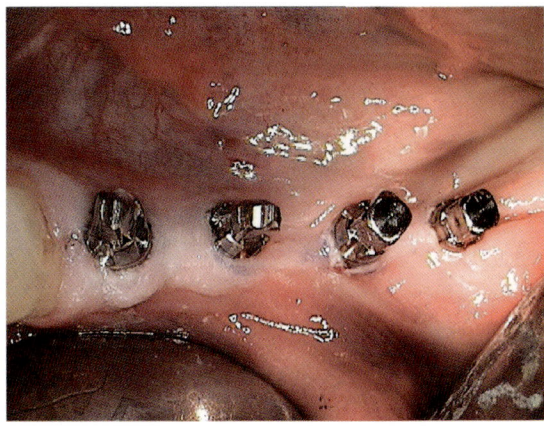

Preparation of implant heads, occlusal view

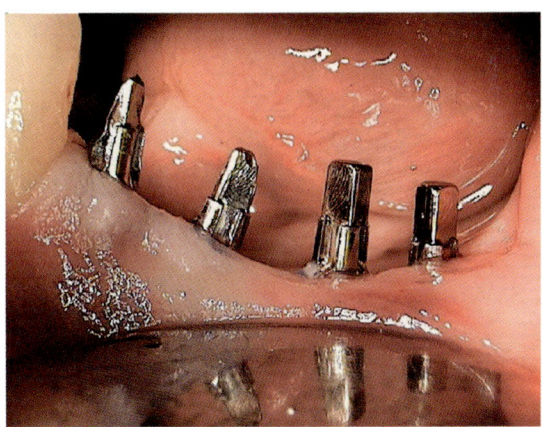

...lateral view

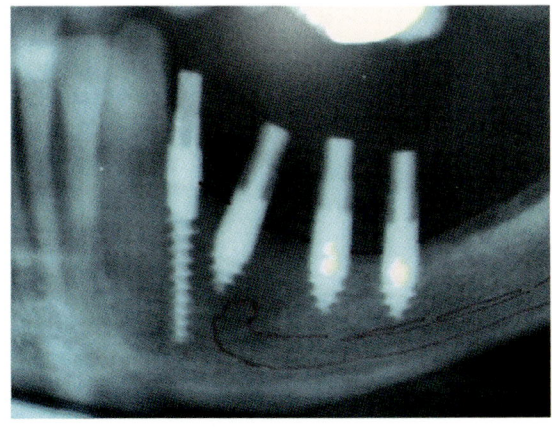

Panoramic radiographic control

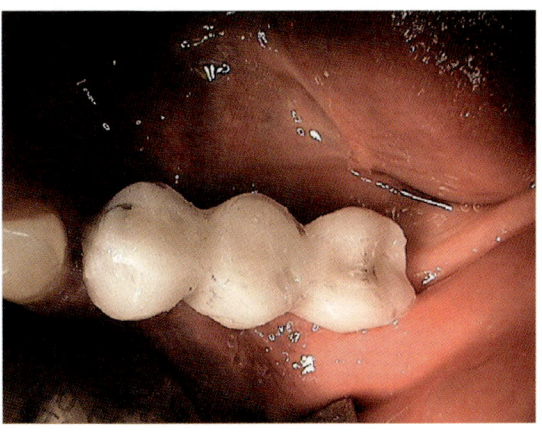

Dental provisional prosthesis, occlusal view

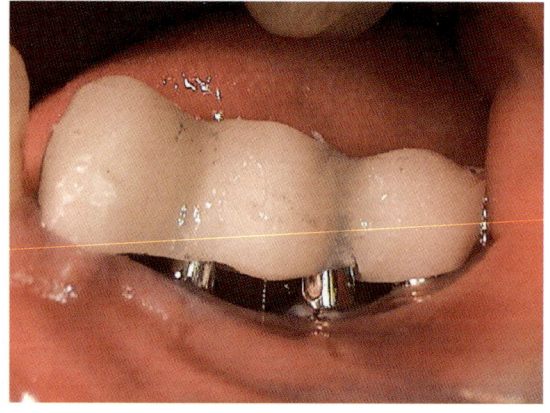

Dental provisional prosthesis, lateral view

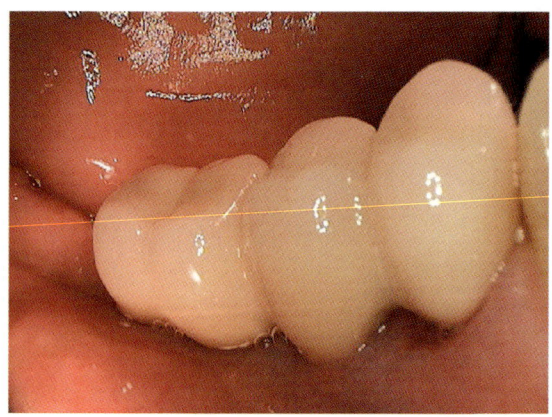

Cemented splinted crown, lingual view

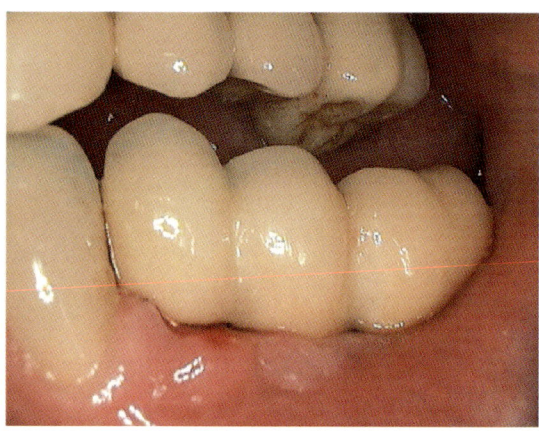

Cemented splinted crown, lateral view

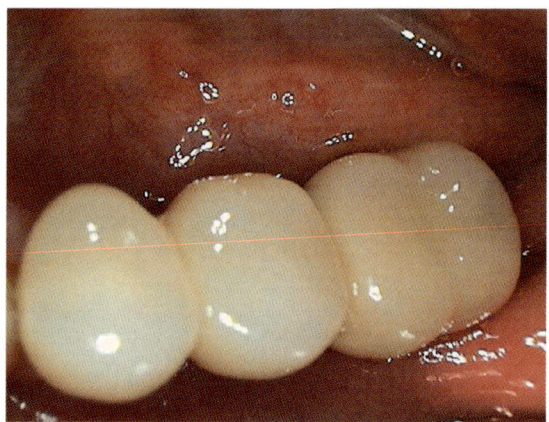

Cemented splinted crown, occlusal view

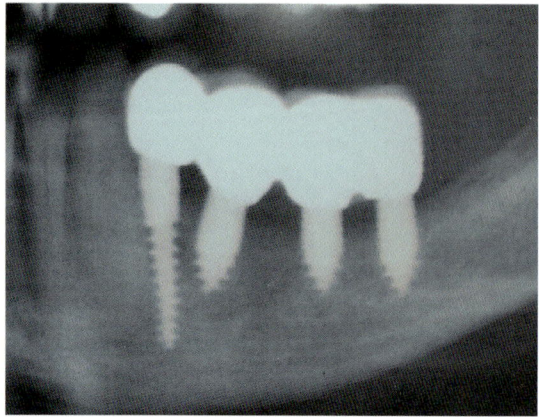

Final radiograph control, zoomed detail

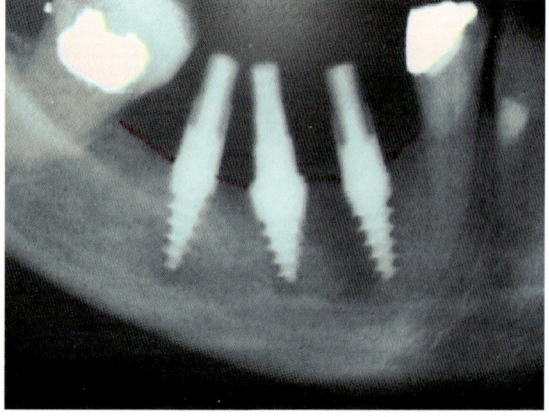

Lower jaw right side, implant placement 15 months ago

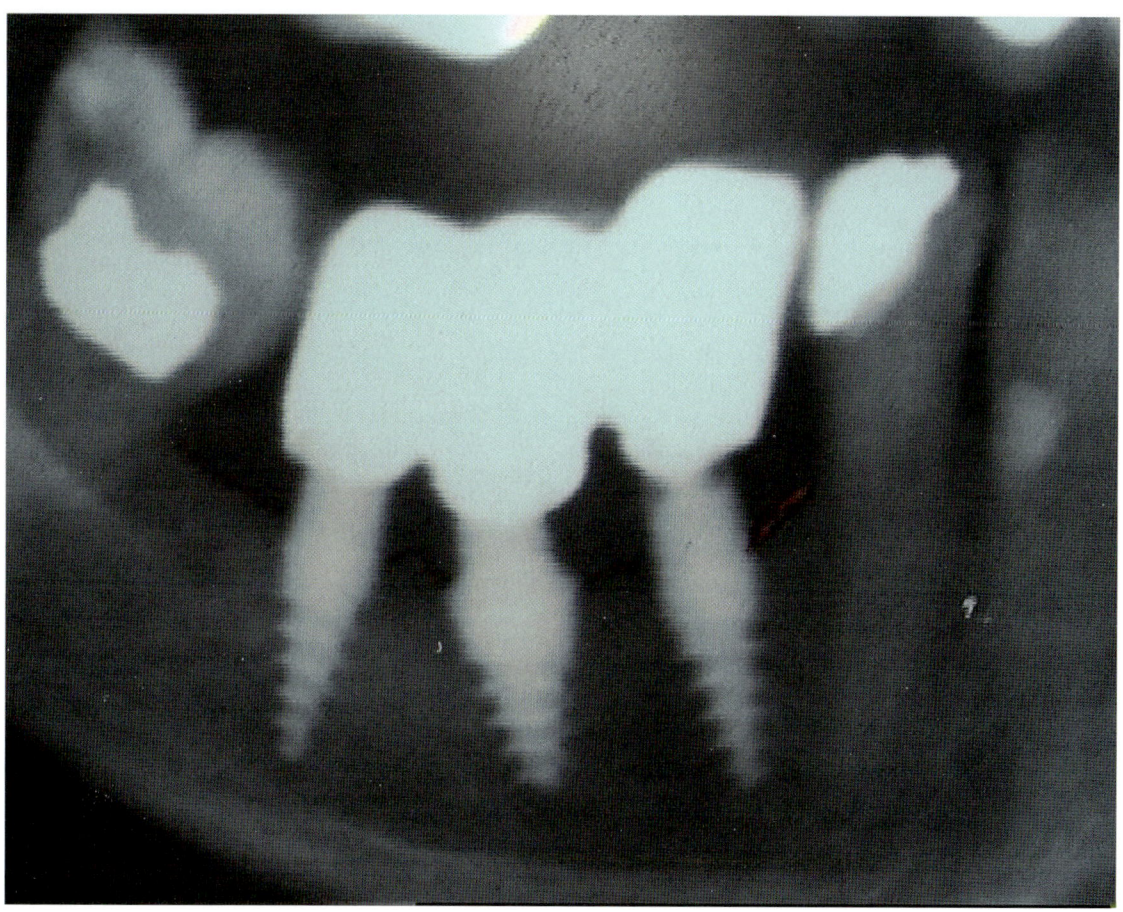

Lower jaw right side, radiographic control after 15 months, zoomed detail

Patient: female, 36 years old

**45-47 implant placement,
augmentation, splinted crown**

21/12/2010	45,46	extraction
14/04/2011	45	Champions® implant Ø 3.5 x 14 mm, 60 Ncm
	46m	Champions® implant Ø 3.5 x 10 mm, >20 Ncm
	46d	Champions® implant Ø 4.5 x 10 mm, 20 Ncm
	47	Champions® implant Ø 3.5 x 8 mm, 40 Ncm
		augmentation with native bone and absorbable membrane
		dentist made temporary
22/08/2011		Impression
07/09/2011	45- 47	cemented zirconium dioxide bridge, panoramic radiograph

Treatment period:

5 months

Remarks:

Extremely anxious, endotracheal anaesthesia
Very slim lower jaw
Longer waiting time between the implant placement and the
prosthesis completion to achieve a secure osseointegration
Late implant placement
Immediate restoration
Late loading

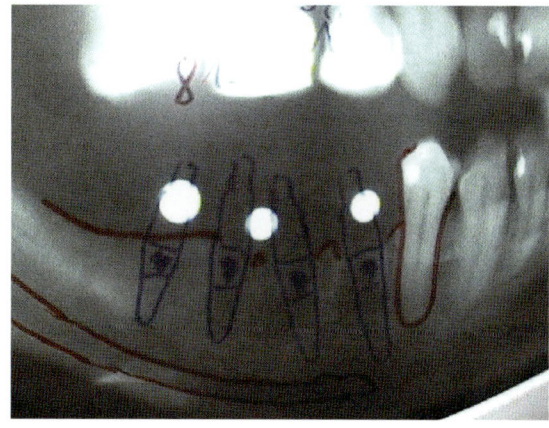

Panoramic radiograph for planned treatment

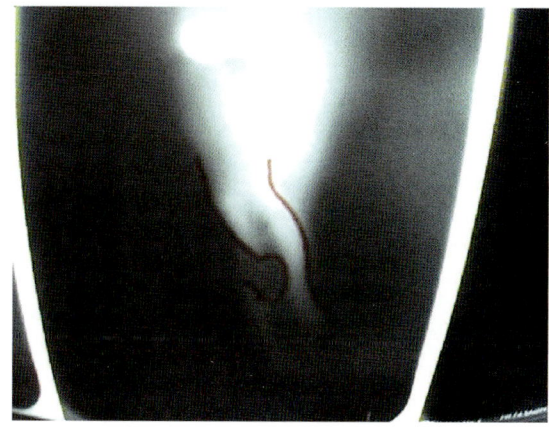

Cross-sectional radiography, right side

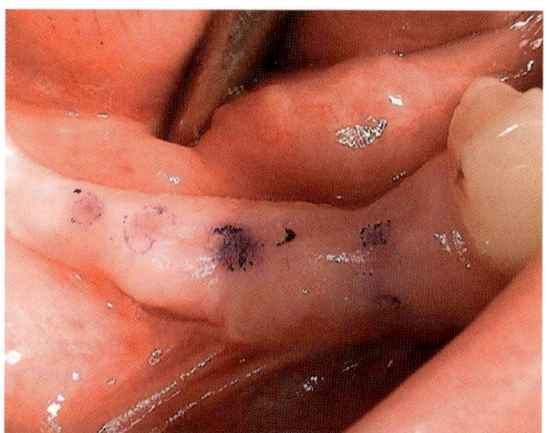

Clinical initial situation

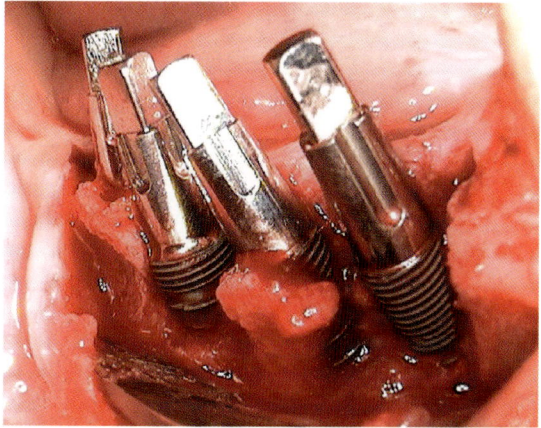

Minimally invasive method of implant placement was not possible in this case!

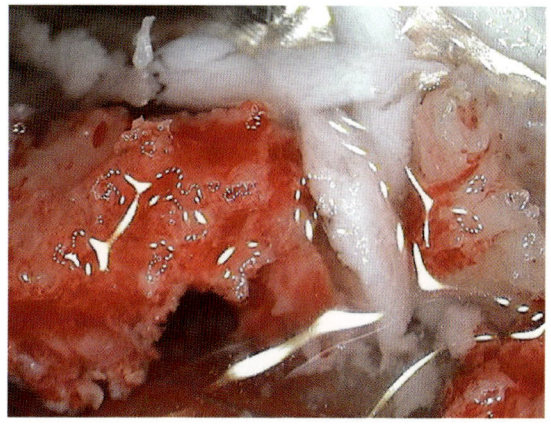

Autologous bone

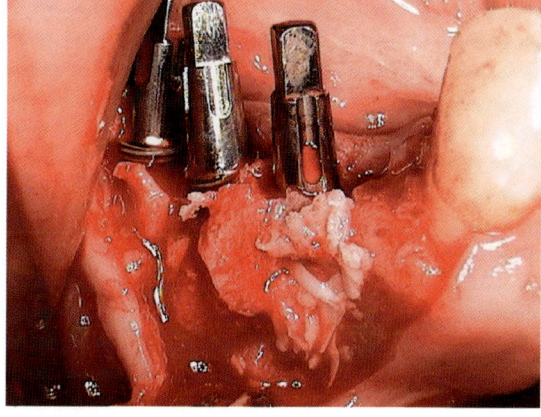

Bone augmentation

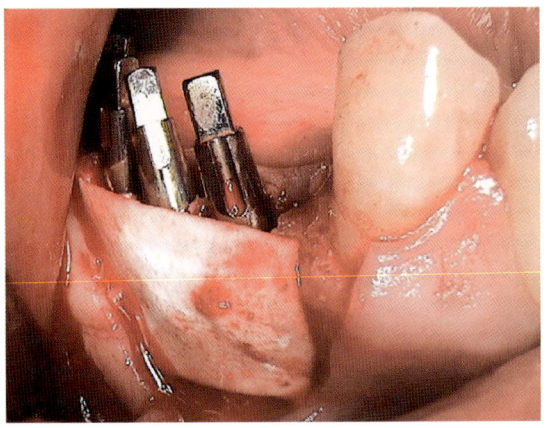

Absorbable membrane

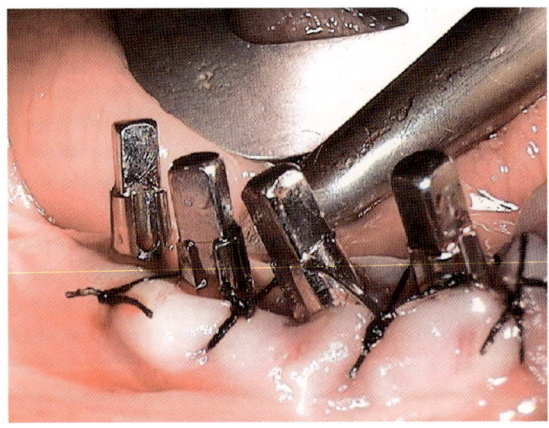

Wound closure

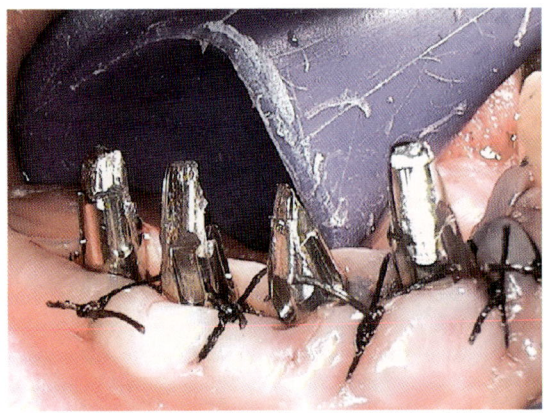

Preparation of implant heads

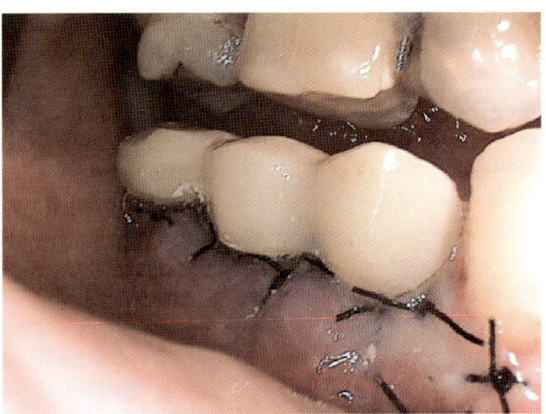

Cemented dentist made temporary

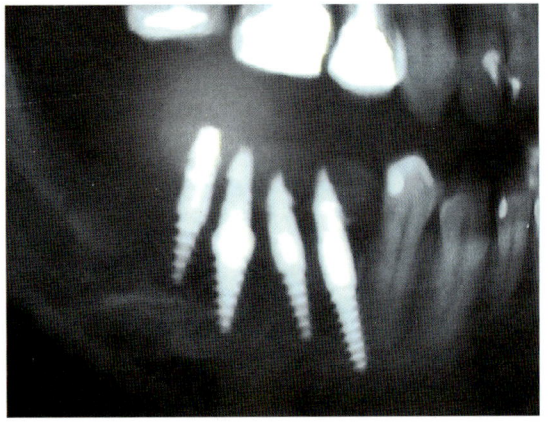

Panoramic radiographic control

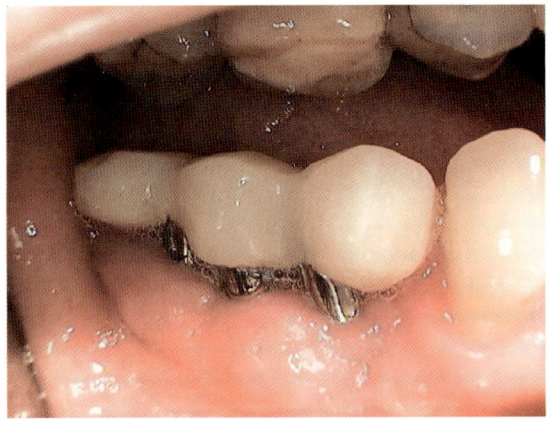

Clinical situation before final impression taking

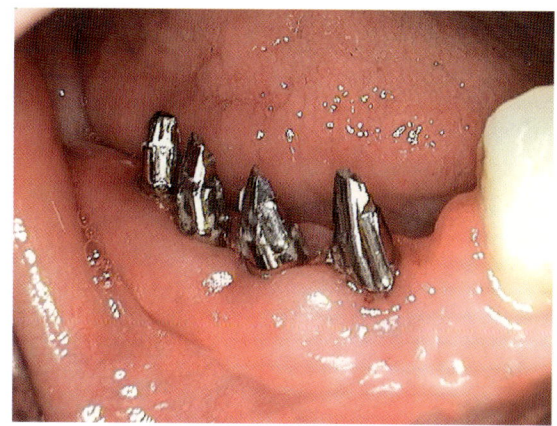

Clinical situation before final impression taking, lateral view

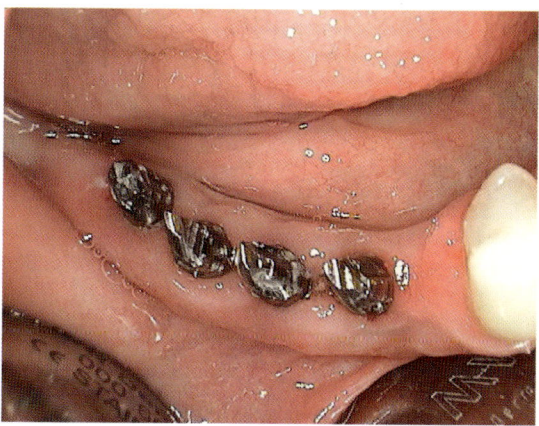

Clinical situation before final impression taking, occlusal view

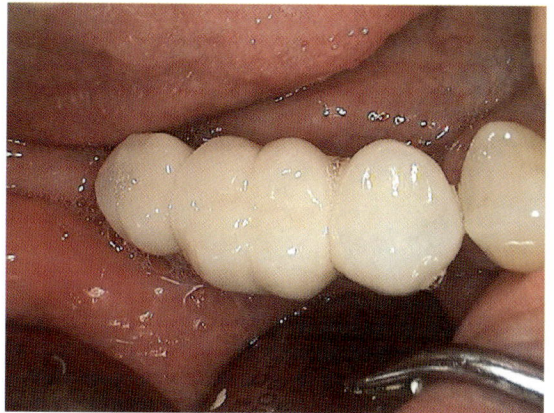

Final cemented splinted crown, occlusal view

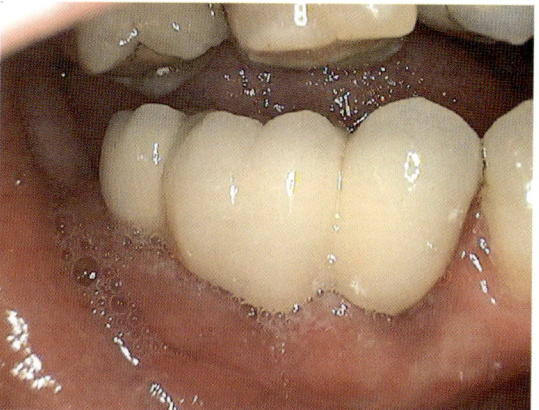

Final cemented splinted crown, lateral view

Patient: female, 60 years old

13 extraction with Benex, 13-16 implants with splinted crowns

---

19/04/2010	13	extraction with Benex
	13	Champions® implant Ø 4.5 x 16 mm, 60 Ncm
	14	Champions® implant Ø 4.5 x 14 mm, 30 Ncm
	15	Champions® implant Ø 3.5 x 10 mm, 30 Ncm
	16	Champions® implant Ø 3.5 x 8 mm, 30 Ncm
	13-16	cemented dentist made temporary
10/08/2010		Implant head preparation
		Impression
24/08/2010	13-16	cemented zirconium dioxide crown
05/10/2011		Panoramic radiographic control due to an additional implant placement in the anterior maxillary region
		No bone loss!

Treatment period:

4 months

Remarks:

Indirect sinus lift
Radiographic control after one year due to an additional implant placement in the anterior maxillary region

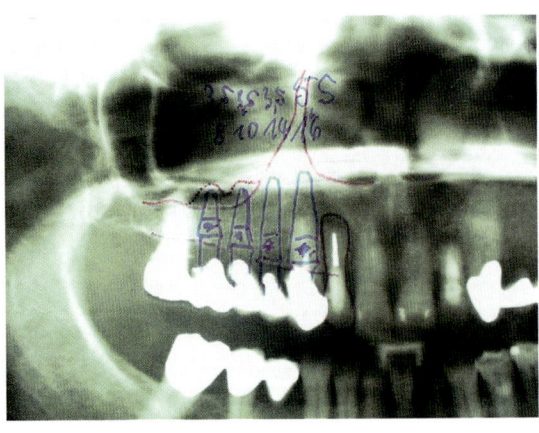

Planned implant placement, initial panoramic radiograph

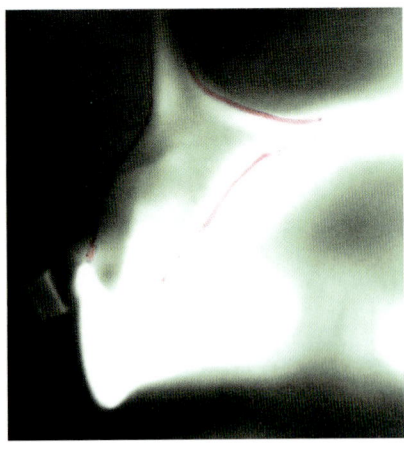

Cross-sectional image

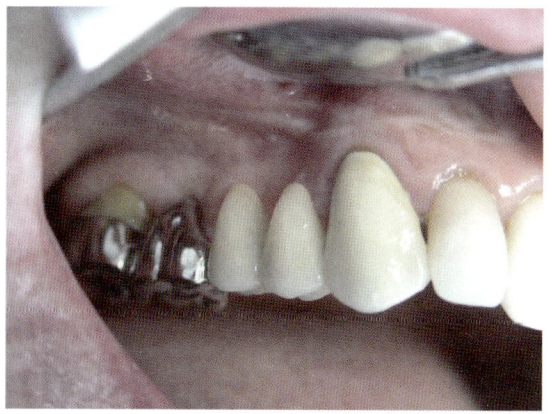

Clinical initial situation

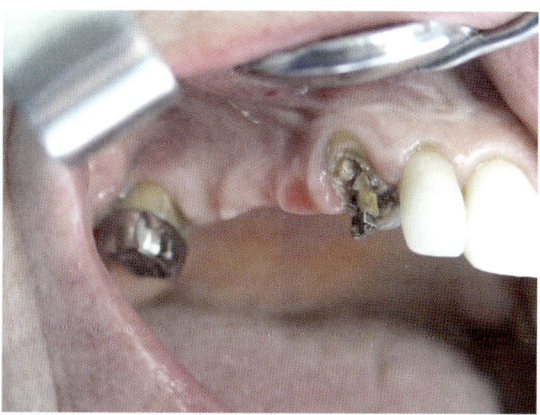

Ruined tooth 13

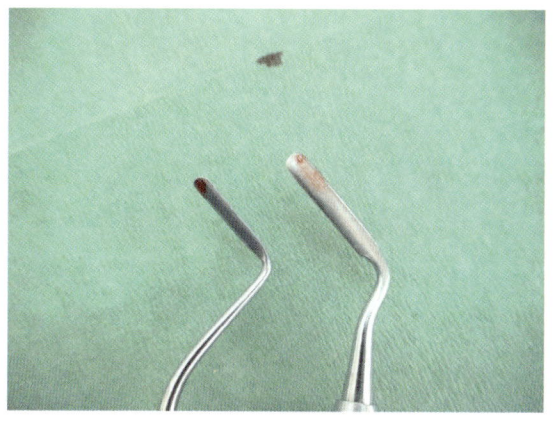

Periotomes in order to gently remove the gingiva

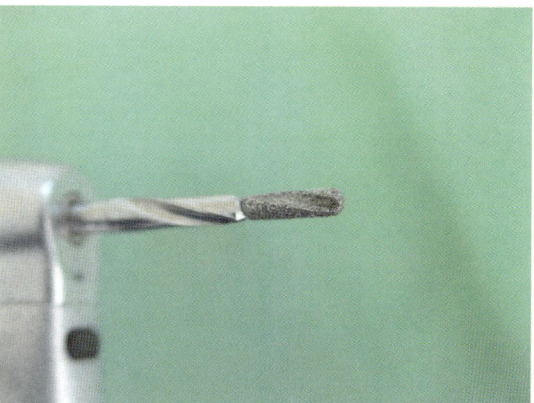

Benex twist drill

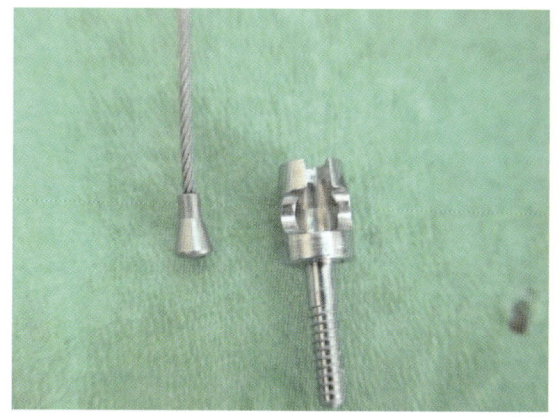

Benex extraction screw

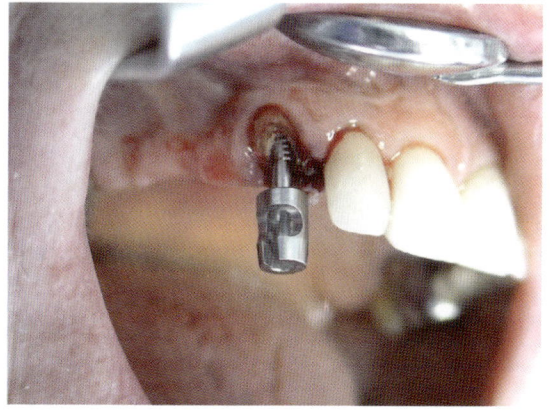

Inserted extraction screw

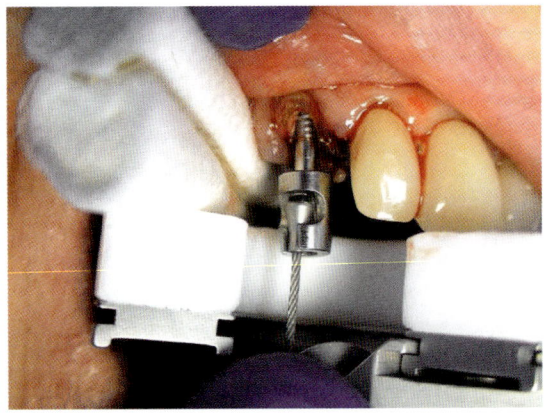

Positioned extractor tool

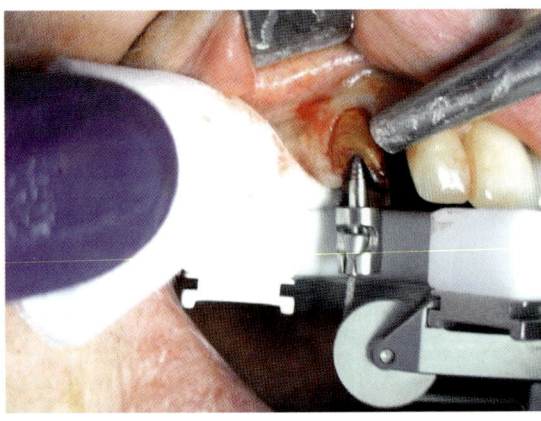

Controlled and gentle...

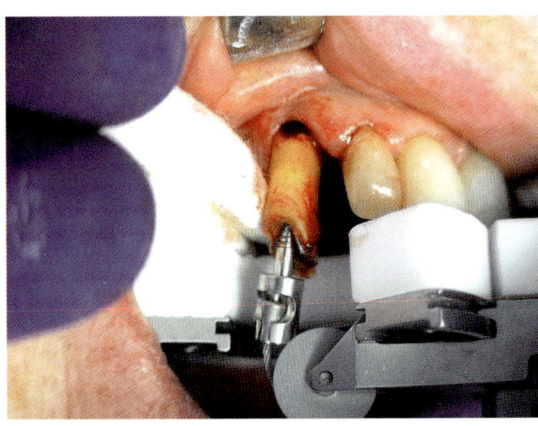

...turning of the hand screw

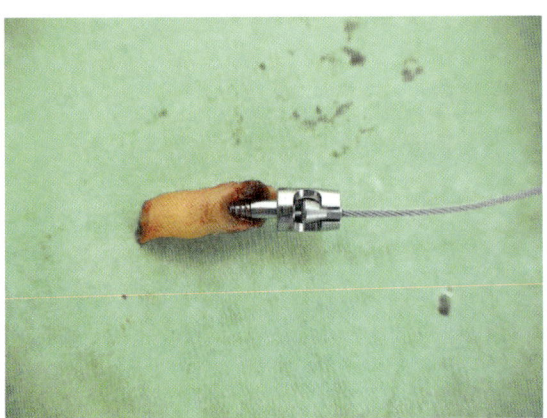

...leads to a luxated tooth

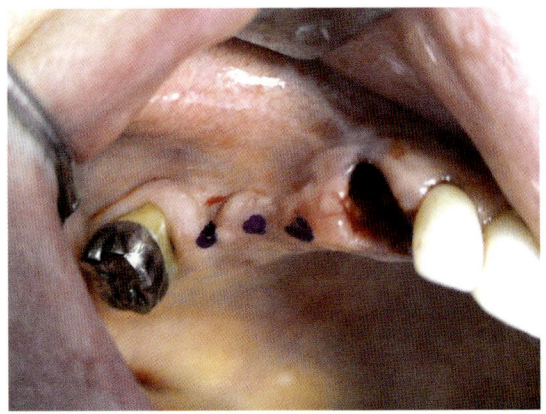

Initial situation for implant placement

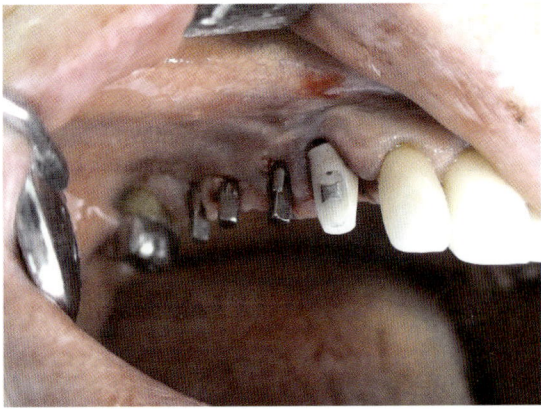

Completed insertion and Prep-Cap, 13 lateral view

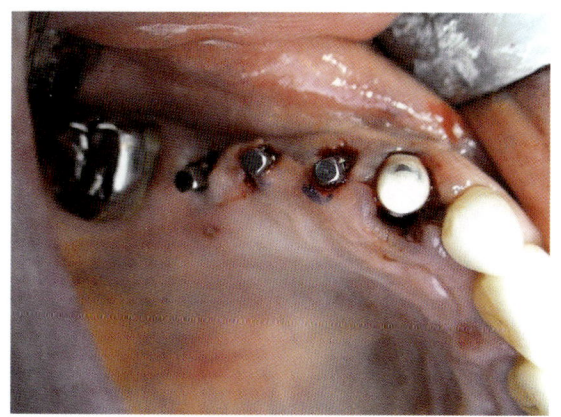

Completed insertion and Prep-Cap 13, occlusal view

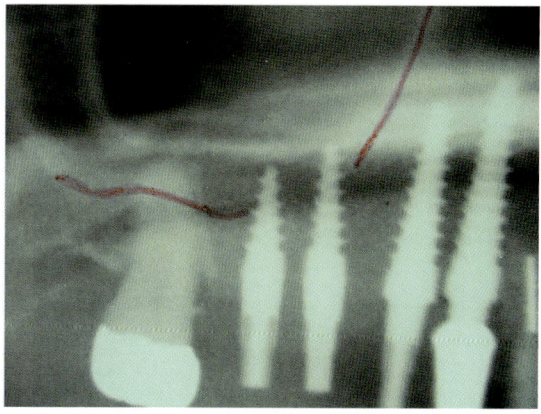

Panoramic radiographic control, indirect sinus lift

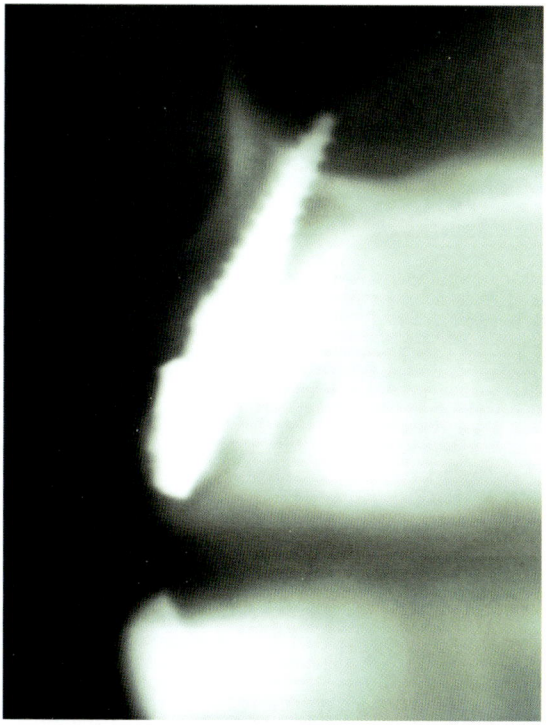

Cross-sectional image

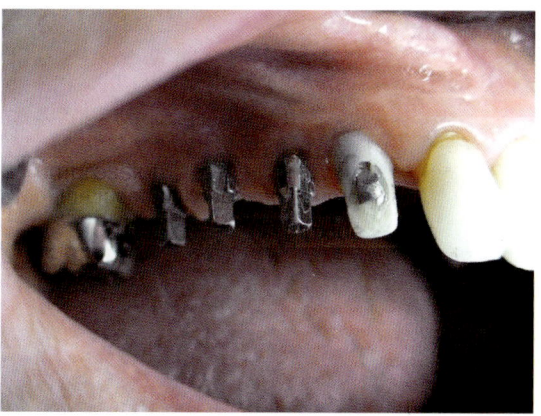

Before impression taking

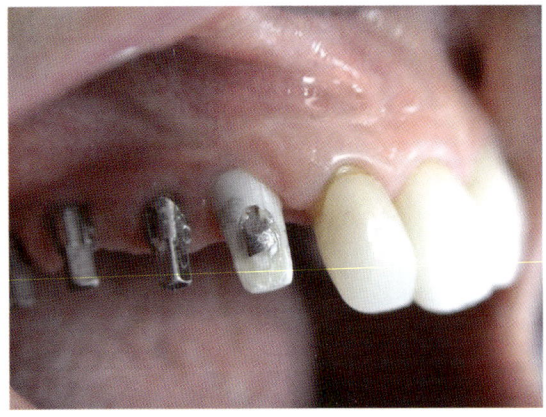

Before impression taking, macro image

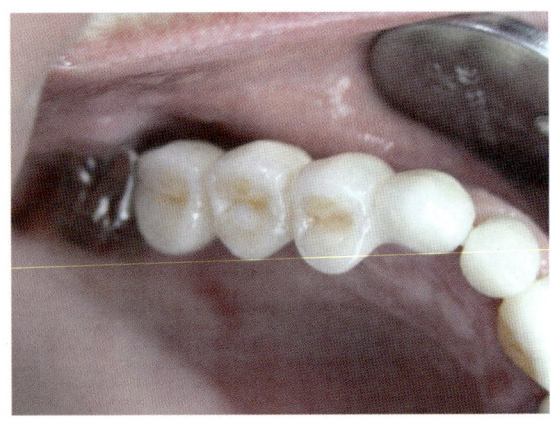

Cemented splinted crown, occlusal view

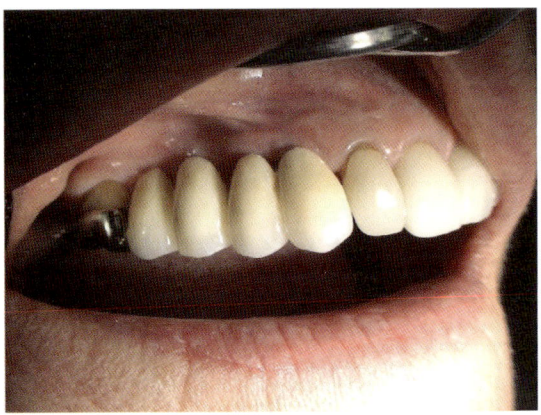

Cemented splinted crown, lateral view

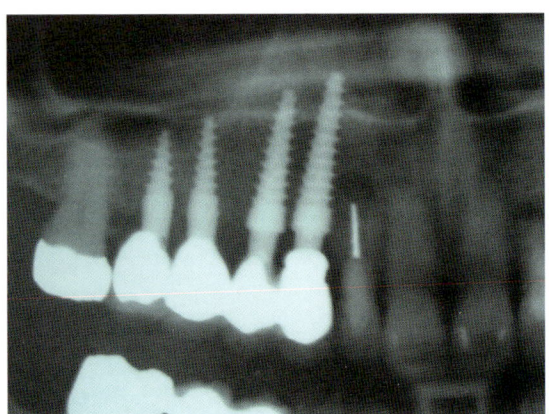

After more than one year...

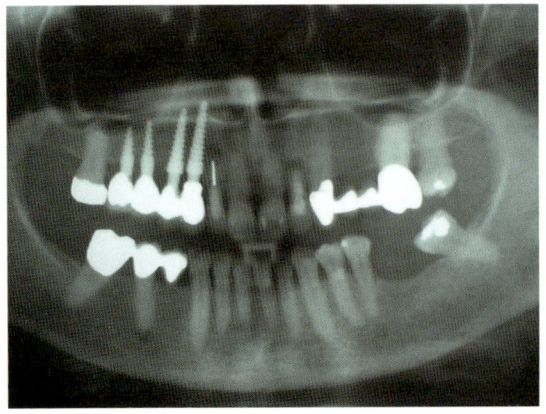

...new panoramic radiograph due to a planned implant placement...

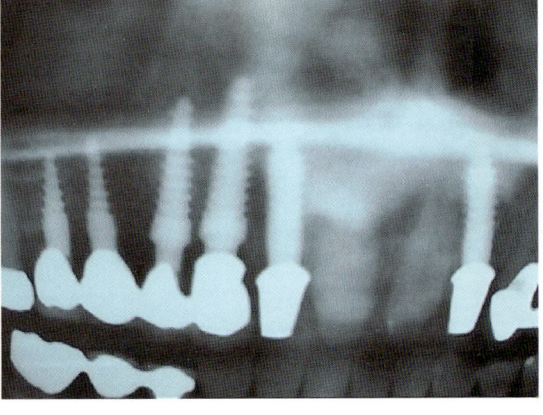

...in the anterior maxillary region, no bone loss is detected

5 - 8 implants

7.3.1/Case 25

Patient: male, 46 years old

35-38 5 implants,
zirconium dioxide splinted crown

13/12/2010	35,36,37,38	5 Champions® implants implant stump preparation cemented dentist made temporary
15/02/2011	38	Periotest -2 impression
01/03/2011	35- 38	cemented zirconium splinted crown
Treatment period:		**2.5 months**
Remarks:	38	when we insert only with a torque of 20 Ncm due to limited space, we spared the 6th implant. late implant placement, late loading

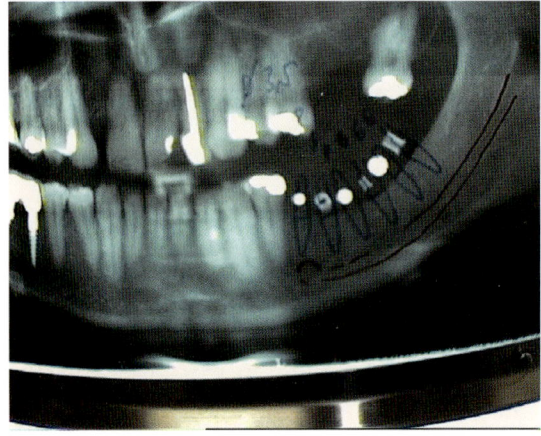

Panoramic radiograph for planned treatment

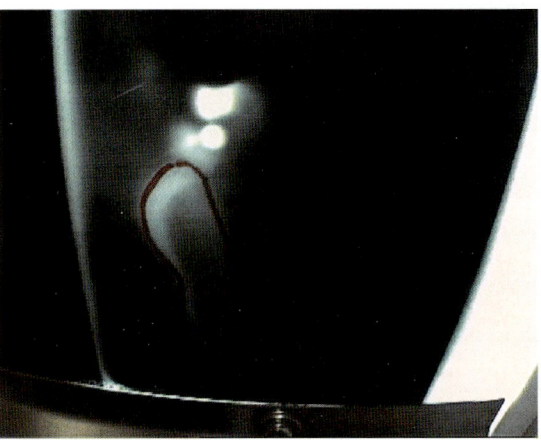

X-ray, cross-sectional image

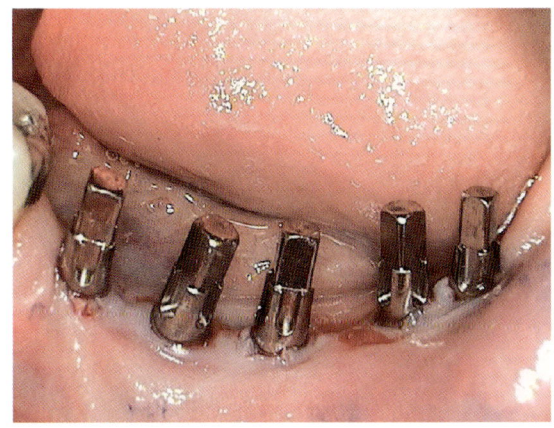

Completed implant placement

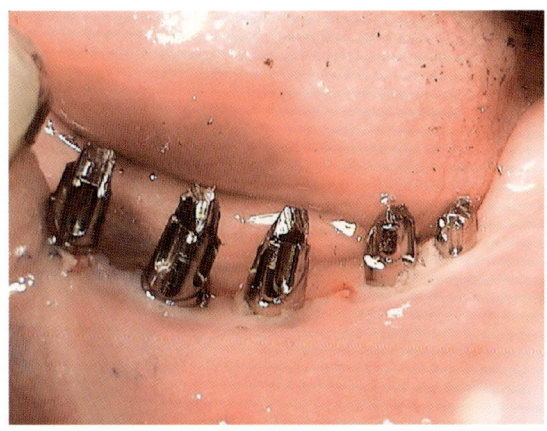

Prepared implant heads in regio 12

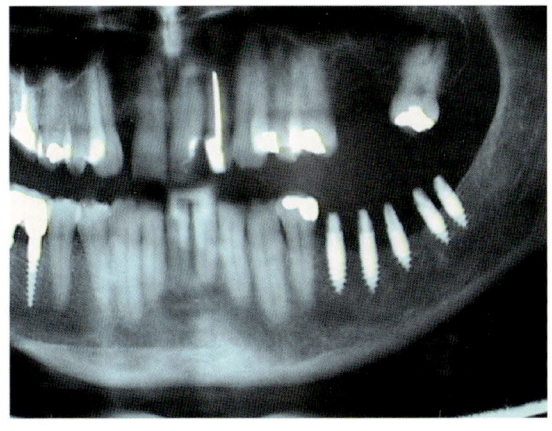

Panoramic radiographic control

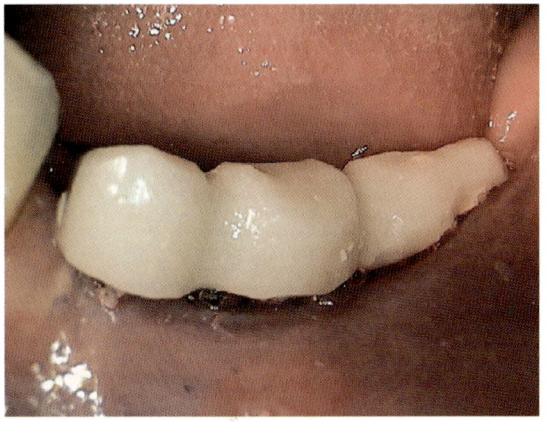

Cemented dentist made temporary, lateral view

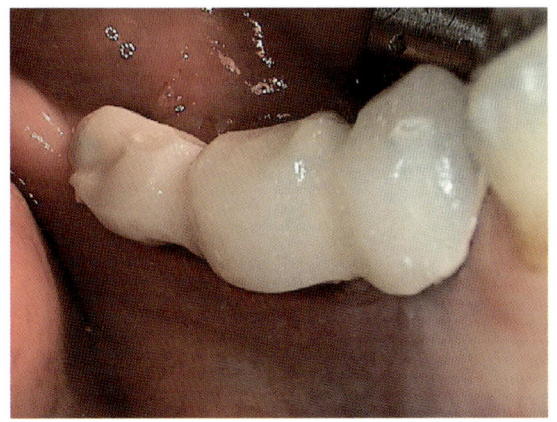

Cemented dentist made temporary, lingual view

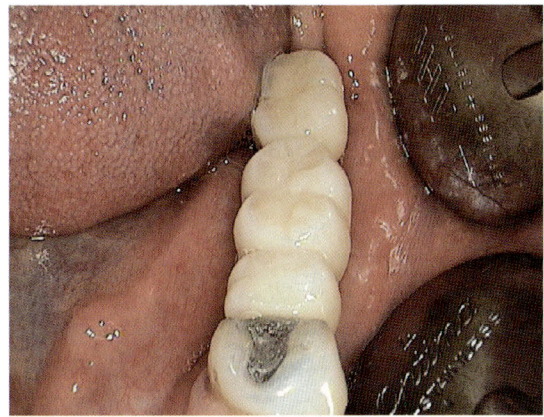

Final cemented splinted crown, occlusal view

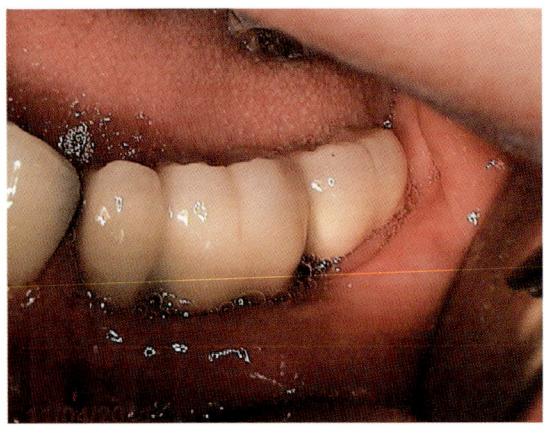

Final cemented splinted crown,
lateral view

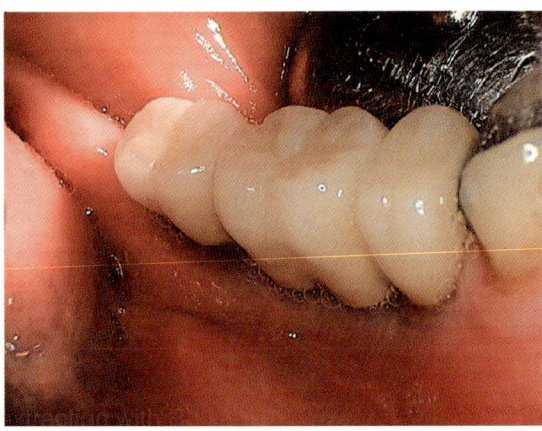

Final cemented splinted crown,
lingual view

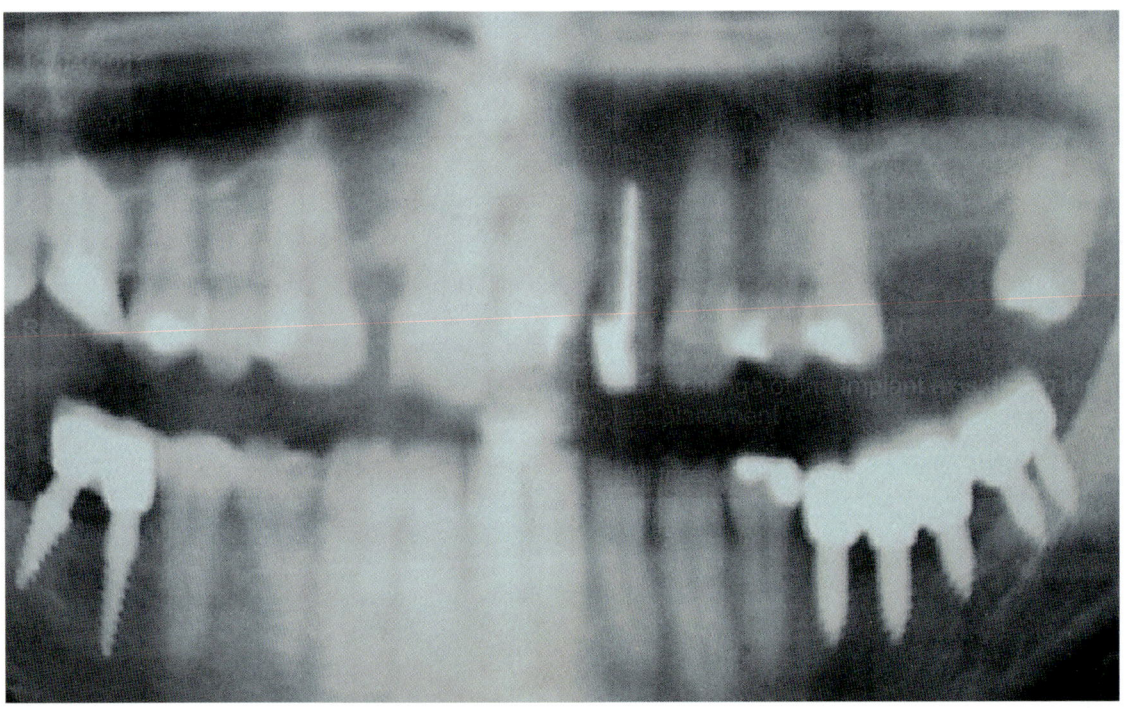

Final cemented splinted crown, panoramic
radiographic control

7.3.2/Case 26

Patient: male, 50 years old

35 -37 5 implants with early loading

30/05/2011	35,36,37	5 Champions® implants Ø 3.5 x 10, 12 mm, >40 Ncm - >60 Ncm preparation impression cemented dentist made temporary
09/09/2011	35- 37	cemented zirconium dioxide splinted crown
Treatment period:		**1 week**
Remarks:		Late implant placement Immediate restoration Early loading No cleaning gaps between the implants since the gingiva "loves" ceramic!

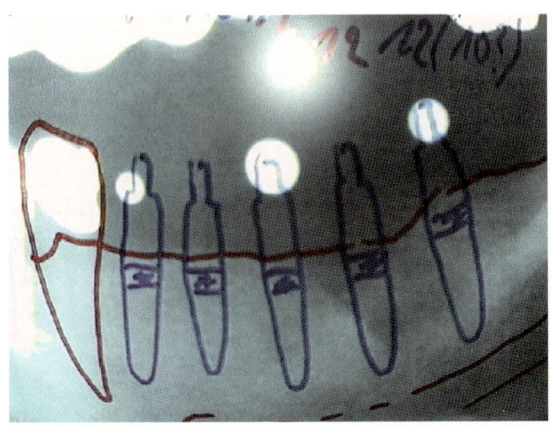

Panoramic radiograph for planned treatment

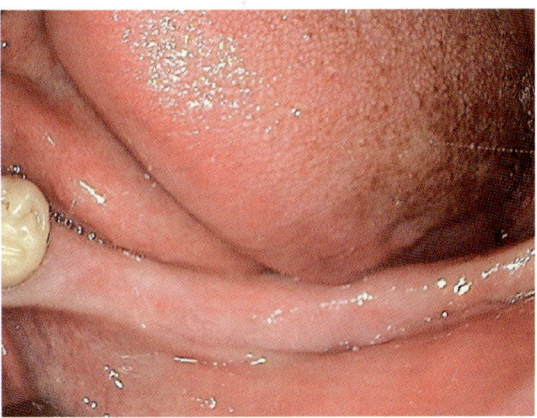

Clinical initial situation...

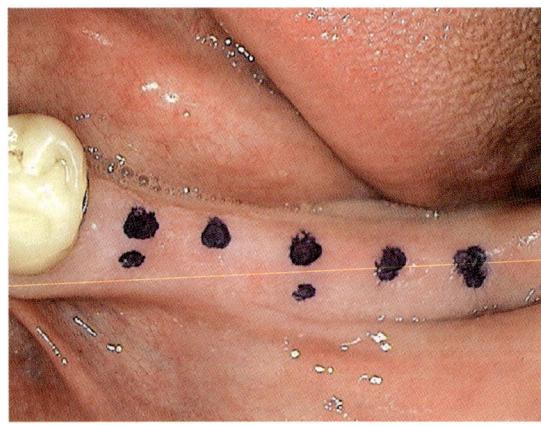

...with marked insertion points...

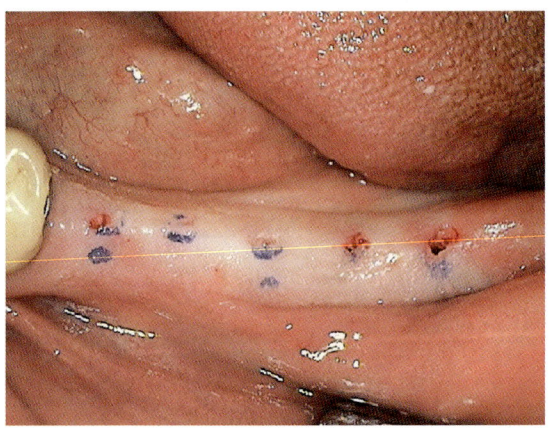

...initial pilot hole preparation...

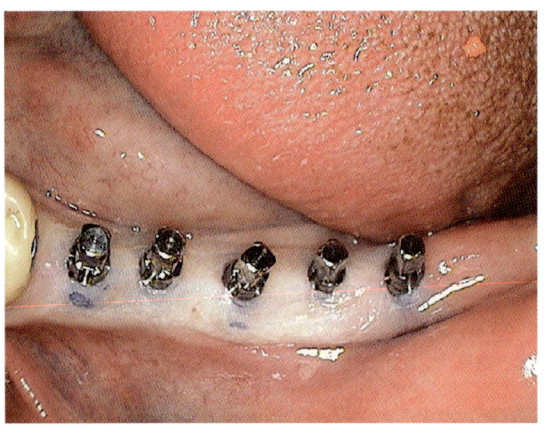

...and completed implant placement, occlusal view

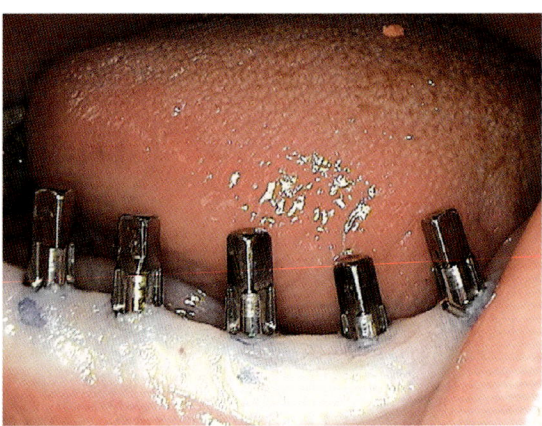

Lateral view

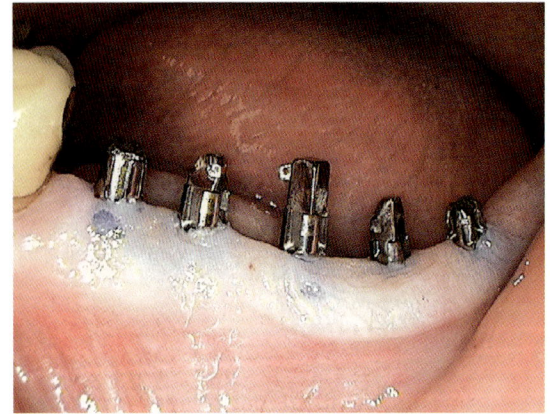

Clinical situation after preparation of implant heads, lateral view...

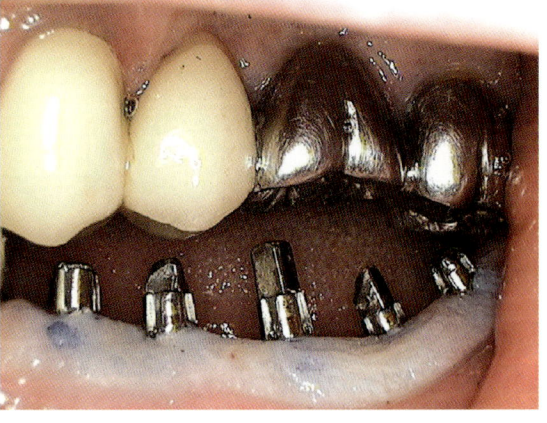

...and in habitual occlusion

138

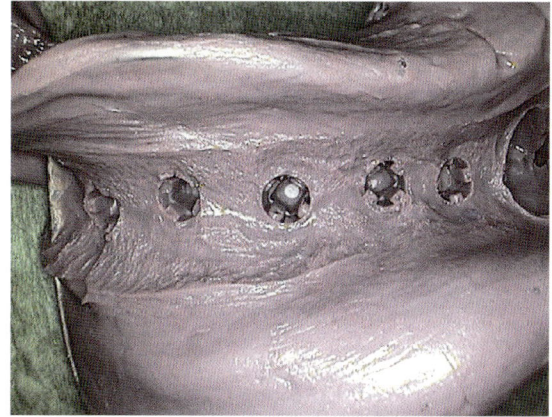

Impression

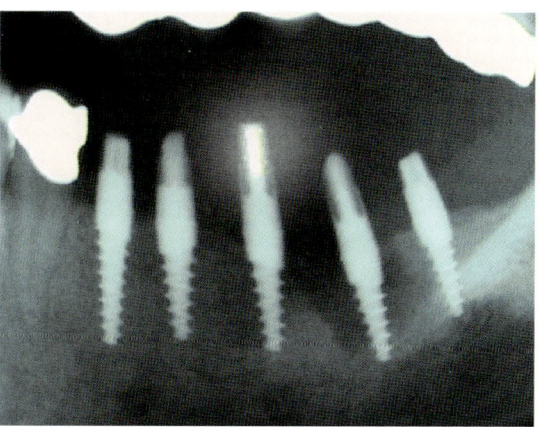

Panoramic radiographic control

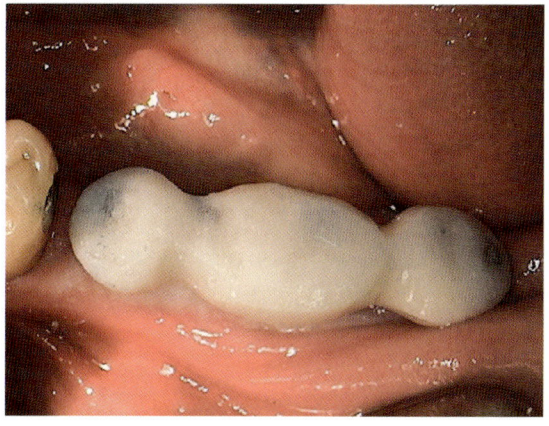

Cemented dentist made temporary,
occlusal view

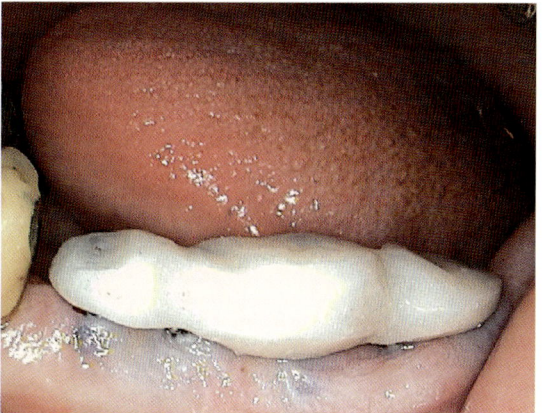

Cemented dental provisional prosthesis,
lateral view

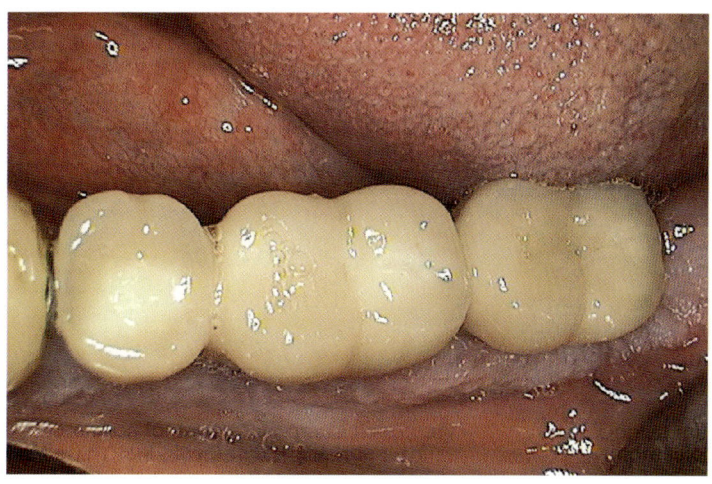

Final cemented splinted crown,
occlusal view

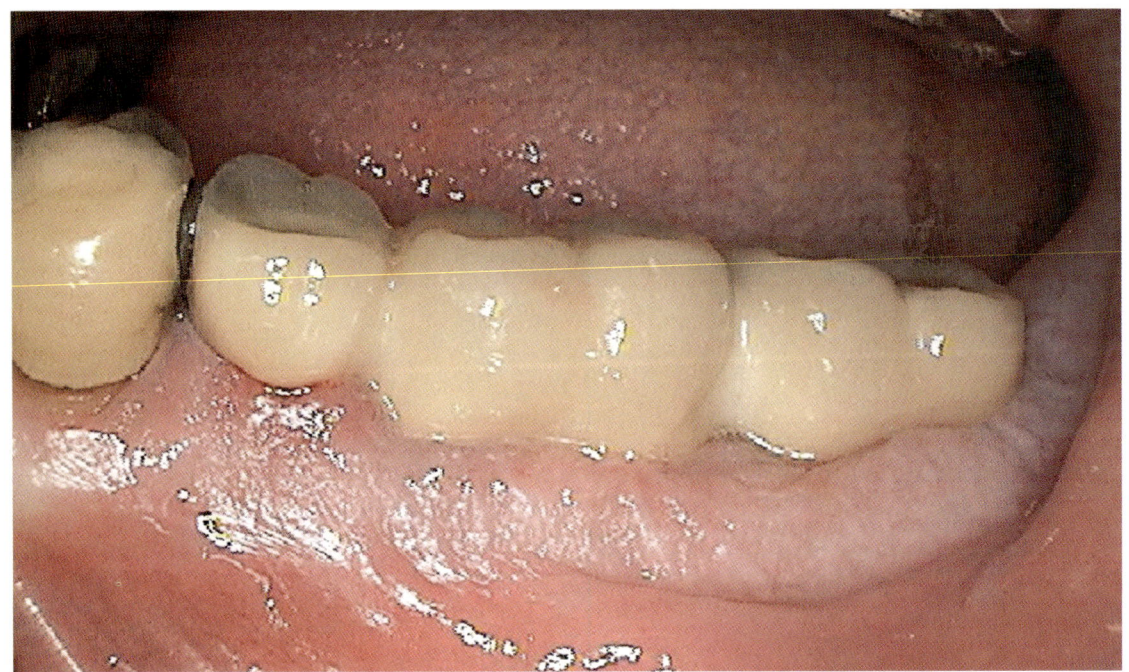

Final cemented splinted crown,
lateral view

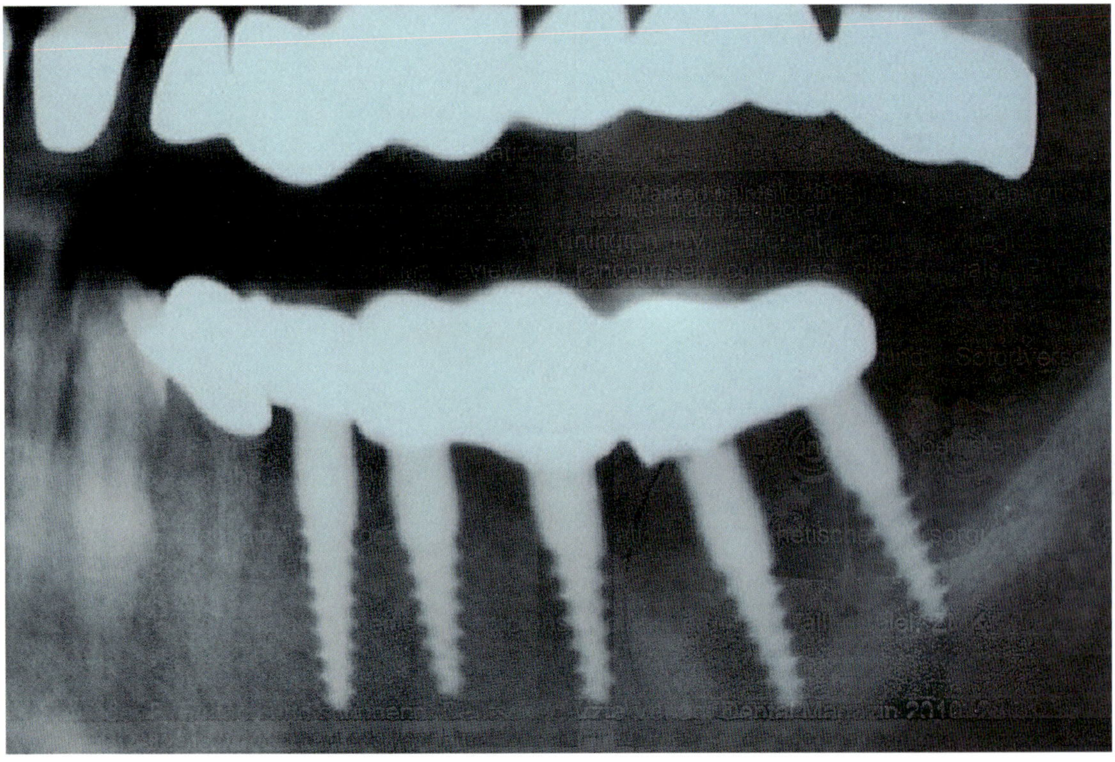

Panoramic radiographic control

7.3.3/Case 27

Patient: female, 58 years old

14 -17 implants, tooth preparation zirconium dioxide splinted crown

---

28/04/2011	15	crown removal, preparation
	14	Champions® implant Ø 3.5 x 12 mm, 50 Ncm, Periotest +3
	16 m	Champions® implant Ø 3.5 x 10 mm, 40 Ncm, Periotest -1
	16 d	Champions® implant Ø 3.5 x 8 mm, 20 Ncm, Periotest +5
	17 m	Champions® implant Ø 3.5 x 6 mm, 15 Ncm, Periotest +5
	17 d	Champions® implant Ø 3.5 x 8 mm, 15 Ncm, Periotest +9 preparation cemented dentist made temporary
08/08/2011		Impression Periotest: 14 +2, 16 m -2, 36d 16, 37 -2 17 m +1, 17 d +2
22/08/2011	14-17	cemented zirconium dioxide splinted crown
Treatment period:		**4 months**
Remarks:		Avoiding an open sinus lift The patient refused a gingival correction at tooth 12

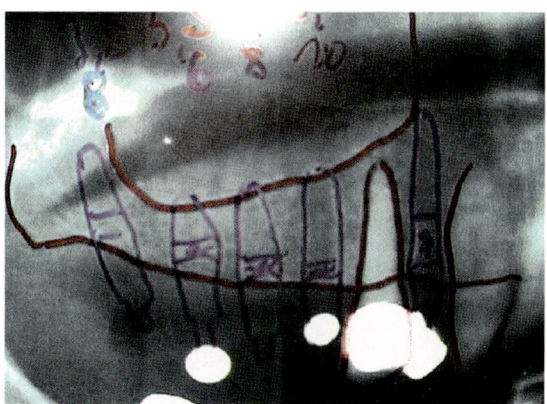

Planned treatment, initial panoramic radiograph

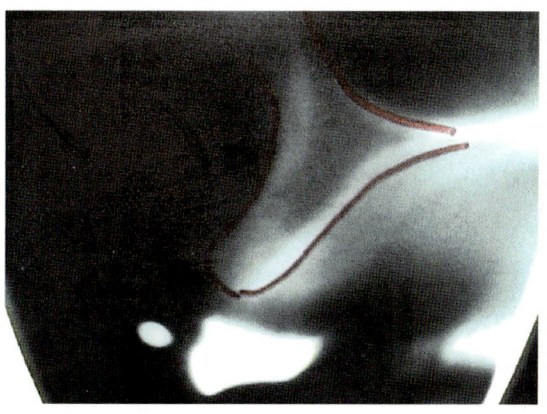

Cross-sectional image in regio 15

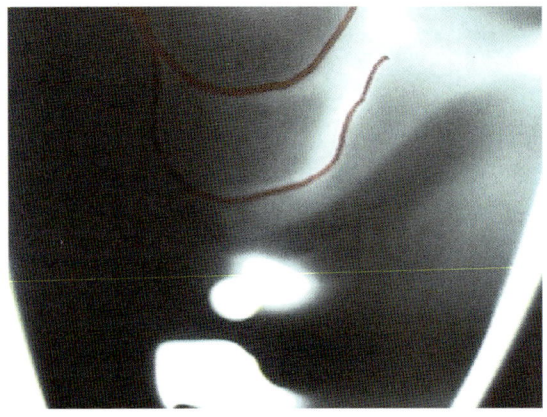

Cross-sectional image in regio 16, 17

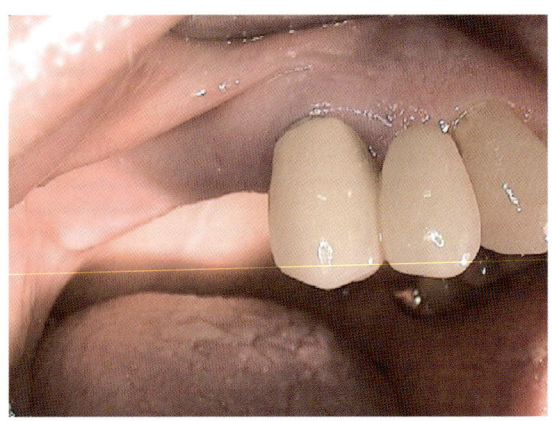

Clinical initial situation,
lateral view

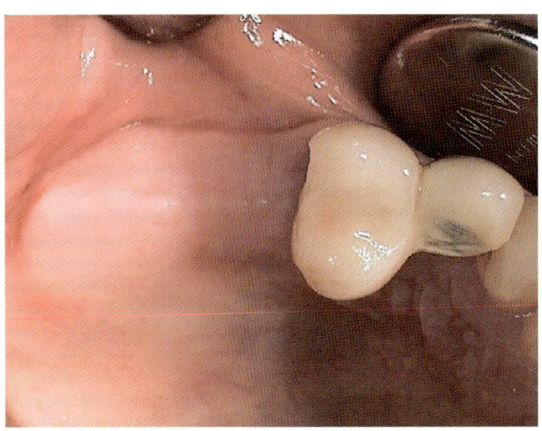

Clinical initial situation,
occlusal view

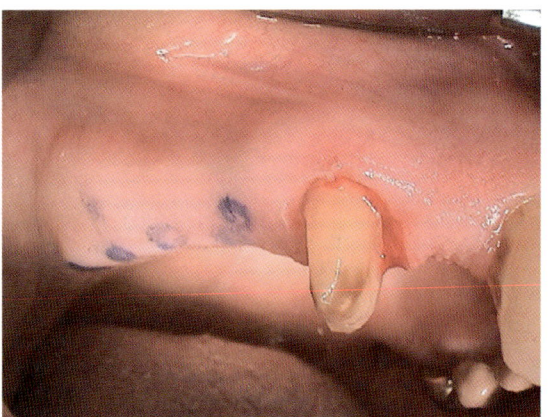

Preparation of tooth 15,
lateral view

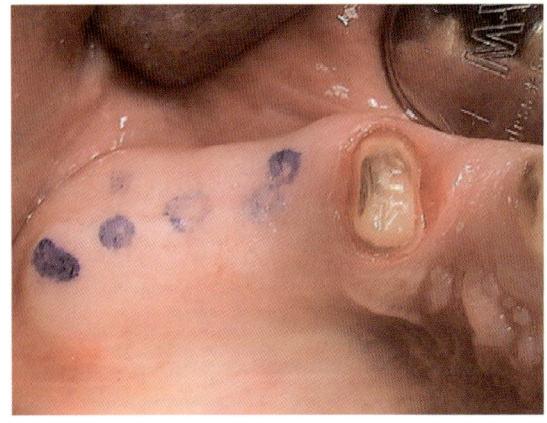

Preparation of tooth 15,
occlusal view

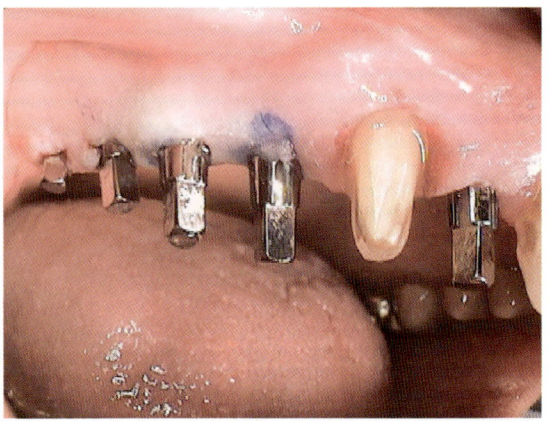

Situation after implant placement,
lateral view

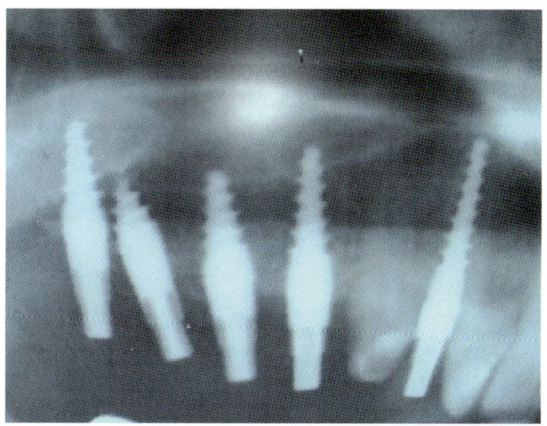

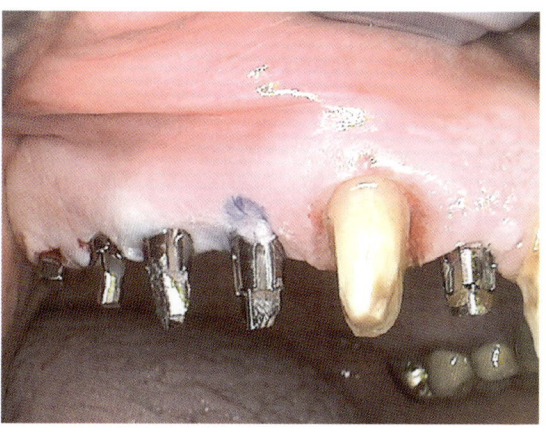

Situation after implant placement,
occlusal view

Panoramic radiographic control after implant placement,
indirect sinus lift

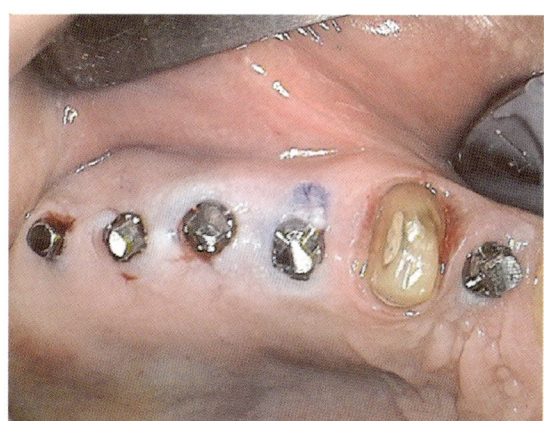

Implant stump preparation,
lateral view

Implant stump preparation,
occlusal view

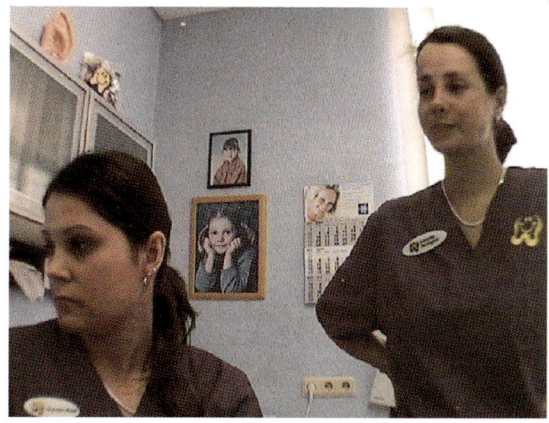

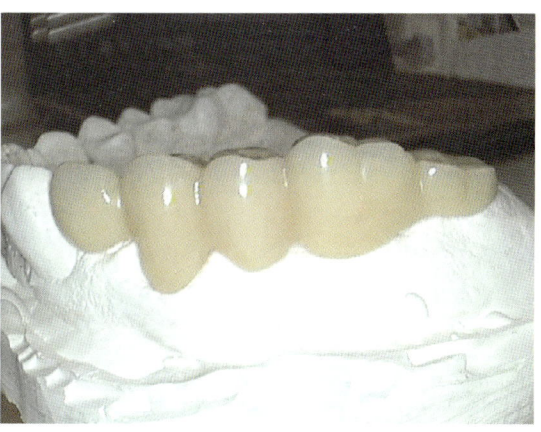

Image control performed by my employees

Laboratory made temporary, lateral view

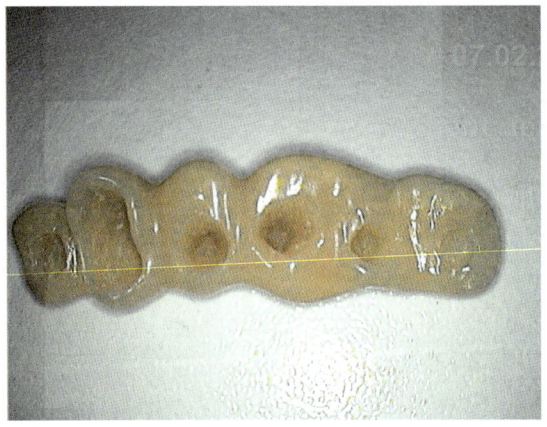

Laboratory made temporary, basal view

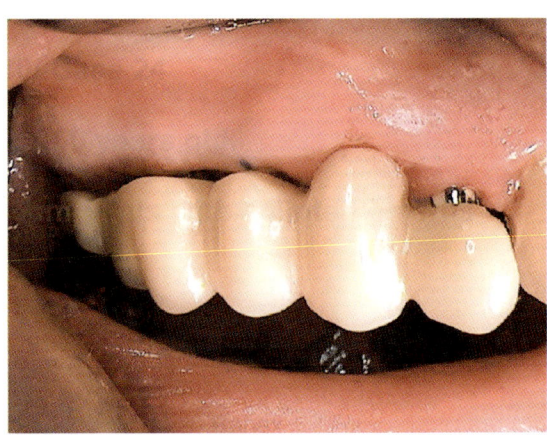

Try-in of the laboratory made temporary

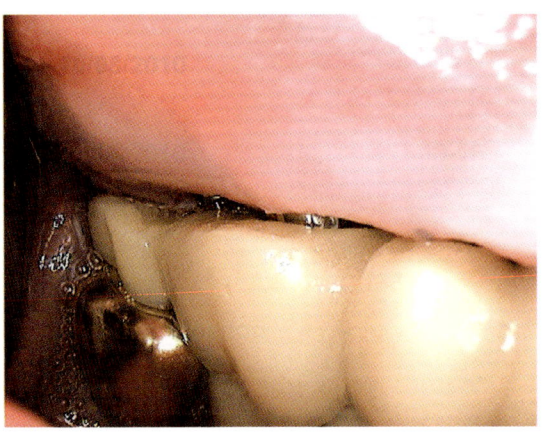

Close-up view of the "dirt niches"

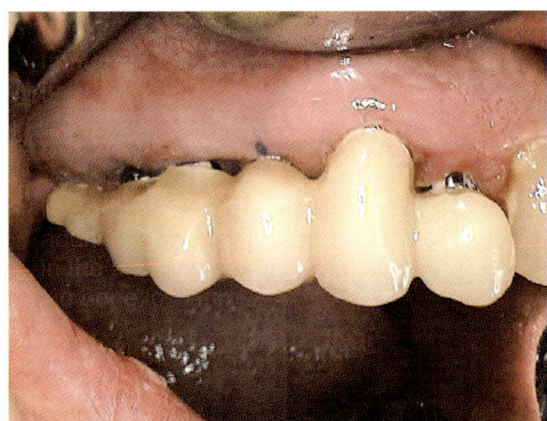

Reduction of the "dirt niches"

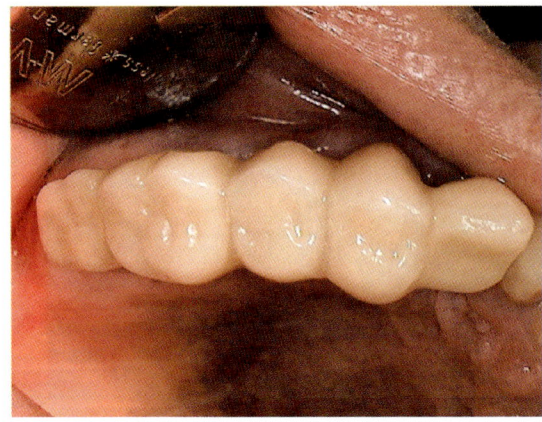

Before impression taking, occlusal view

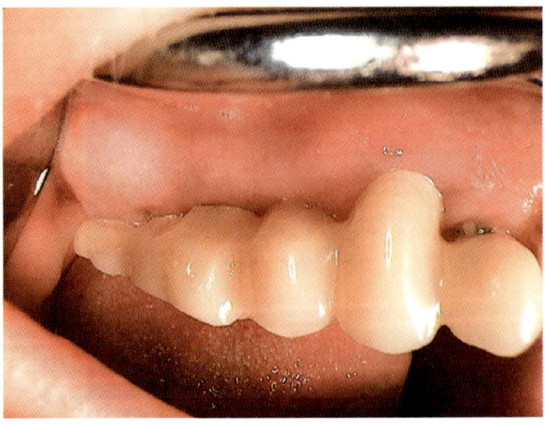

Before impression taking, lateral view

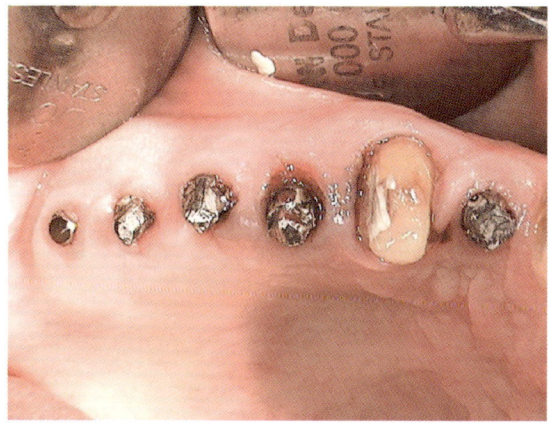

Situation before impression taking

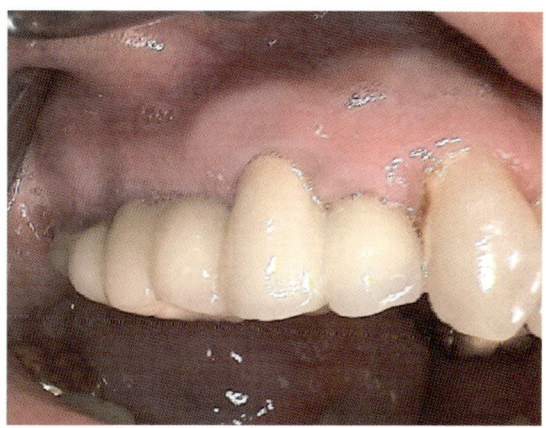

Final cemented splinted crown,
lateral view

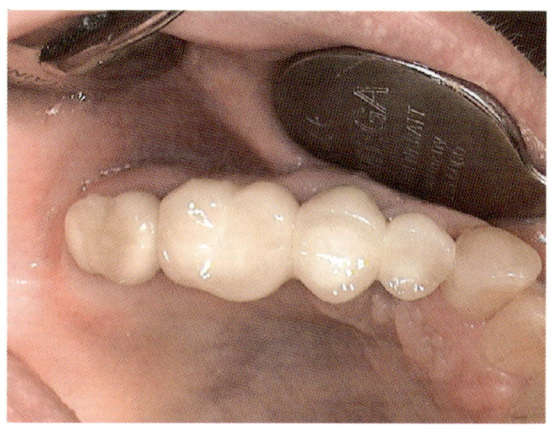

Final cemented splinted crown,
occlusal view

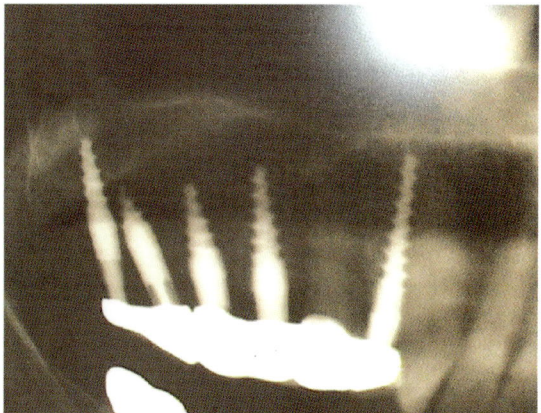

Final cemented splinted crown,
Panoramic radiographic control

7.3.4/Case 28

Patient: male, 61 years old

24-27 implant placement, 26 immediate implant placement, augmentation,
23-27 splinted crown

01/02/2011	26	extraction
	23	tooth preparation
	24	Champions® implant Ø 3.5 x 12 mm, >40 Ncm, Periotest -2
	25	Champions® implant Ø 3.5 x 10 mm, >30 Ncm, Periotest -2
	26 m	Champions® implant Ø 3.0 x 10 mm, >30 Ncm, Periotest +5
	26 d	Champions® implant Ø 3.5 x 10 mm, >30 Ncm, Periotest +3
	27	Champions® implant Ø 3.5 x 10 mm, >20 Ncm, Periotest +6
	26	augmentation implant stump preparation cemented dentist made temporary
02/02/2011	23-27	laboratory made temporary
27/04/2011		Impression Periotest: 24 -6, 25 -1, 26 m +4, 26 d +5, 27 0
11/05/2011	23-27	cemented zirconium dioxide splinted crown
Treatment period:		**3.3 months**
Remarks:	26	Indirect sinus lift Immediate implant placement Augmentation with bone chips Immediate restoration, late loading

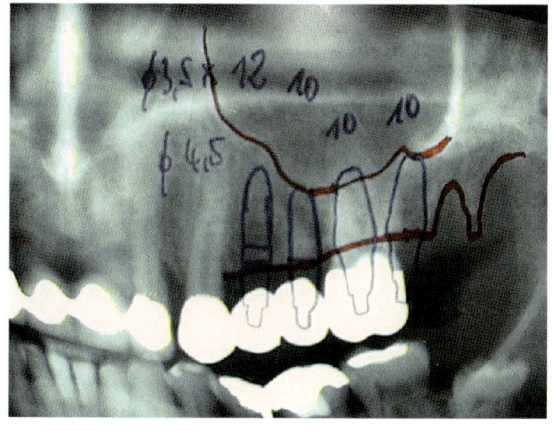

Panoramic radiograph for planned treatment

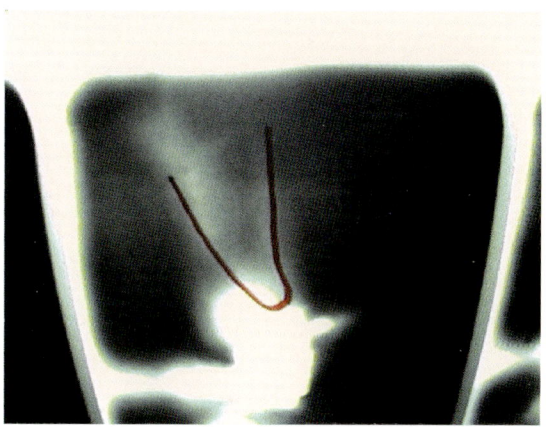

Cross-sectional image

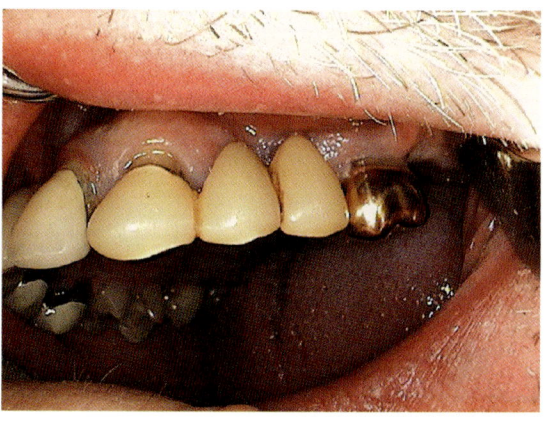

Clinical initial situation, lateral view

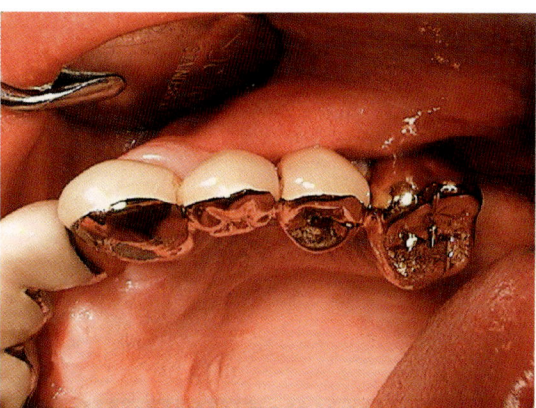

Clinical initial situation, occlusal view

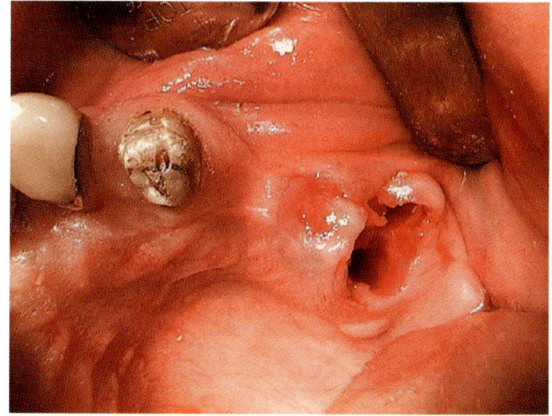

Extracted tooth 26

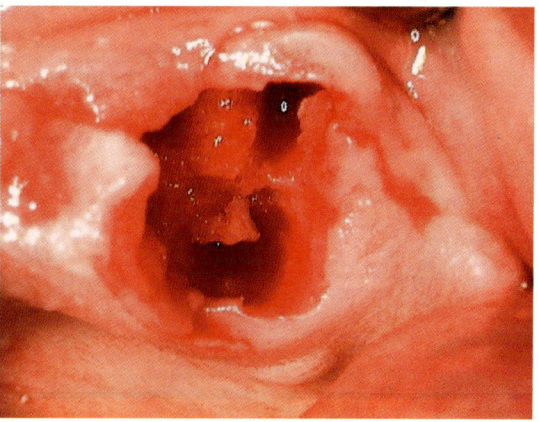

26 close-up view of the alveolus

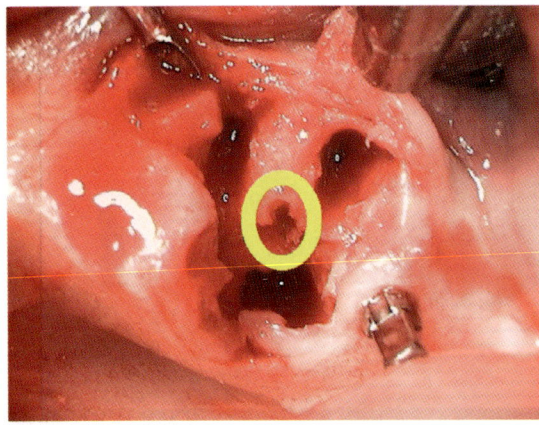

Pre-drilled hole for the implant in region 26

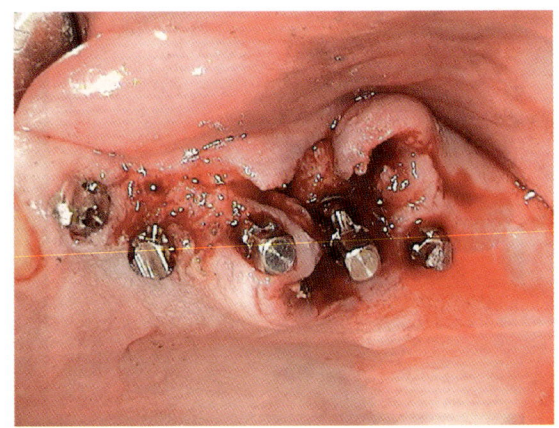

Completed implant placement

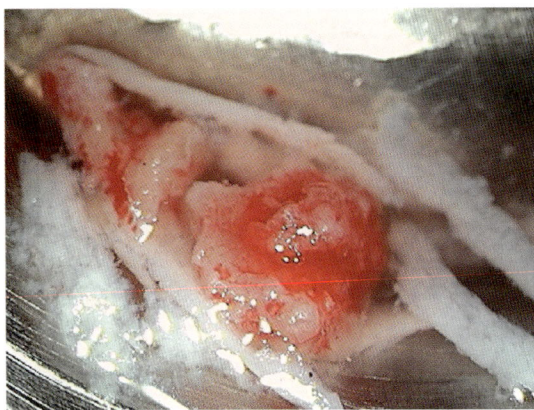

Collected bone chips

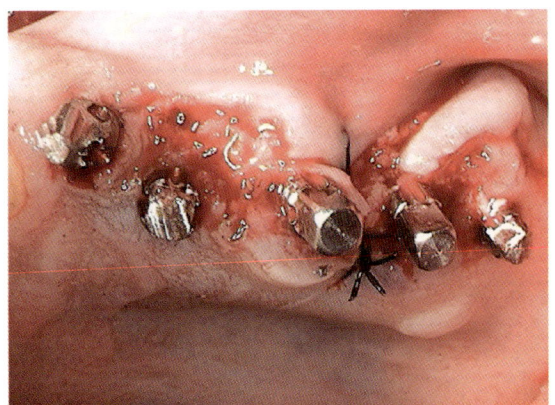

Wound healing after augmentation

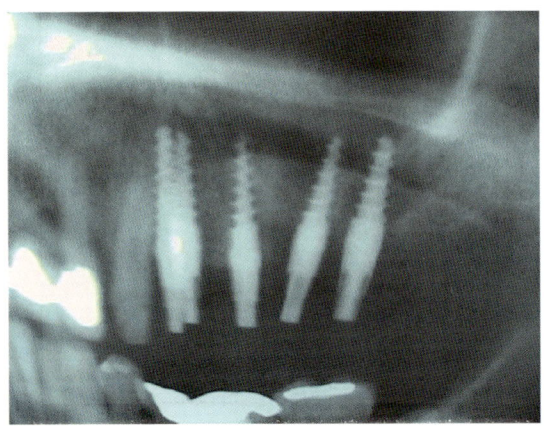

Radiographic control, panoramic radiograph

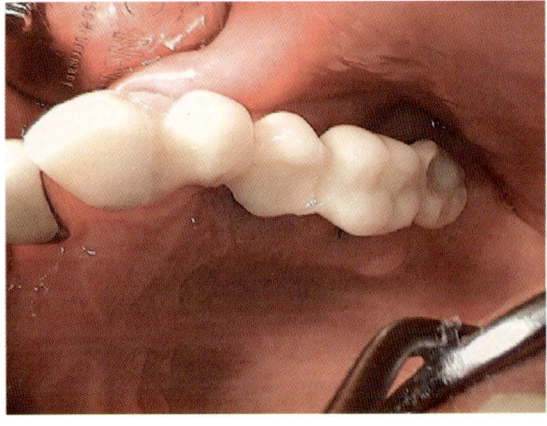

Cemented laboratory made temporary, occlusal view, 1st postoperative day

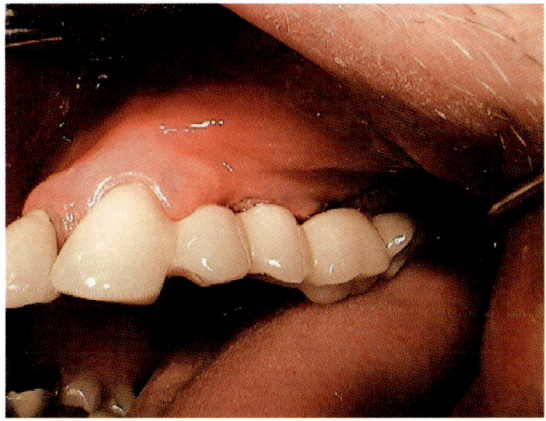

Cemented laboratory made temporary,
occlusal view, 1st postoperative day

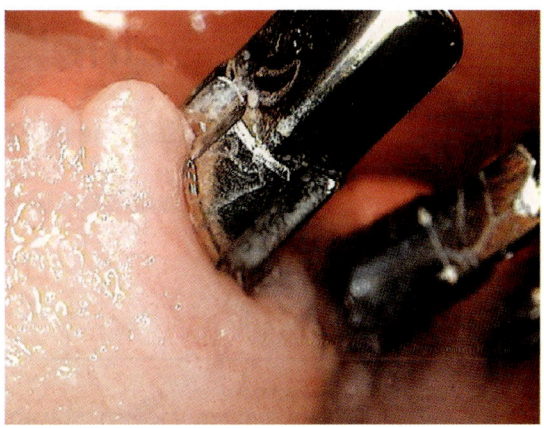

Irritation-free gingiva before impression taking

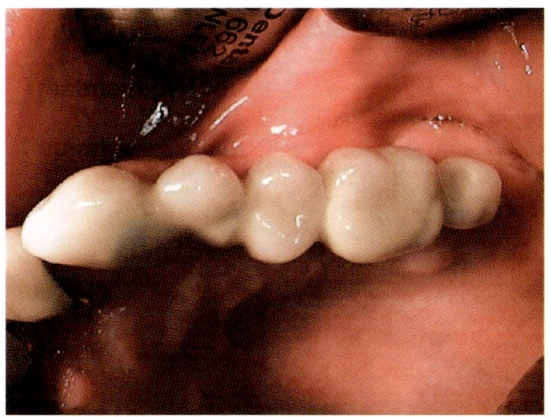

Final cemented splinted crown,
occlusal view

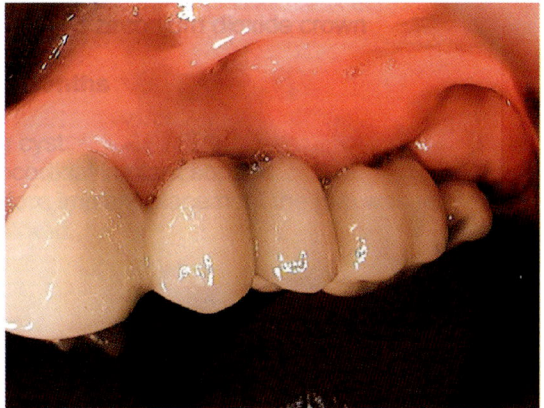

Final cemented splinted crown,
lateral view

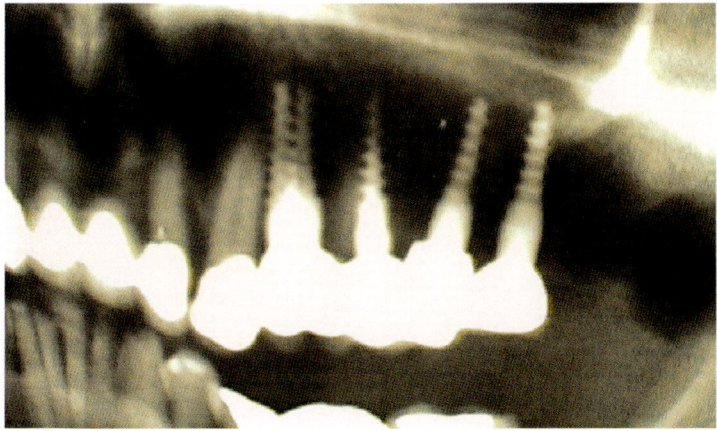

X-ray final control, zoomed panoramic radiographic detail

7.3.5/Case 29

Patient: female, 49 years old

14-18 implant placement, 13 tooth preparation
13-18 splinted crown

26/05/2011	14	Champions® implant Ø 3.5 x 12 mm, >50 Ncm, Periotest 0
	15	Champions® implant Ø 3.5 x 6 mm, >20 Ncm, Periotest +2
	16	Champions® implant Ø 3.5 x 6 mm, 30 Ncm, Periotest 0
	17	Champions® implant Ø 3.5 x 6 mm, 30 Ncm, Periotest +2
	18	Champions® implant Ø 3.5 x 8 mm, 15 Ncm, Periotest +6
	13	tooth preparation preparation of implant heads cemented dentist made temporary
30/08/2011		Impression Periotest: 14 -2, 15 -3 16 -2, 17 +1,18 +2
07/09/2011	13-18	cemented zirconium dioxide splinted crown
Treatment period:		**3.5 months**
Remarks:		Avoiding a direct sinus lift which as been declared as inevitable by 2 oral surgeons.

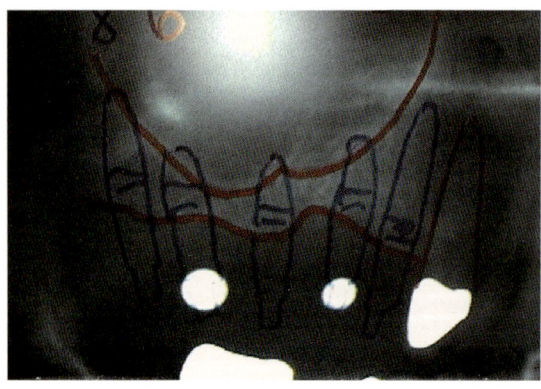

Planned treatment, initial panoramic radiograph

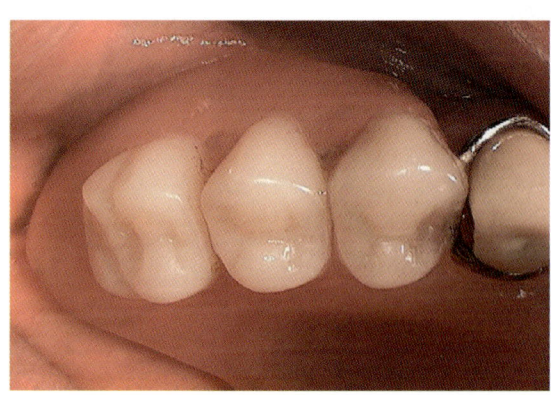

Existing prosthesis in situ

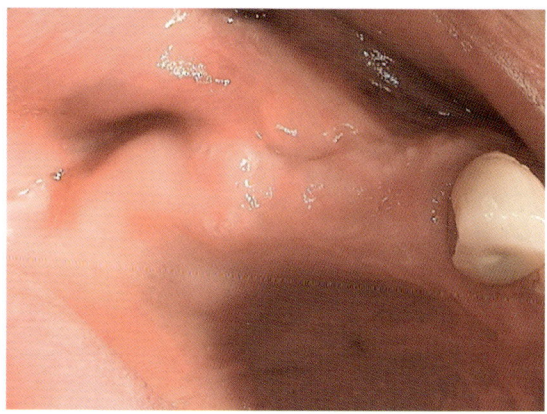

Clinical initial situation,
occlusal view

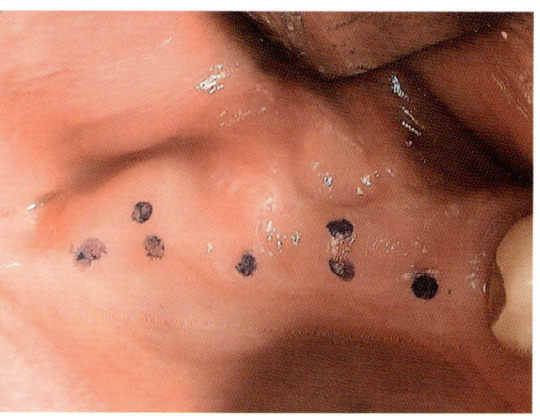

Marked insertion points

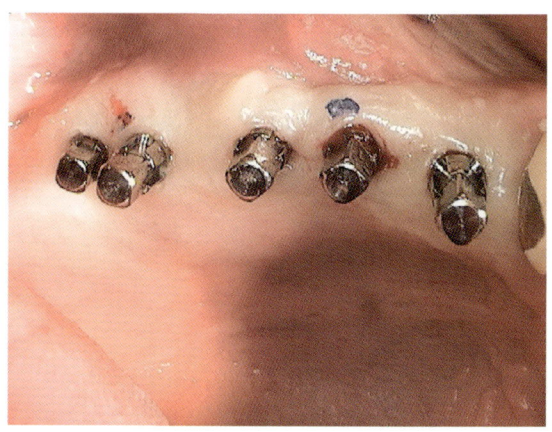

Completed implant placement,
occlusal view

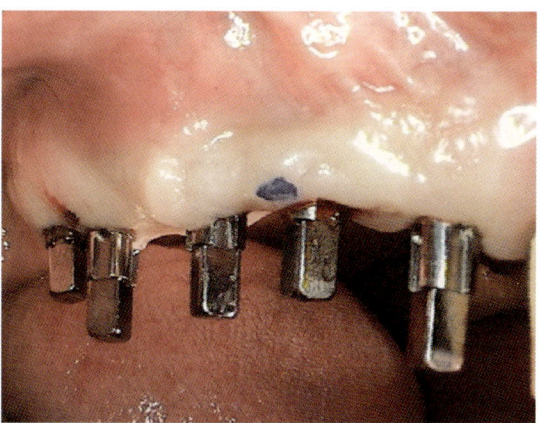

Completed implant placement,
lateral view

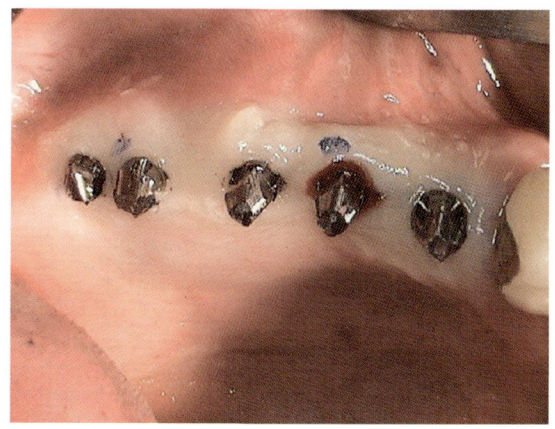

Implant head preparation,
occlusal view

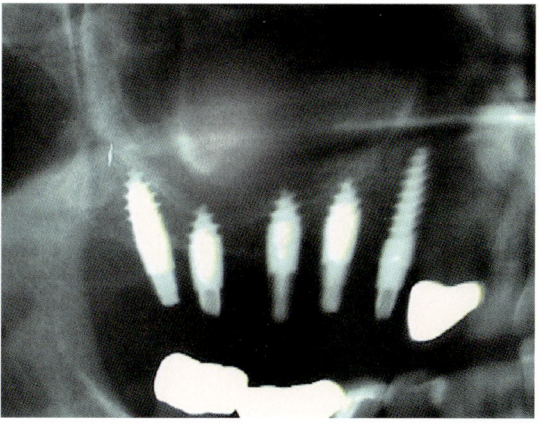

Panoramic radiographic control, detail

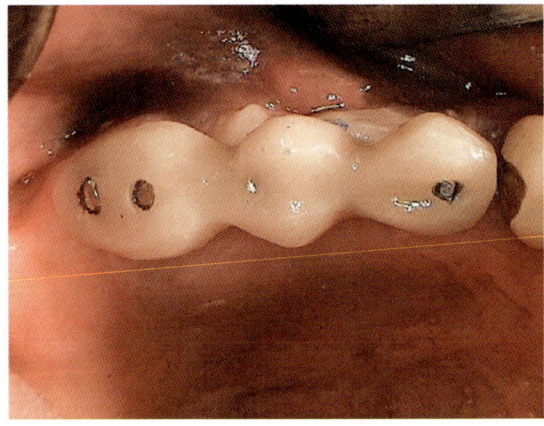

Dentist made temporary, occlusal view

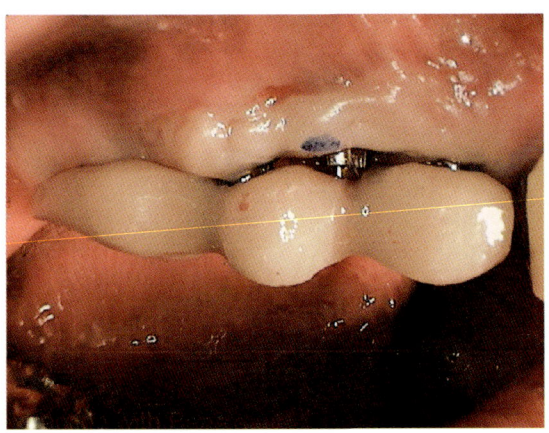

Dentist made temporary, lateral view

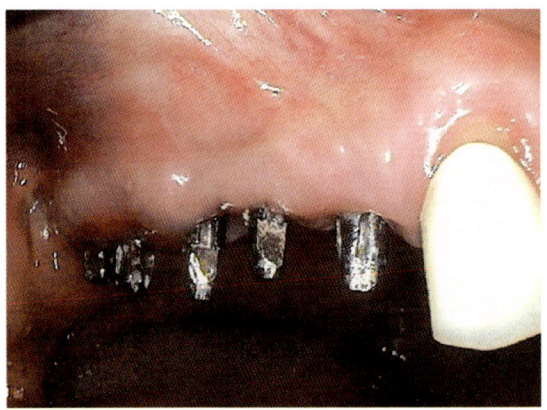

Before impression

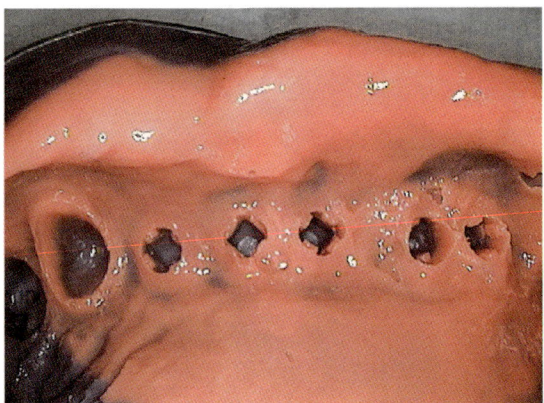

Impression taking

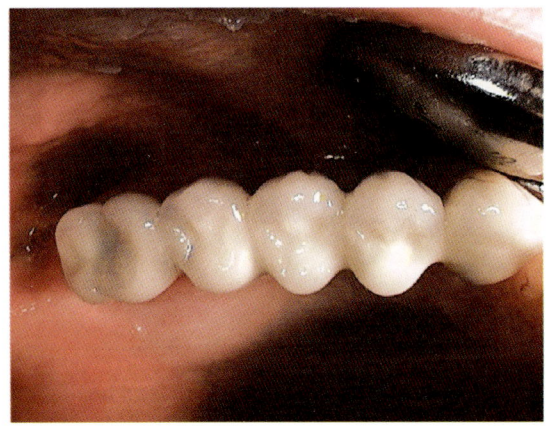

Final cemented splinted crown,
occlusal view

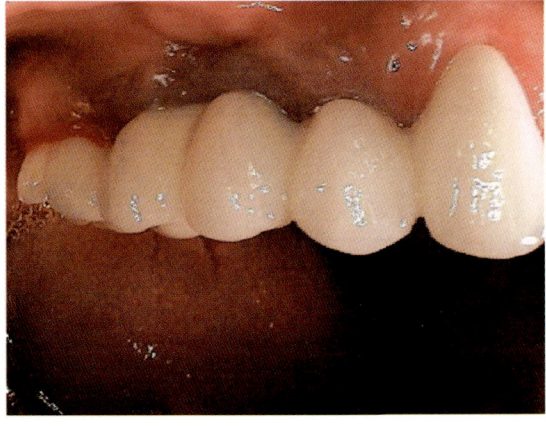

Final cemented splinted crown,
lateral view

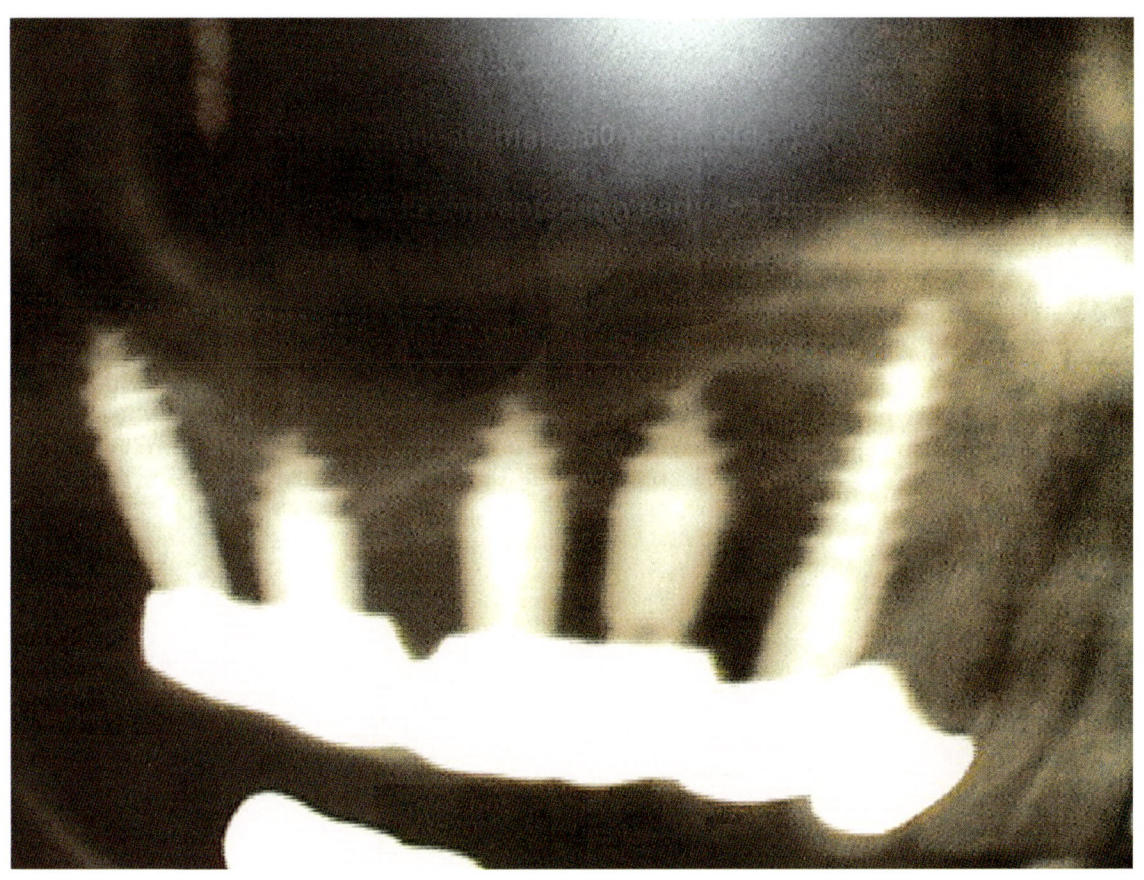

Final cemented splinted crown, panoramic radiographic control, zoomed detail

Patient: female, 48 years old

**35-37, 44-46   6 implants,
plastic caps, 2 splinted crowns**

11/12/2007	Upper jaw	implant placement
15/07/2008	Upper jaw	bridge restoration

Treatment period: **7 months (KIV)**

09/02/2010	35	Champions® implant Ø 3.5 x 10 mm, 80 Ncm
	36	Champions® implant Ø 3.5 x 10 mm, 80 Ncm
	37	Champions® implant Ø 3.3 x 8 mm, 80 Ncm
	44	Champions® implant Ø 3.0 x 14 mm, 60 Ncm
	45	Champions® implant Ø 3.5 x 8 mm, 80 Ncm
	46	Champions® implant Ø 3.5 x 8 mm, 80 Ncm

11/10/2011		Post-control, panoramic radiograph, image

18/02/2010	35-37	cemented zirconium dioxide splinted crown
	44-46	cemented zirconium dioxide splinted crown

Treatment period: **1 week (MIMI)**

Remarks: Primary stability 40-70 Ncm!
Today, we would lightly relieve the implants,
stronger spread or prepare greater pilot holes,
20 months after implant placement, no bone loss!

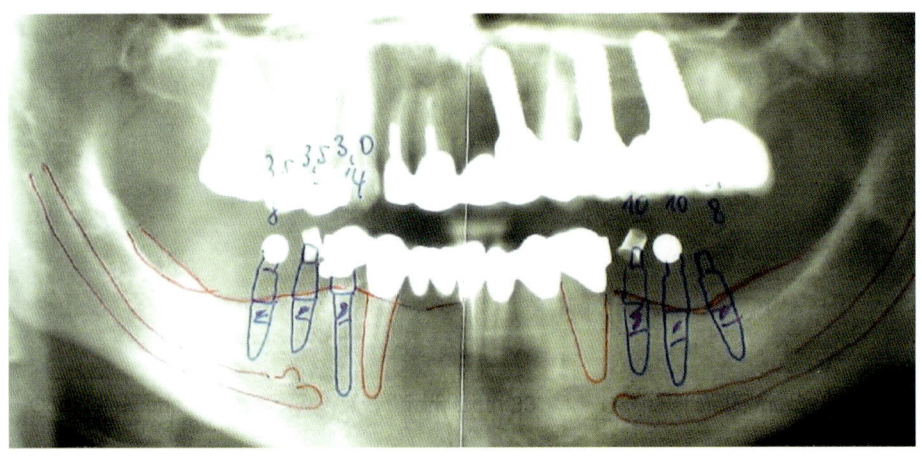

Panoramic
radiograph for
planned
treatment

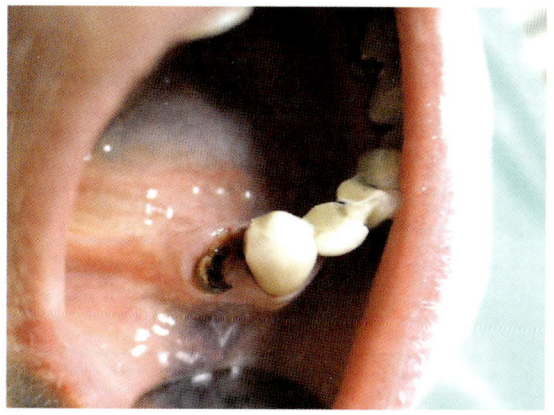

Clinical situation, right side

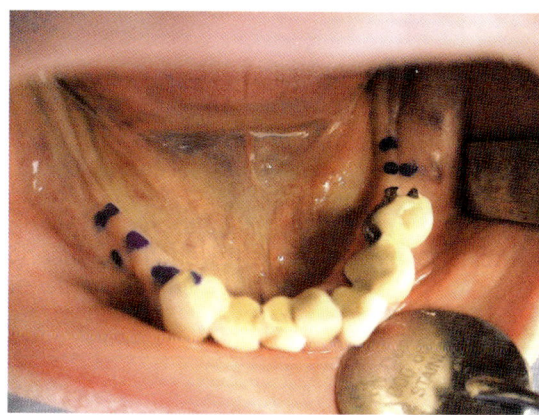

Clinical situation

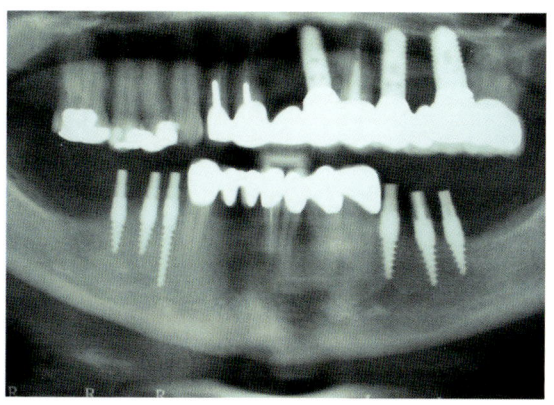

Radiographic control after implant placement

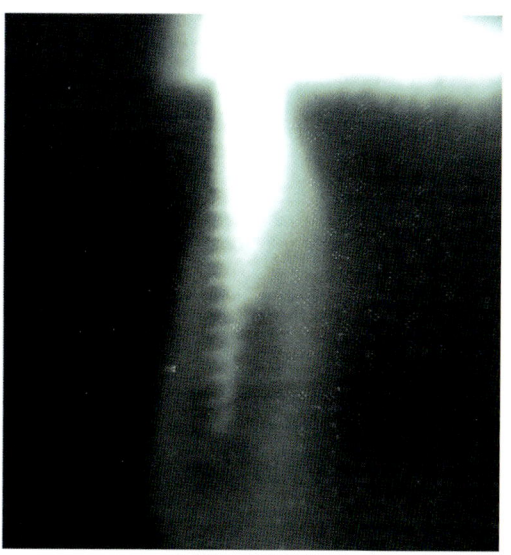

Cross-sectional image

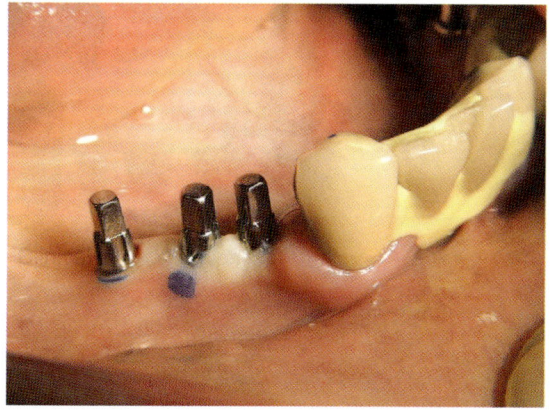

After implant placement, right side

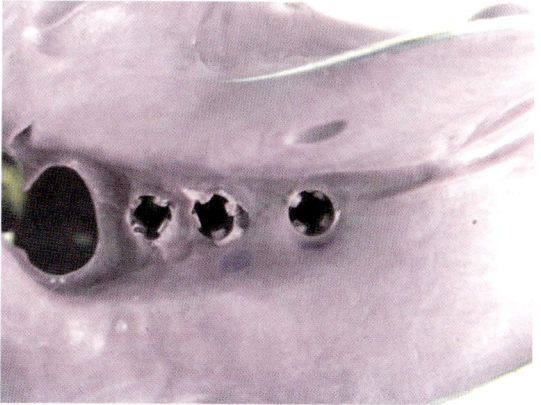

Impression

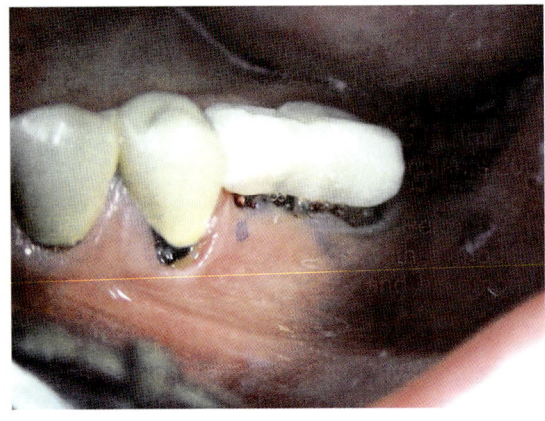

Dentist made temporary

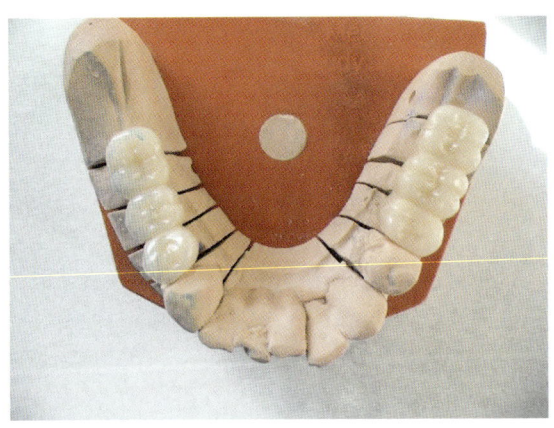

Final splinted crowns onto the cast

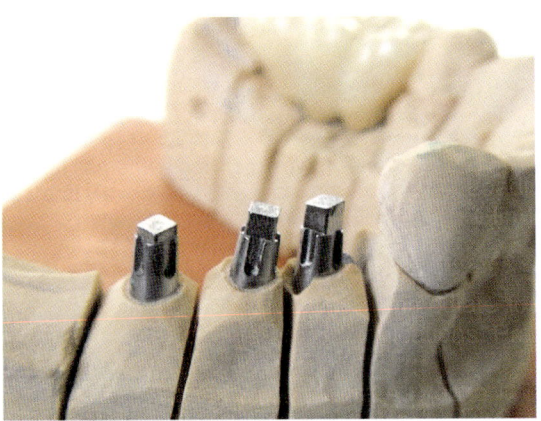

Prepared laboratory analogues, right side

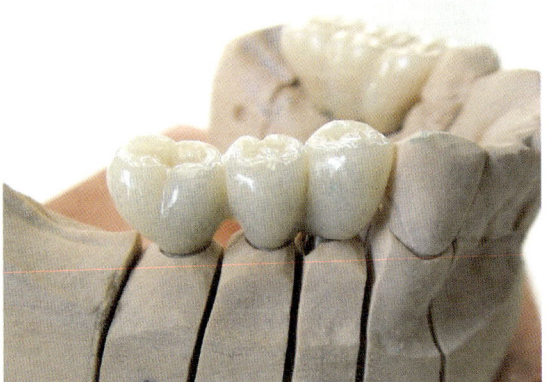

Final splinted crown, right side

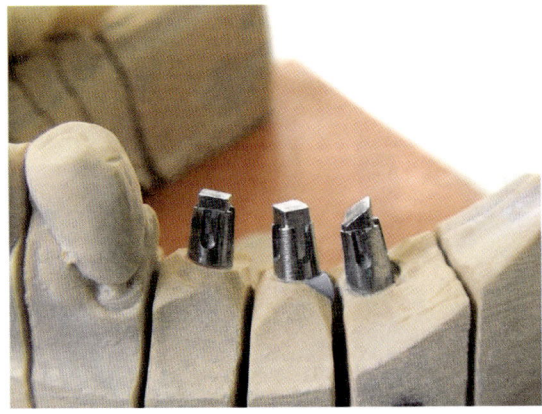

Prepared laboratory analogues, left side

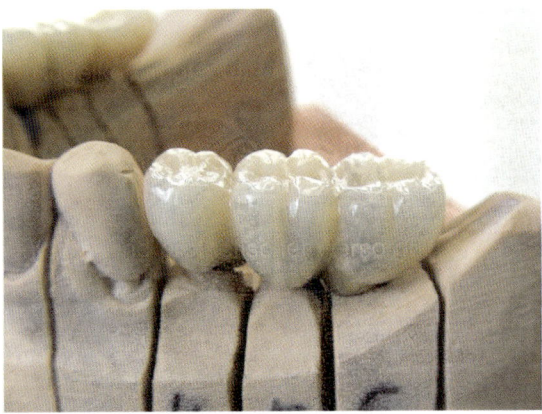

Final splinted crown, left side

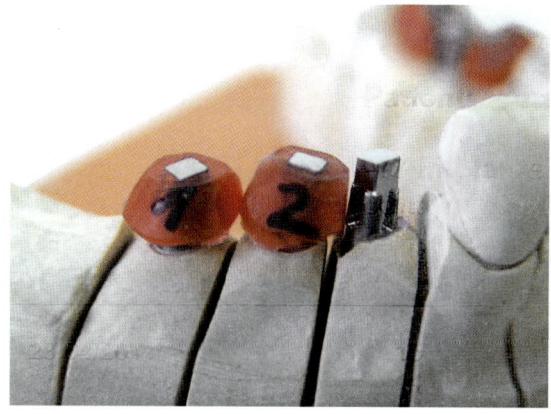

Stump preparation caps, right side

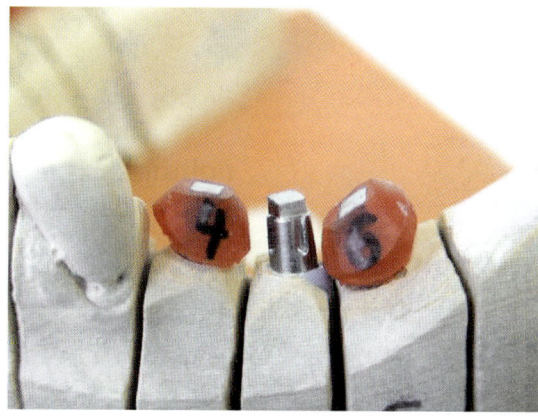

Stump preparation caps, left side

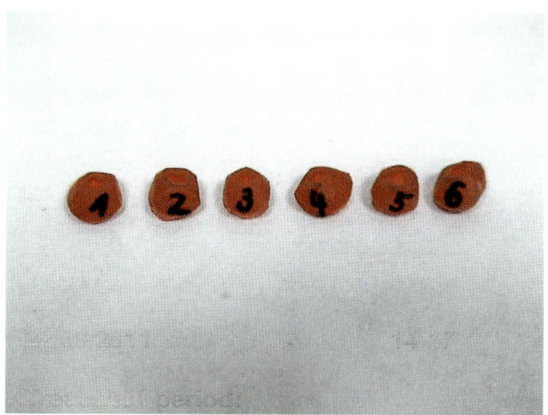

All plastic caps

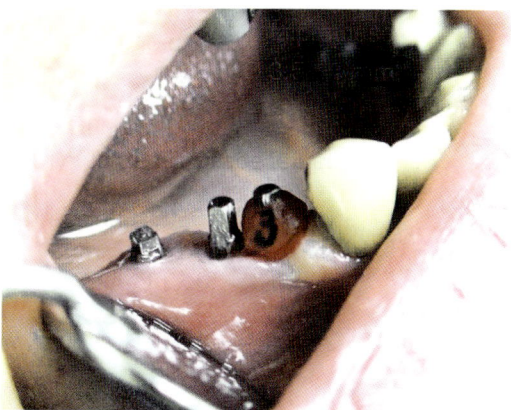

Procedure: Attach the caps...

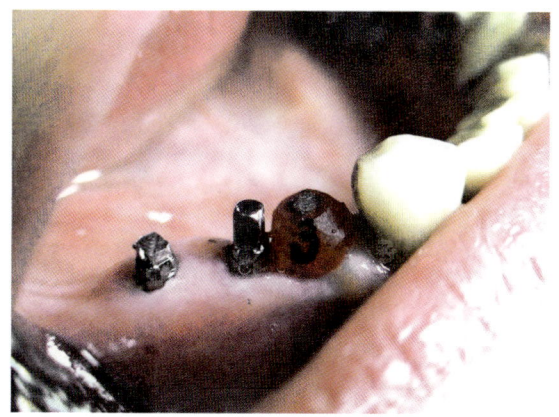

... prepare the overhanging parts...

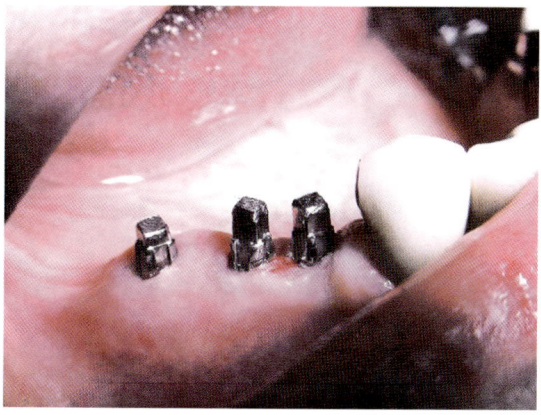

...and finished

157

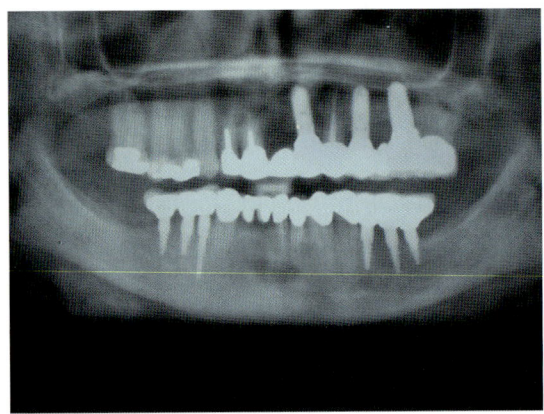

Panoramic radiographic control

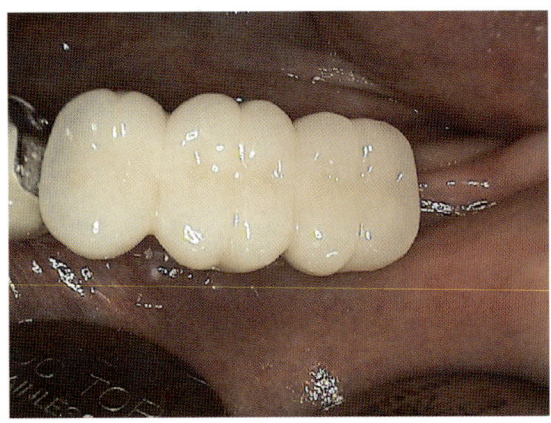

20 months after implant placement, left side, occlusal view

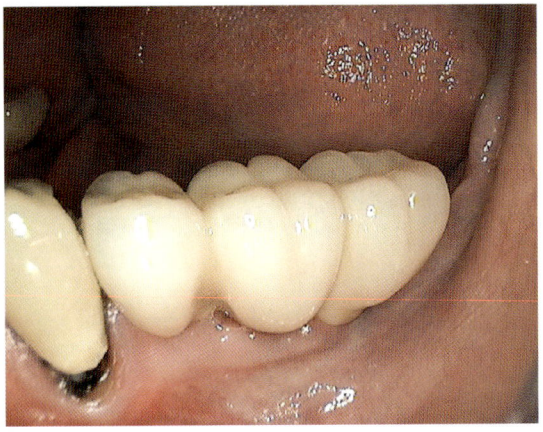

20 months after implant placement, left side, lateral view

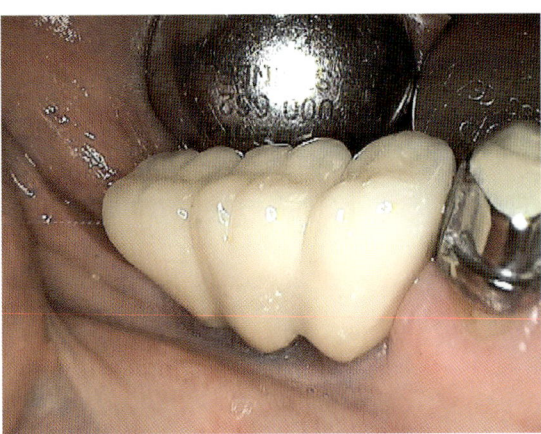

20 months after implant placement, left side, lingual view

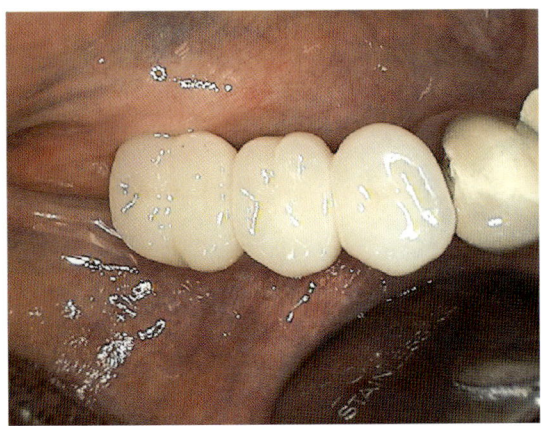

20 months after implant placement, left side, occlusal view

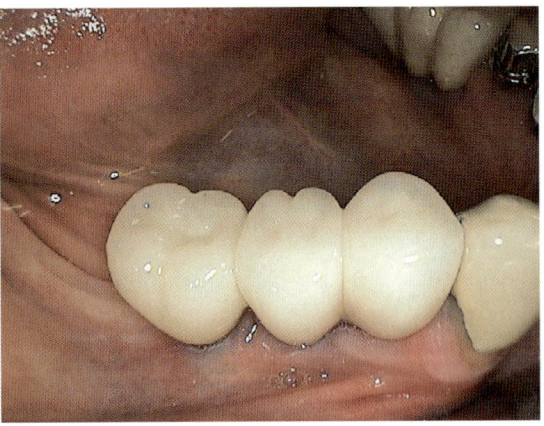

20 months after implant placement, left side, lateral view

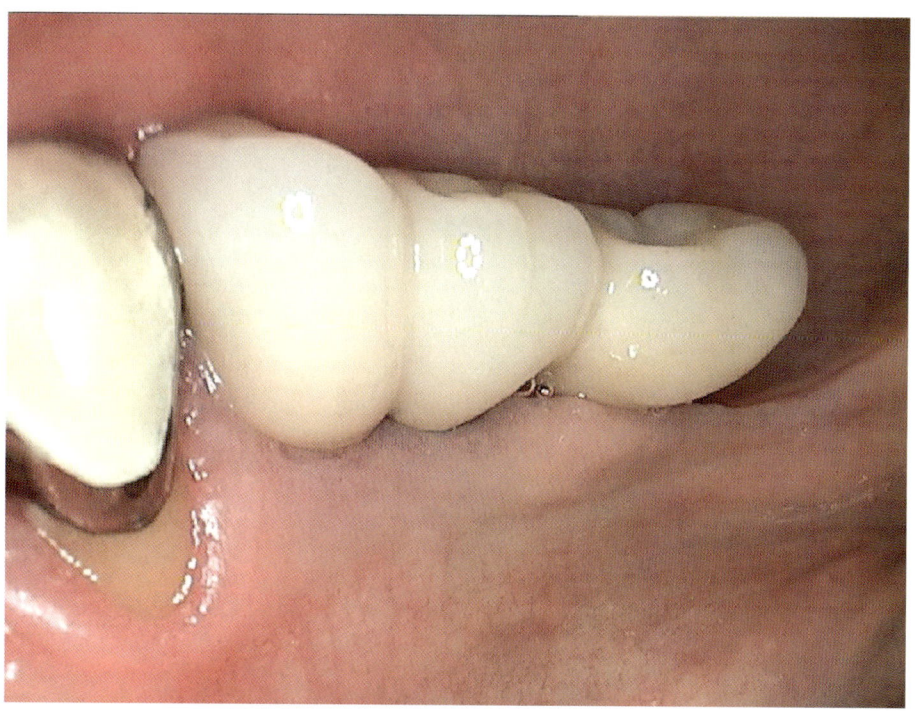

20 months after implant placement, right side, lingual view

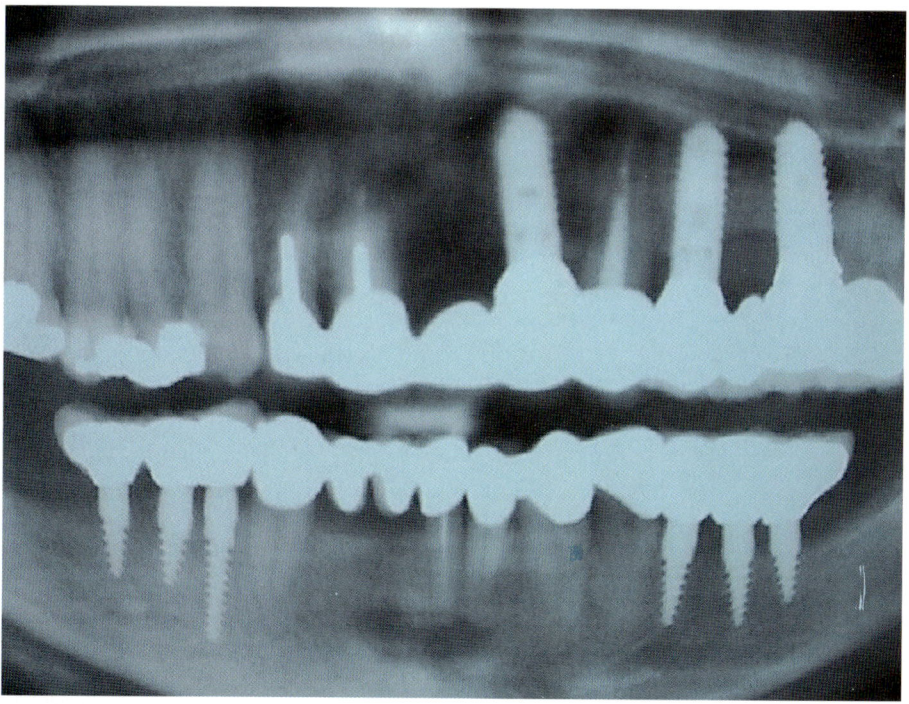

20 months after implant placement,
panoramic radiographic control

7.3.7/Case 31

Patient: female, 51 years old

36, 37 splinted crown, 44-47 splinted crown

18/08/2009	36 m	Champions® implant Ø 3.5 x 12 mm, >40 Ncm
	36 d	Champions® implant Ø 3.5 x 12 mm, 35 Ncm
	37	Champions® implant Ø 3.0 x 12 mm, >40 Ncm
26/08/2009	36,37	cemented zirconium dioxide splinted crown
16/11/2009	44	Champions® implant Ø 3.5 x 16 mm, >40 Ncm
	45	Champions® implant Ø 3.5 x 12 mm, >40 Ncm
	46 m	Champions® implant Ø 3.4 x 14 mm, >60 Ncm
	46 d	Champions® implant Ø 3.5 x 14 mm, >60 Ncm
	47	Champions® implant Ø 3.5 x 14 mm, >40 Ncm
	44-47	impression, cemented dentist made temporary
24/08/2010		Abutment preparation according to the laboratory requirements with plastic transfer caps Cemented zirconium dioxide splinted crown

Treatment period: **in each case 1 week**

Remarks:

Immediate restoration
Early loading

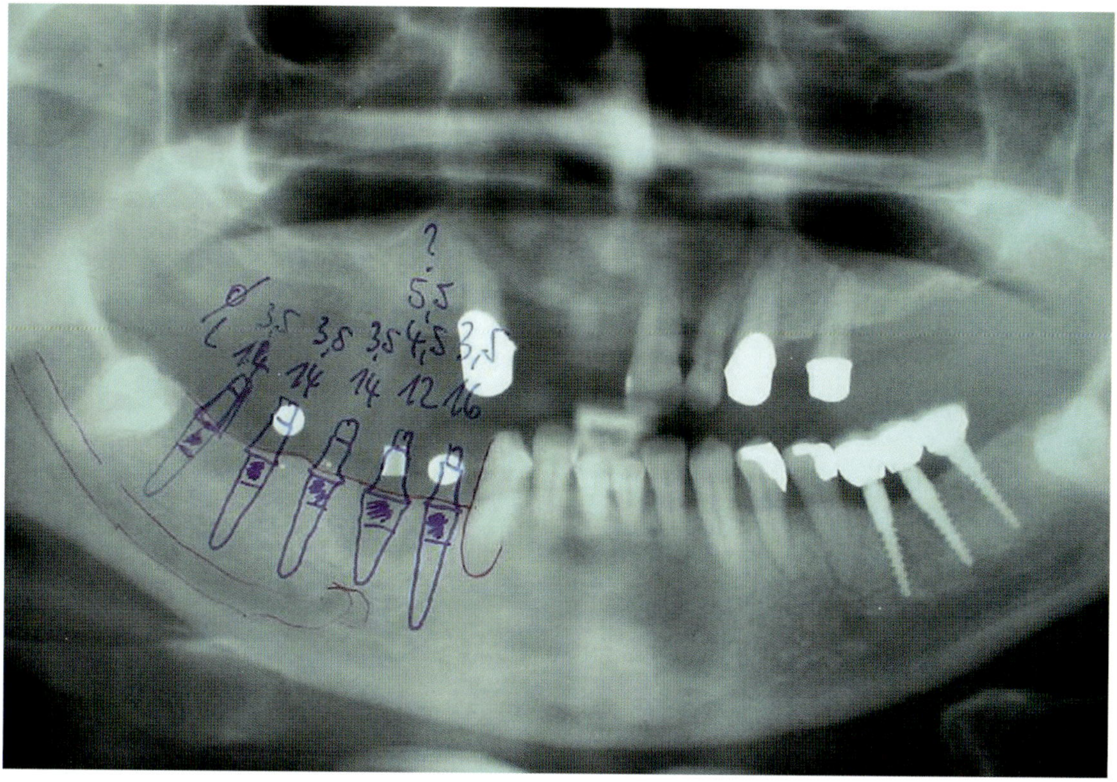

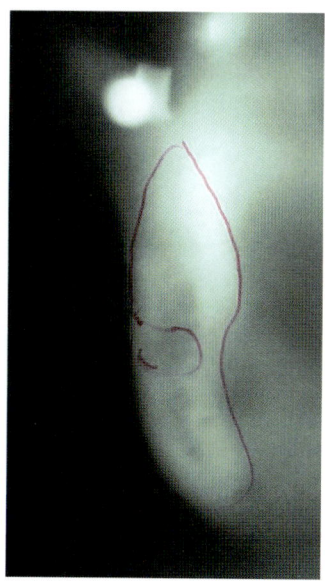

Planned treatment right side lower jaw, panoramic radiograph

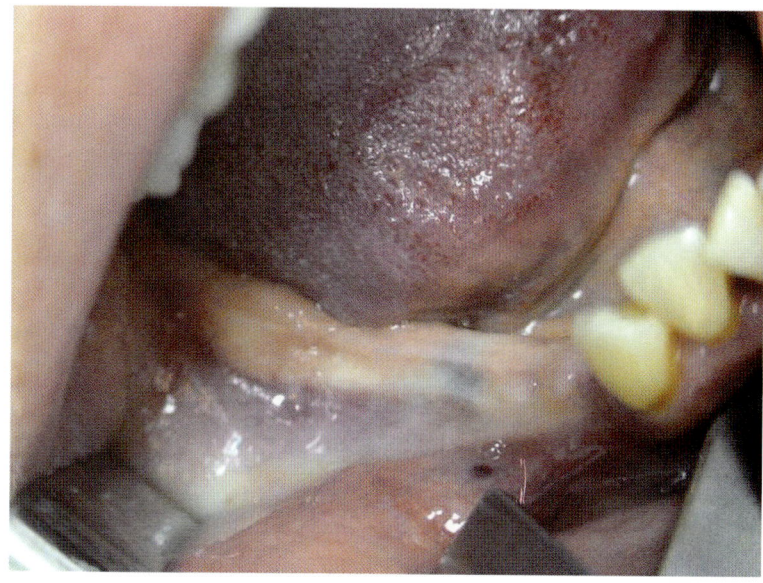

Planned treatment, cross-sectional image

Clinical initial situation

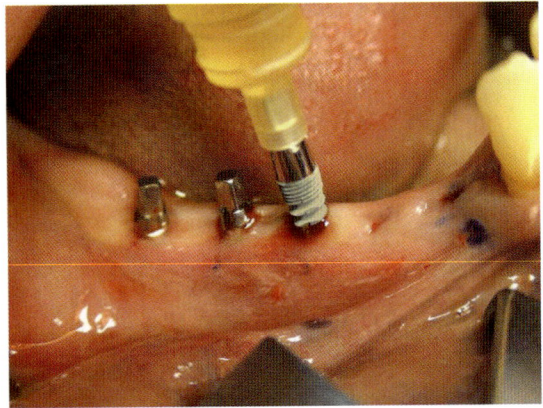

Implant placement

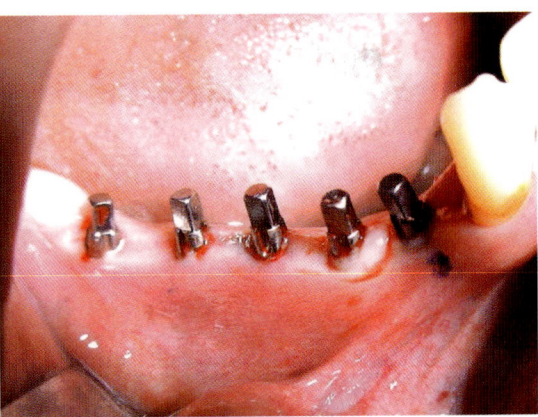

Completed implant placement

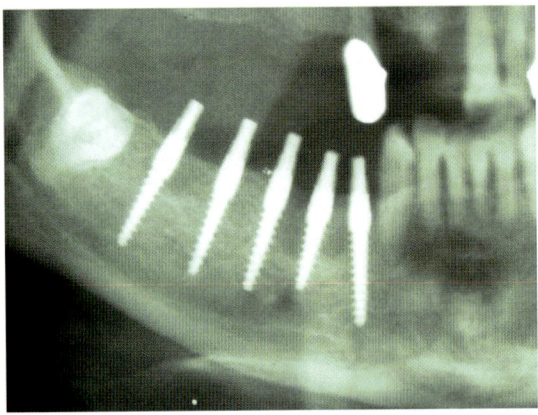

Panoramic radiographic control

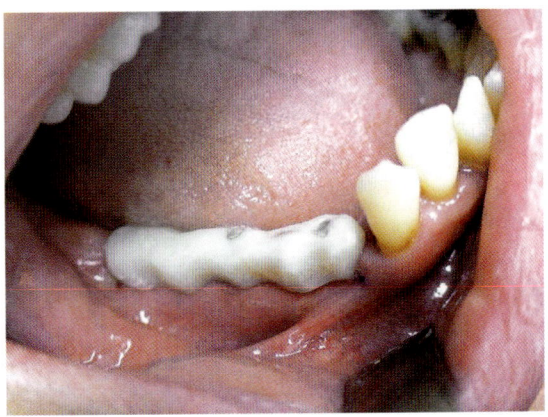

Dentist made temporary

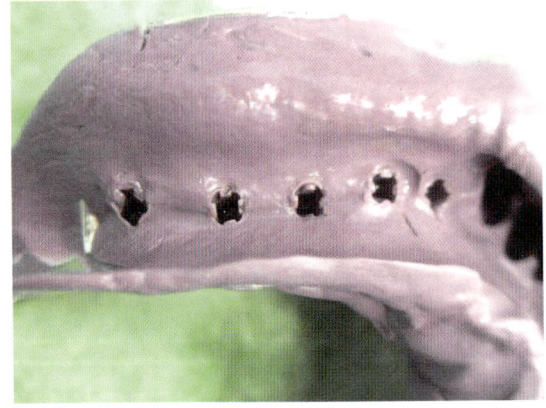

Impression for final dental prosthesis

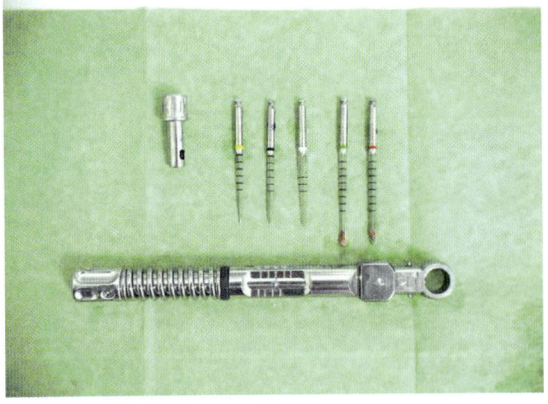

Surgery set

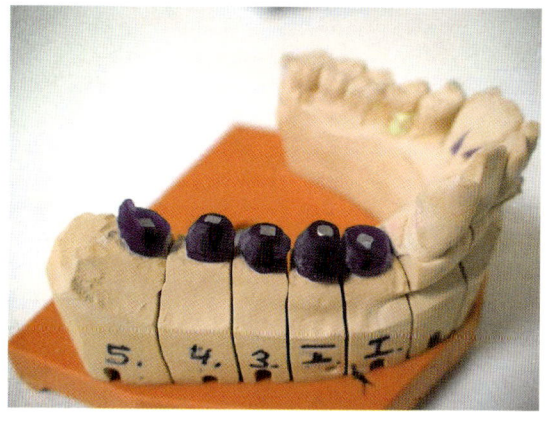

Transfer caps for stump preparation in mouth

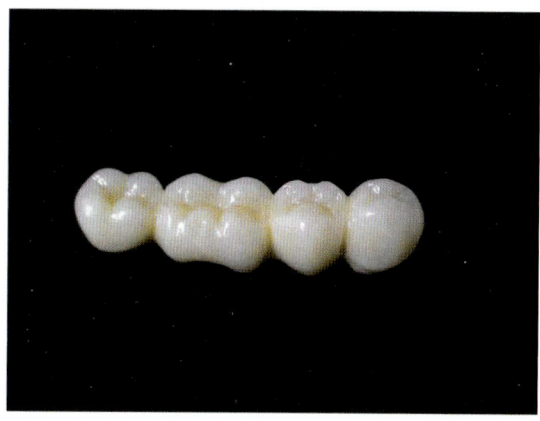

Final splinted crown

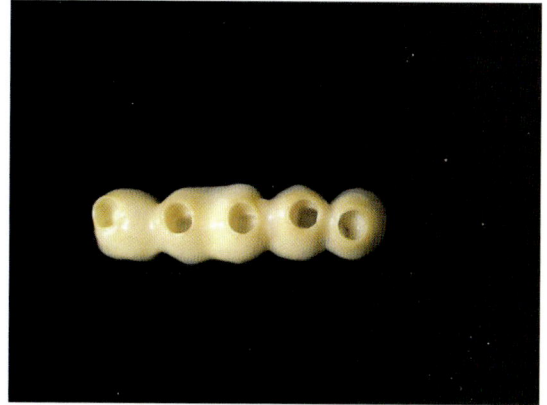

Final splinted crown, basal view

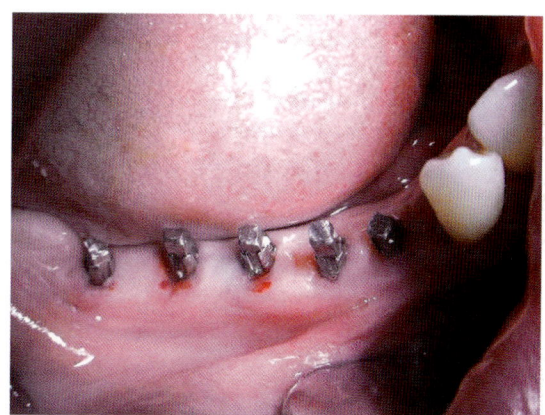

Clinical situation before insertion

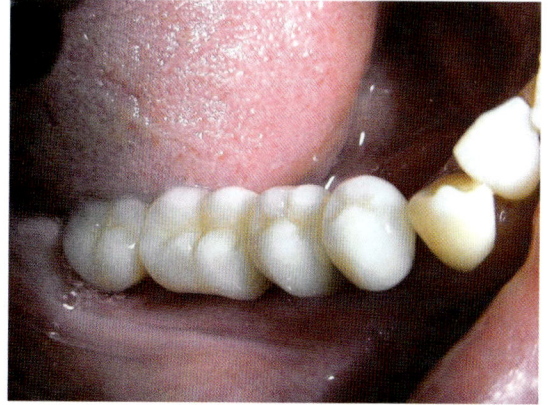

Final image

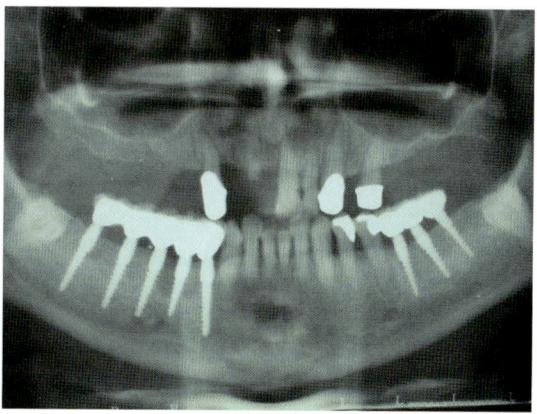

Panoramic radiographic control

7.3.8/Case 32

Patient: female, 56 years old

34-37, 43-46 implants,
paranerval implant placement, 2 zirconium dioxide splinted crowns

---

08/03/2011	43	Champions® implant Ø 3.5 x 10 mm, >60 Ncm
	44	Champions® implant Ø 3.5 x 14 mm, >60 Ncm
	45	Champions® implant Ø 3.5 x 8 mm, >40 Ncm
	46	Champions® implant Ø 3.5 x 8 mm, >40 Ncm
	33	removed attachment
	35	extraction
	34	Champions® implant Ø 3.0 x 14 mm, >60 Ncm
	35	Champions® implant Ø 4.5 x 10 mm, >50 Ncm, Prep-Cap
	36	Champions® implant Ø 3.5 x 10 mm, >60 Ncm
	37	Champions® implant Ø 3.5 x 8 mm, >60 Ncm
		impression
		dentist made temporary
16/03/2011	34-37, 43-46	cemented zirconium dioxide splinted crown
04/04/2011		Final control, image
Treatment period:		**1 week**
Remarks:	35	Immediate implant placement
	45, 46	Paranerval implant placement
		Immediate restoration
		Early loading

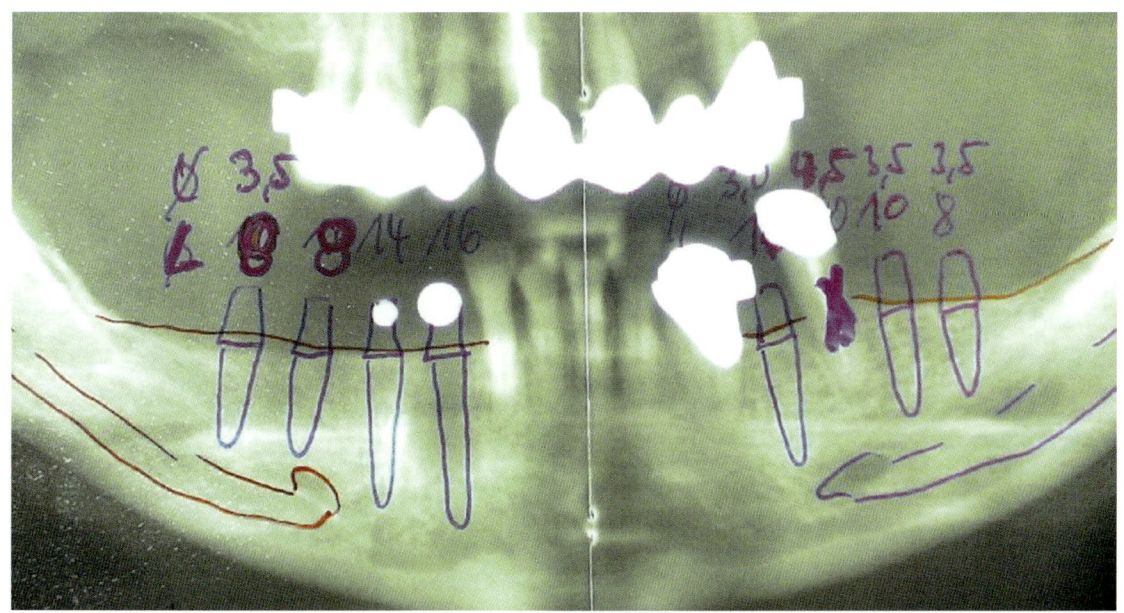

Panoramic radiograph for planned treatment

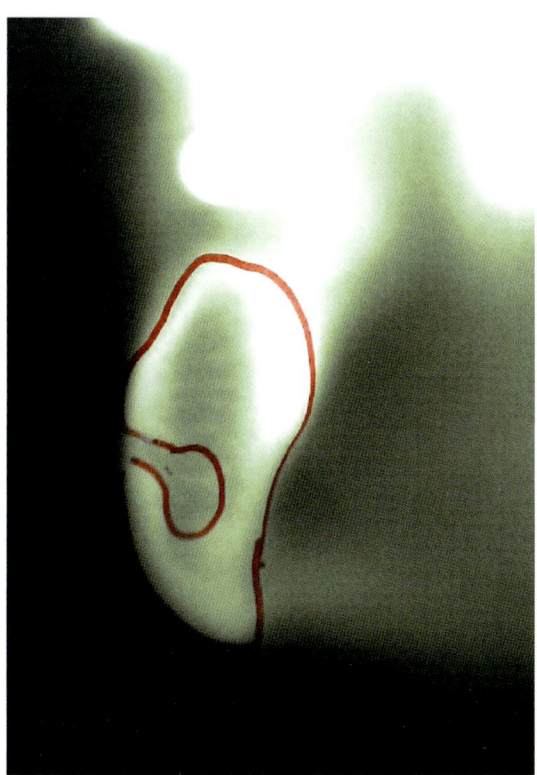

Cross-sectional radiography, right side

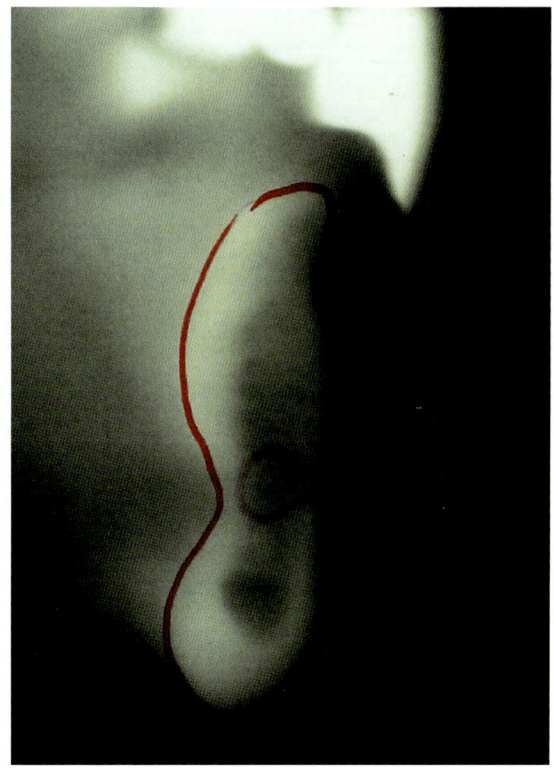

Cross-sectional radiography, left side

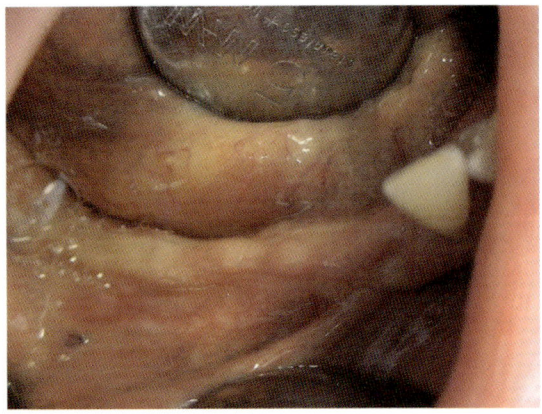

Clinical situation, right side

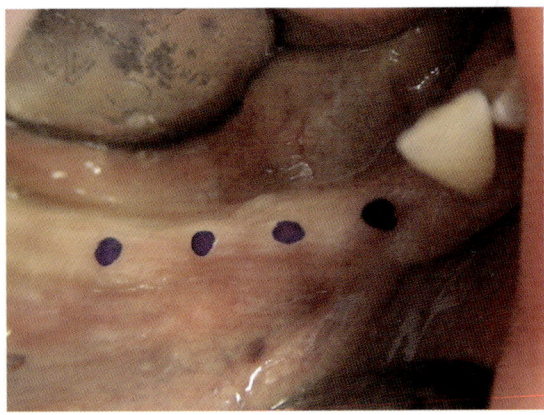

Marked points for initial pilot hole preparation

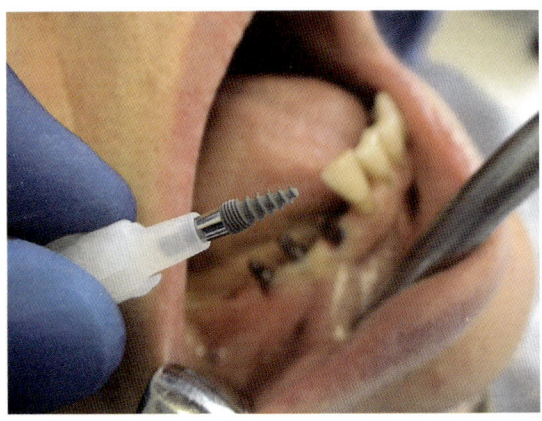

Implant placement, right side

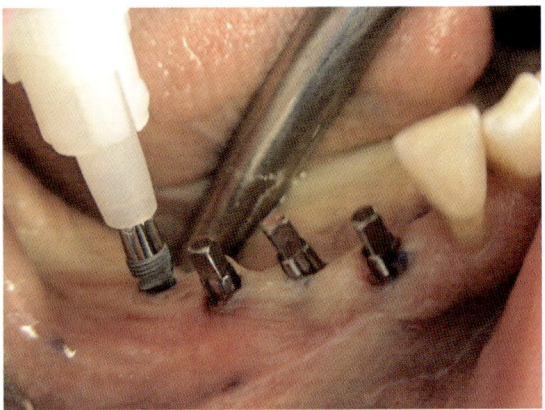

During the Implant placement

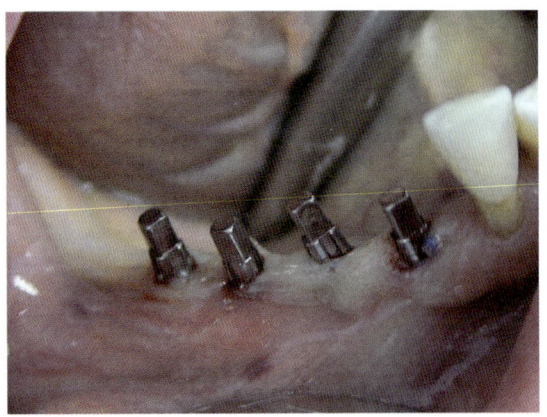

Completed implant placement, occlusal view

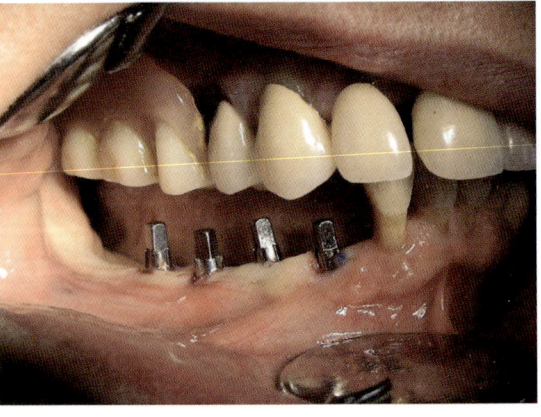

Completed implant placement, lateral view

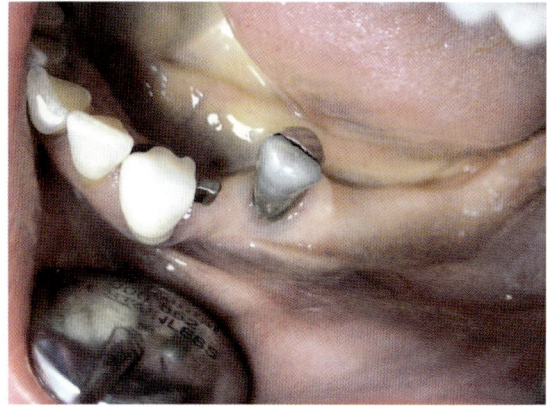

Clinical situation, left side

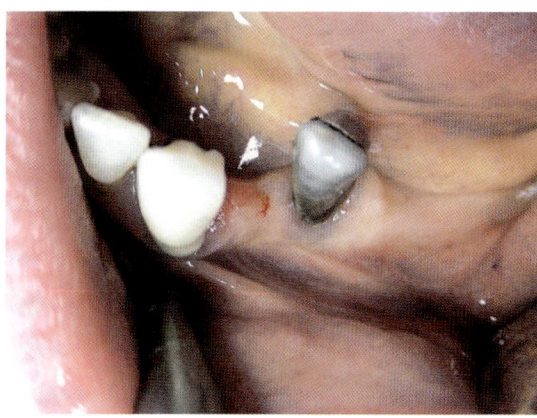

Detached attachment in regio 33

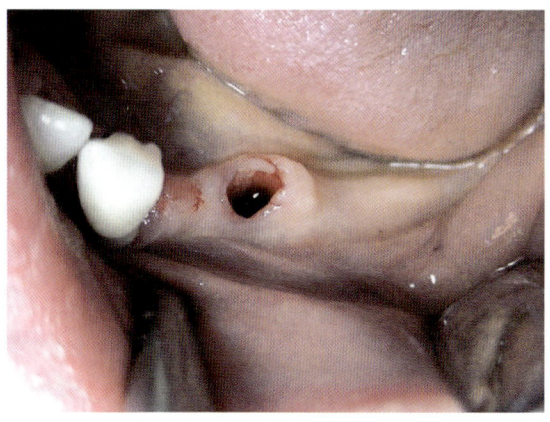

Alveolus after extraction of tooth 35

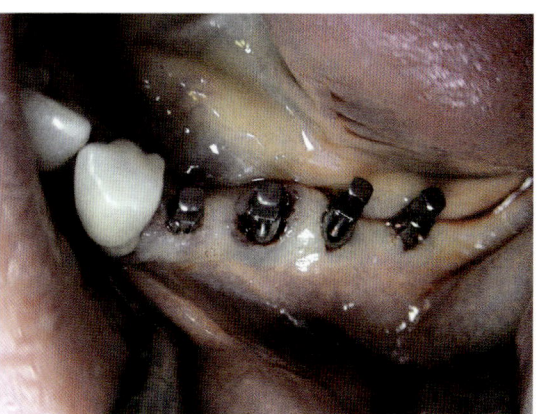

Implant placement, left side

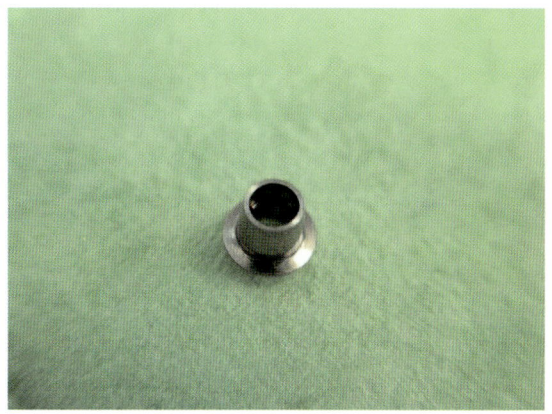

PC for 35

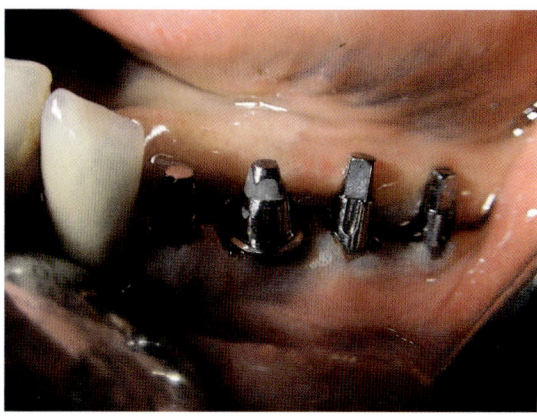

PC for 35 cemented and prepared

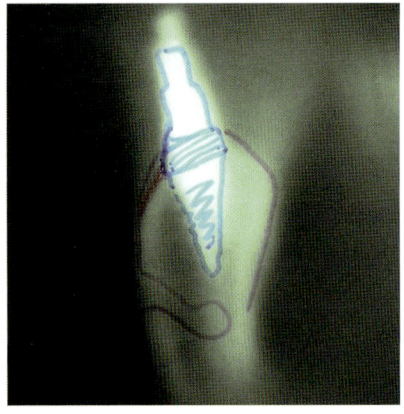

Cross-sectional radiography, paranerval implant placement, right side

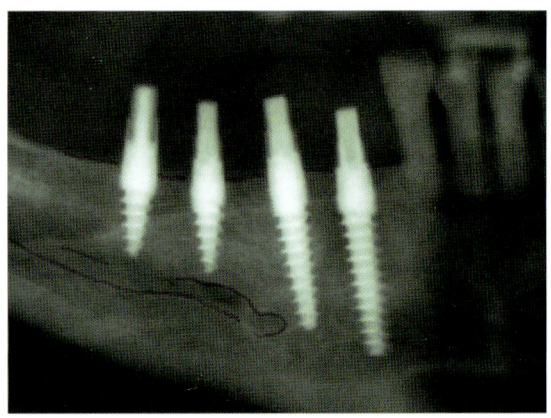

Radiographic control, panoramic radiograph, right side, zoomed detail

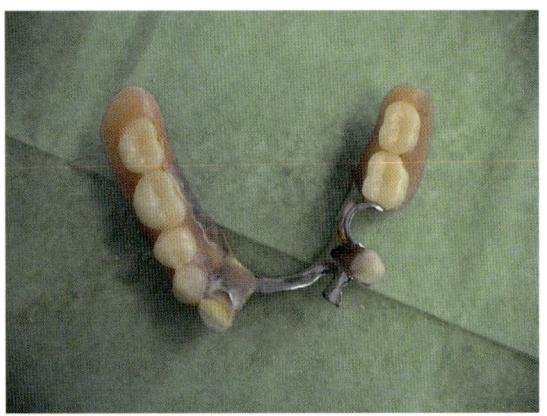

Former model casting prosthesis

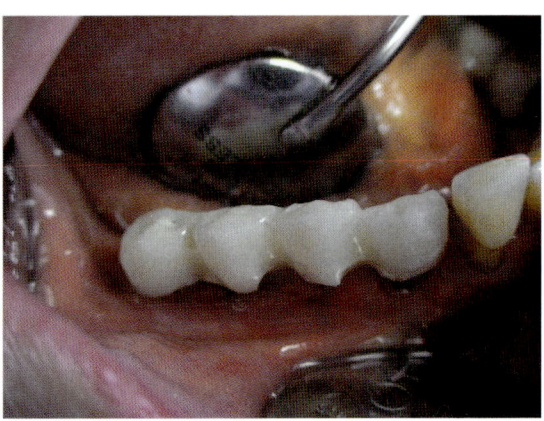

Dentist made temporary, right side

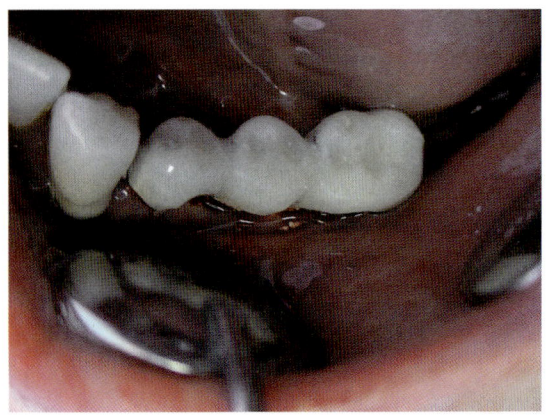

Dentist made temporary, left side

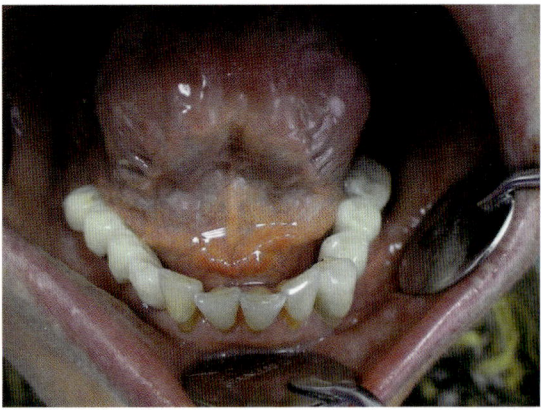

Dentist made temporary, occlusal view

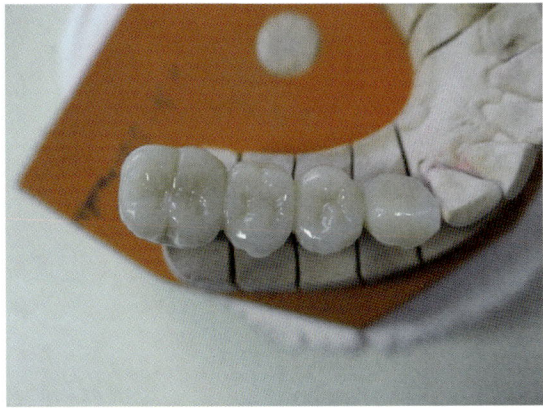

Final splinted crown, cast, right side

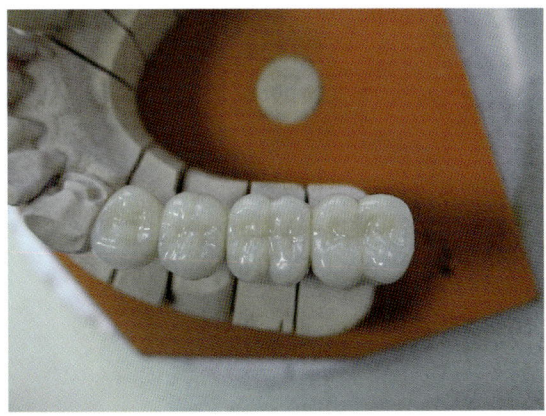

Final splinted crown, cast, left side

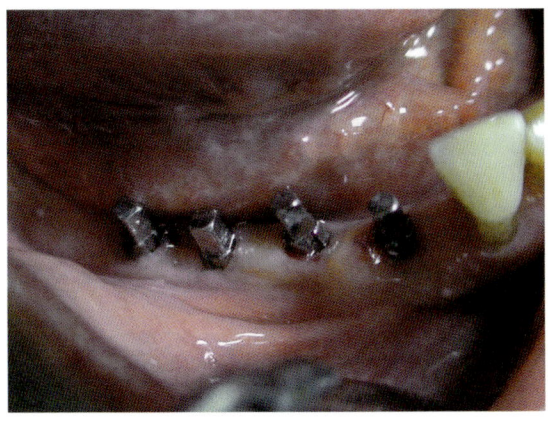

Clinical situation before prosthesis insertion

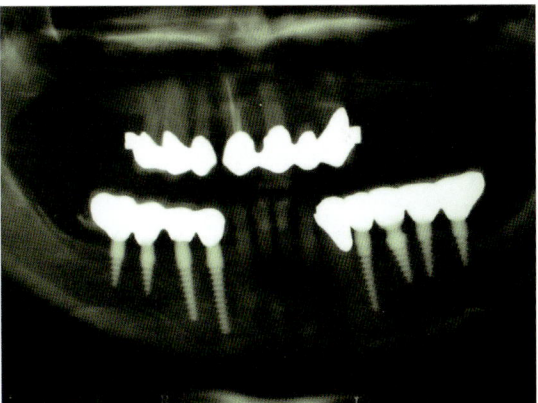

Radiographic control, panoramic radiograph

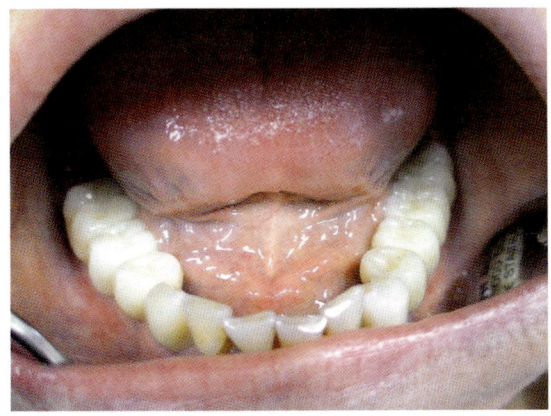

Clinical situation after prosthesis insertion

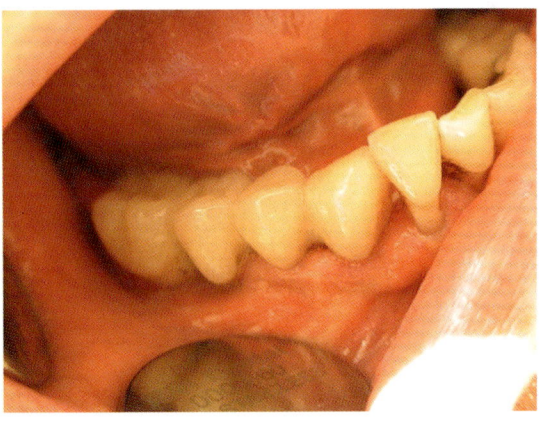

Final control 19 days after prosthesis insertion,
lateral view, right side

9 and more implants

Patient: male, 44 years old

11 implants (upper jaw, lower jaw), 48 osteotomy, augmentation, fracture of an implant, 2 splinted crowns

---

31/05/2011	22,25,26	extraction
	48	osteotomy cystectomy
	36m	Champions® implant Ø 3.5 x 12 mm, >60 Ncm
	36d	Champions® implant Ø 3.5 x 10 mm, >60 Ncm
	37	Champions® implant Ø 3.5 x 12 mm, >60 Ncm
	22	Champions® implant Ø 3.5 x 14 mm, 40 Ncm, cemented Prep-Cap
	23	Champions® implant Ø 3.0 x 10 mm, 30 Ncm
	24m	Champions® implant Ø 3.0 x 10 mm, >40 Ncm
	24d	Champions® implant Ø 4.5 x 10 mm, 25 Ncm
	25	Champions® implant Ø 4.5 x 14 mm, 30 Ncm
	26m	Champions® implant Ø 3.5 x 10 mm, >40 Ncm
	26d	Champions® implant Ø 3.5 x 10 mm, >20 Ncm
	27	Champions® implant Ø 3.5 x 8 mm, >30 Ncm preparation, cemented dentist made temporary
01/06/2011	22-27	laboratory made temporary
17/08/2011		Impression
		Periotest: 36m -7, 36d -6, 37 -4, 22 0, 23 0, 24m +2, 24d -2, 25 -2, 26m -2, 26d -1, 27 +2
31/08/2011	36/37	cemented zirconium dioxide splinted crown
	22-27	cemented zirconium dioxide splinted crown
Treatment period:		**3 months**
Remarks:		Endotracheal anaesthesia
		Fracture of the implant in regio 23!
		Primary stability precedes abutment parallelism!
		For one-piece implants there is no defined interimplant minimum distance.
		The patient refused the removal of the gingival hyperplasia during impression.
	22,25,26	immediate implant placement immediate restoration, late loading

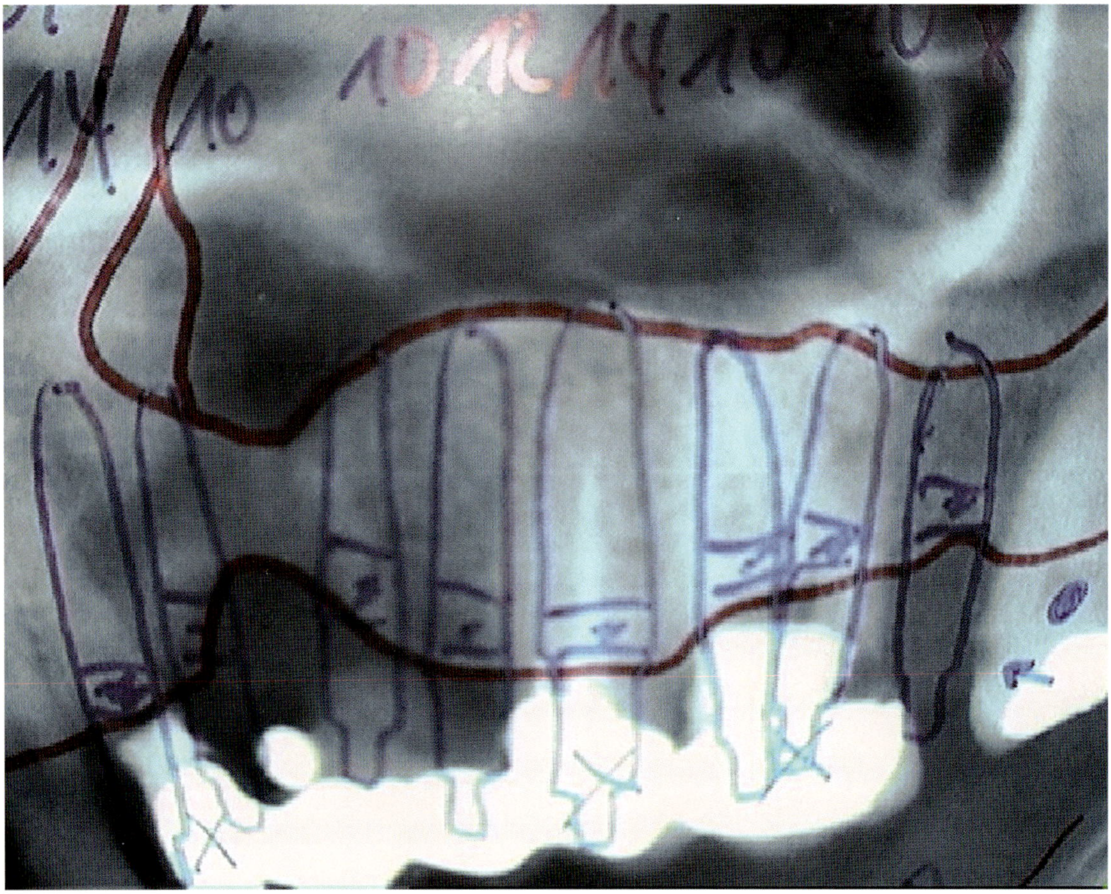

Panoramic radiograph for planned treatment, upper jaw, left

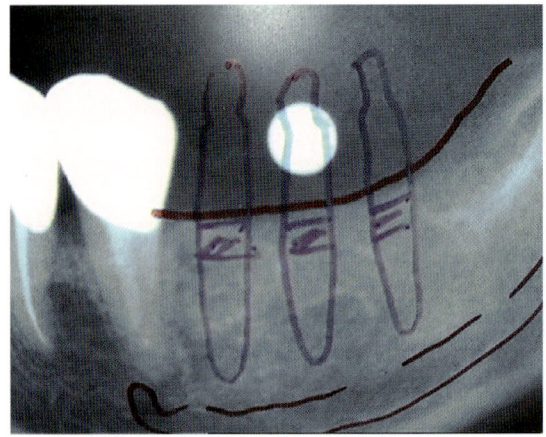

Panoramic radiograph for planned treatment,
lower jaw, left side

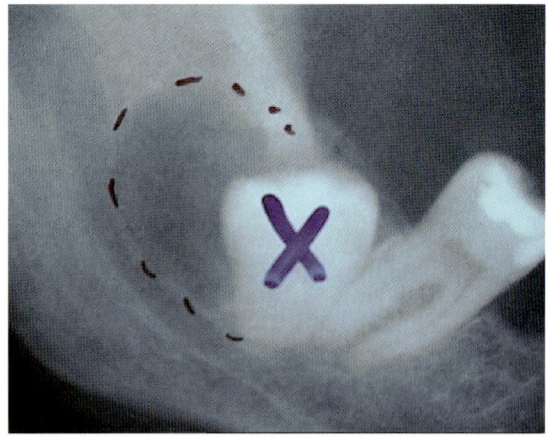

Panoramic radiograph for planned treatment, lower
jaw, right side

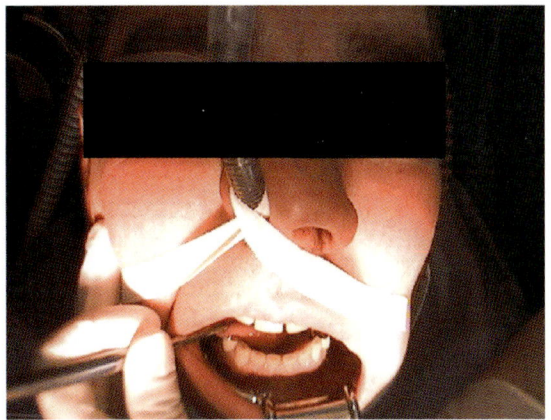

Endotracheal anaesthesia

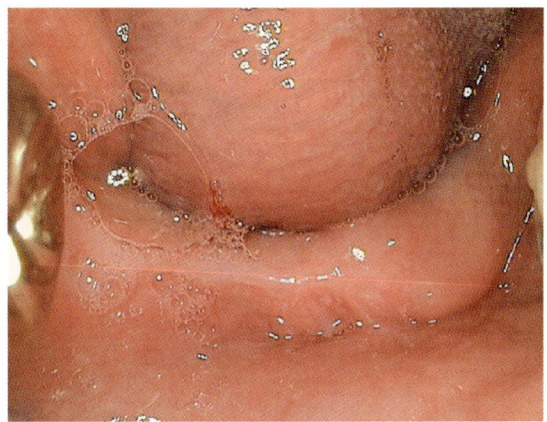

Clinical situation in the left lower jaw

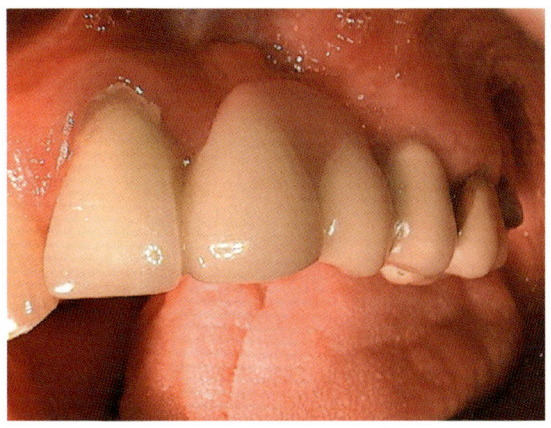

Clinical situation in the left upper jaw, lateral view

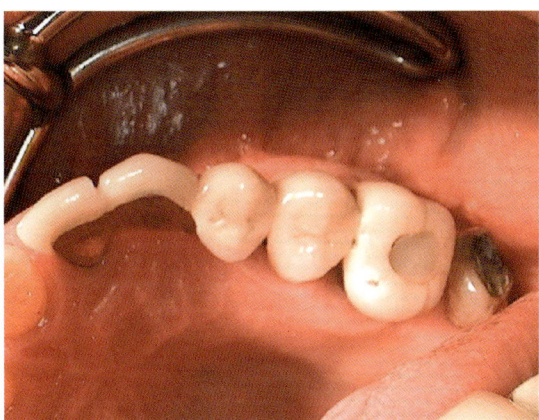

Clinical situation in the left upper jaw, occlusal view

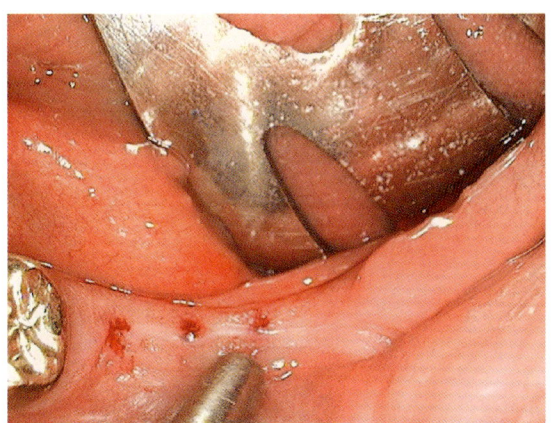

Initial pilot hole preparation in the lower jaw

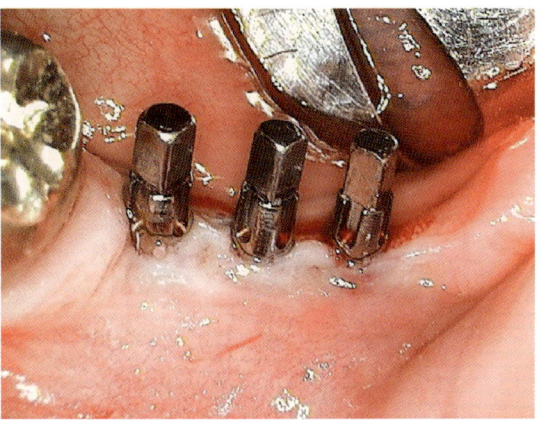

Implant placement in the lower jaw

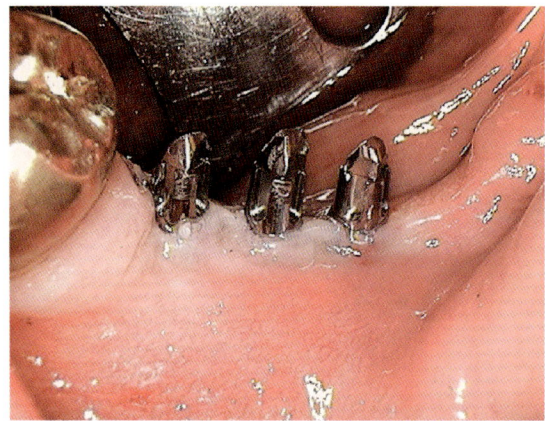

Prepared implant heads

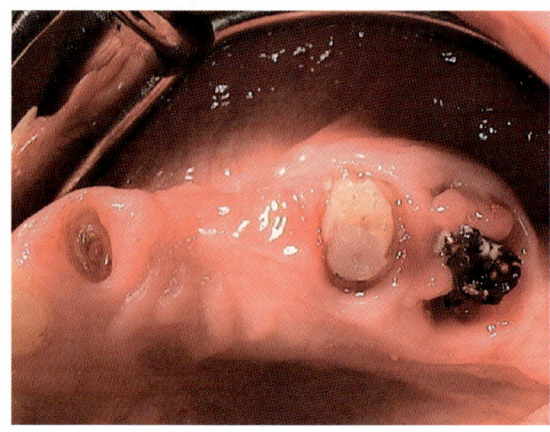

Situation after bridge removal in the upper jaw

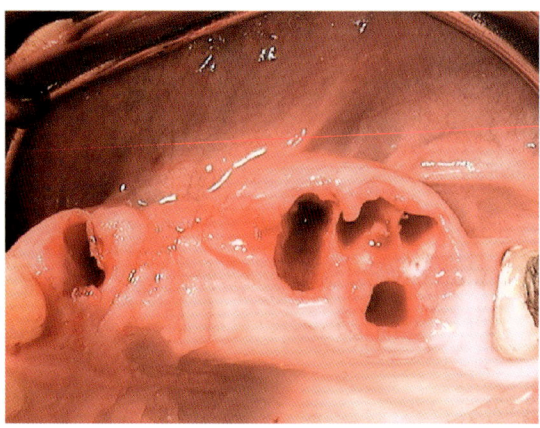

Alveoli after extraction 22, 25, 26

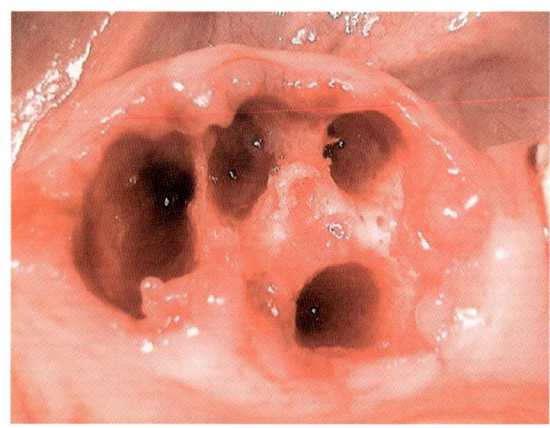

Alveolus 25, 26

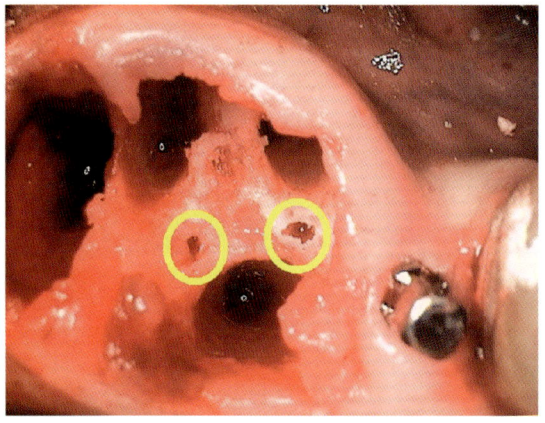

Initial pilot hole preparation for 2 implants at 26

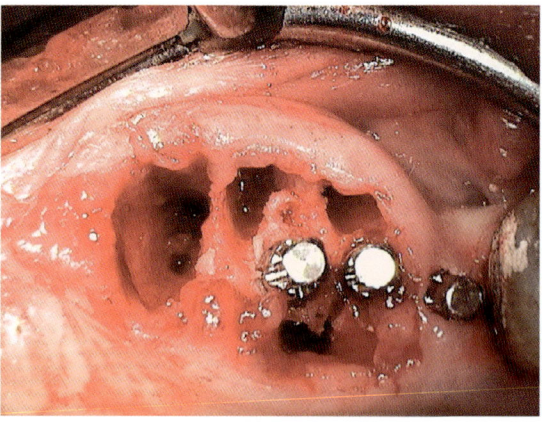

Implant placement 26

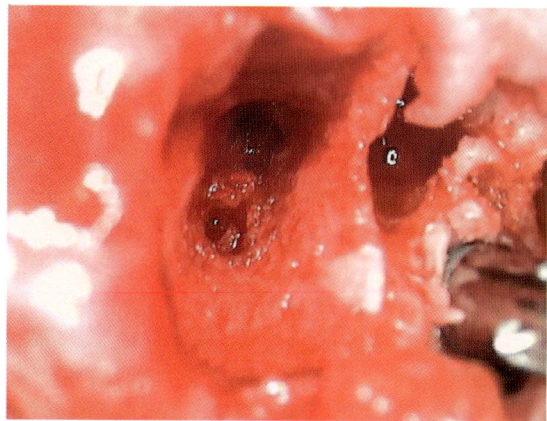

Palatal pilot hole preparation 25

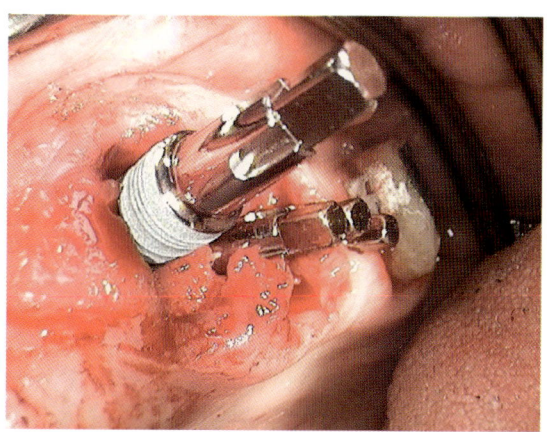

Implant placement in regio 25

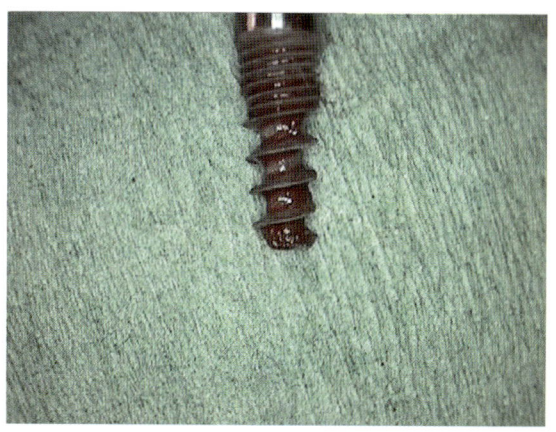

Removed fractured implant in regio 23, 24

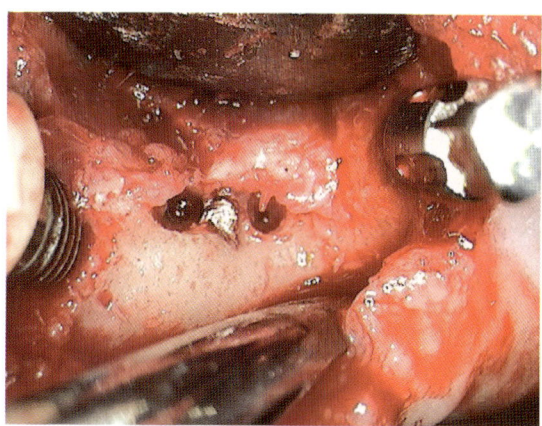

Implant fracture in region 23, 24

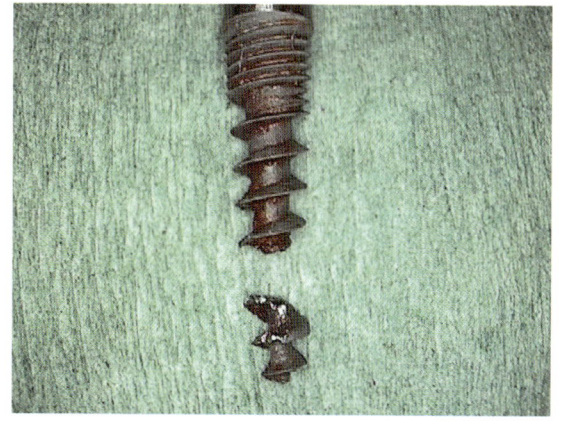

Removed fractured implant apex...

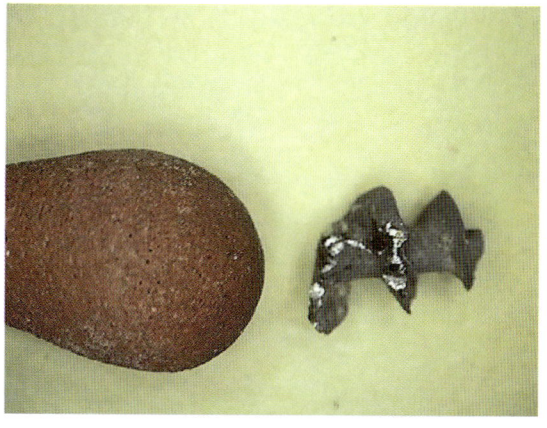

....macro image

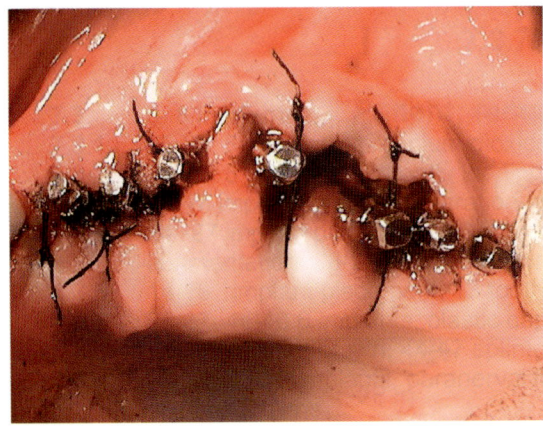

Surgical site with suture closure

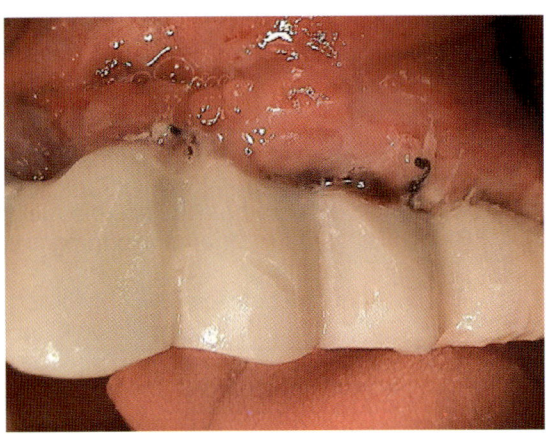

Dentist made temporary, upper jaw

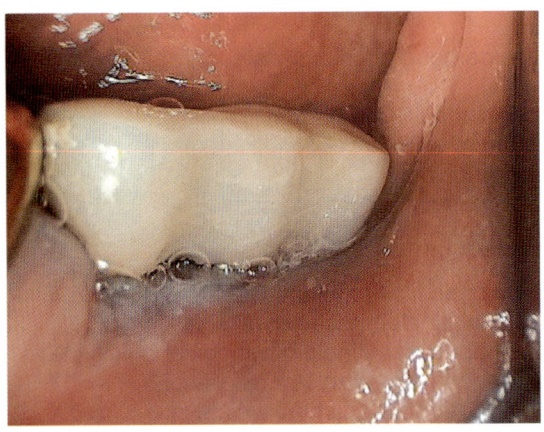

Dentist made temporary, lower jaw

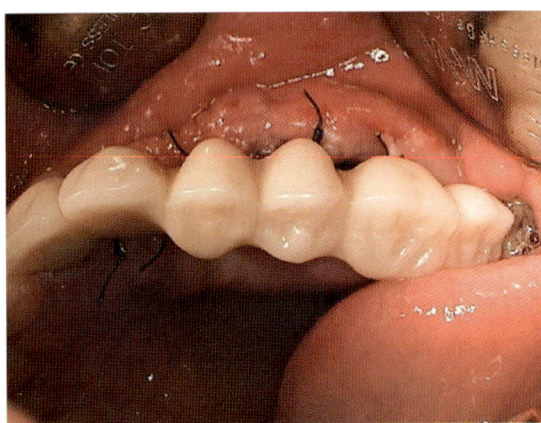

1st postoperative day, laboratory made temporary, occlusal view

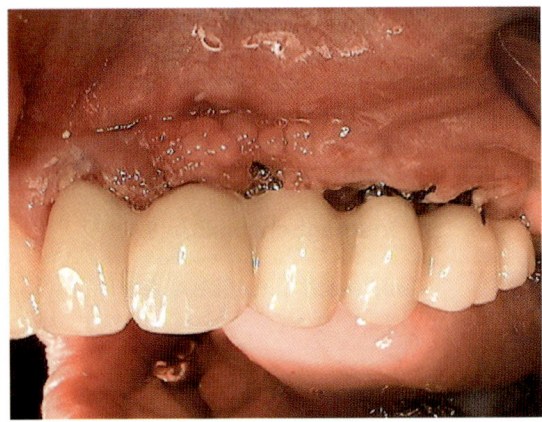

1st postoperative day, laboratory made temporary, lateral view

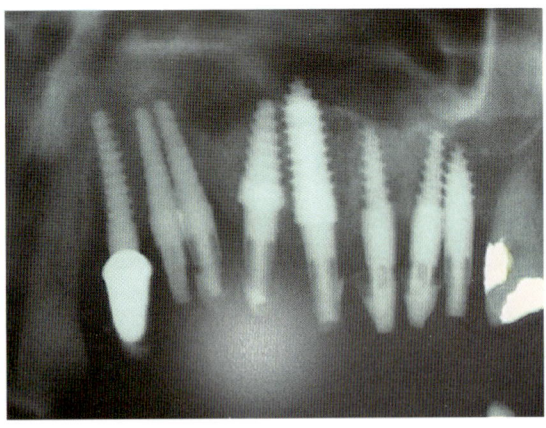

1st postoperative day, radiographic control, panoramic radiograph, detail

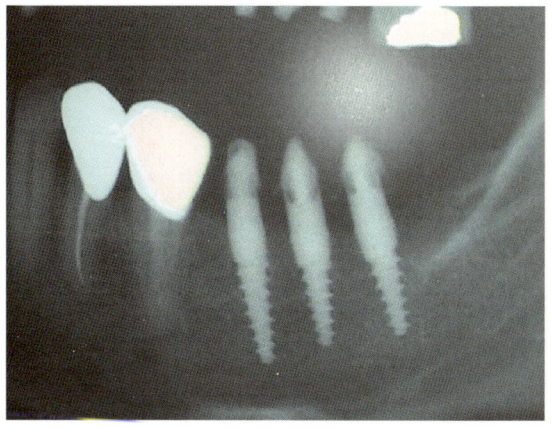

1st postoperative day, radiographic control, panoramic radiograph, detail

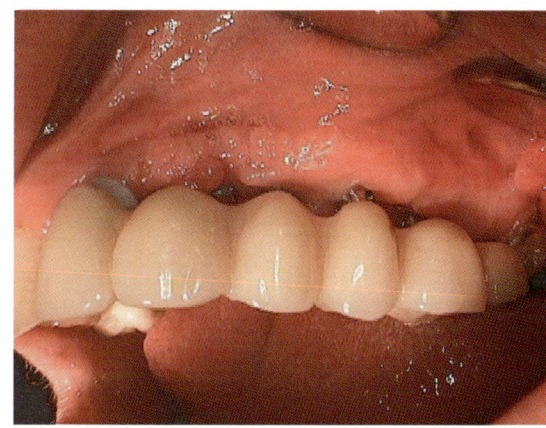

After osseointegration

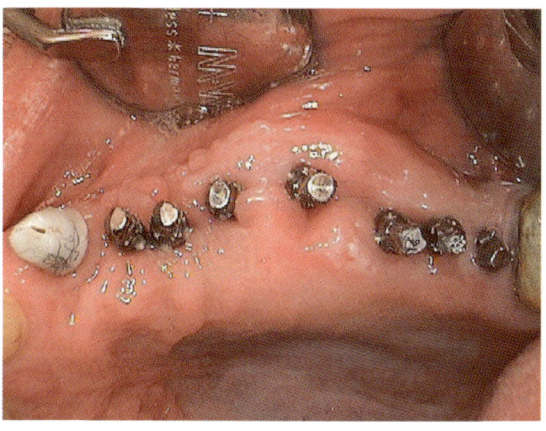

After osseointegration, before impression taking

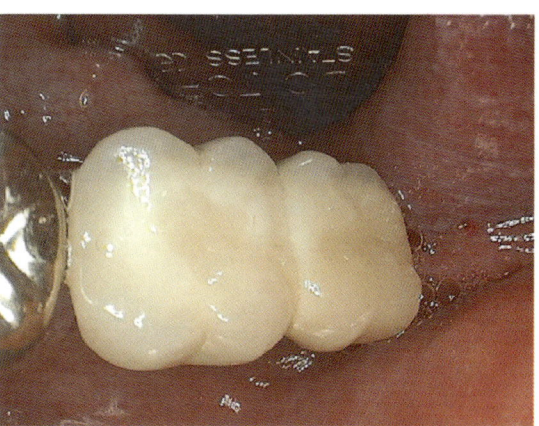

Final cemented splinted crown, occlusal view

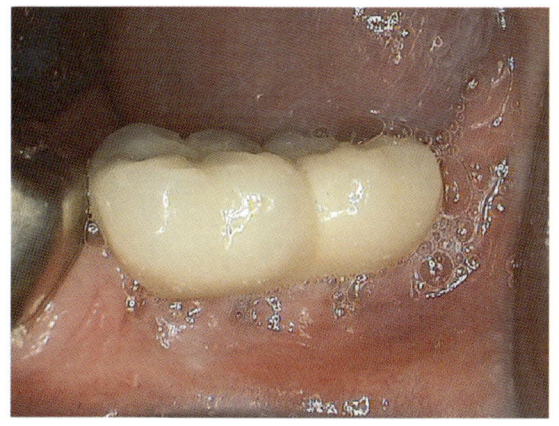

Final cemented splinted crown, lateral view

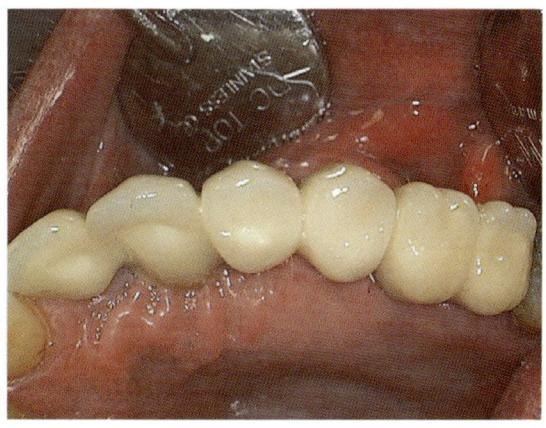

Final cemented splinted crown, occlusal view

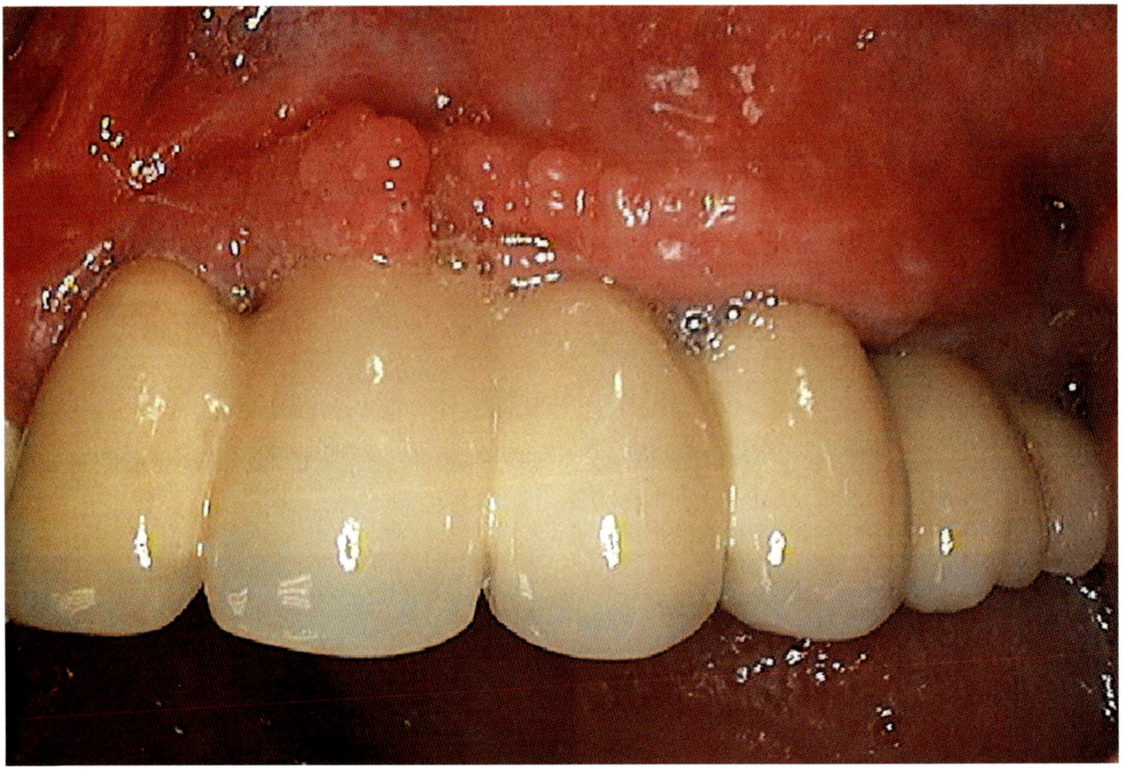

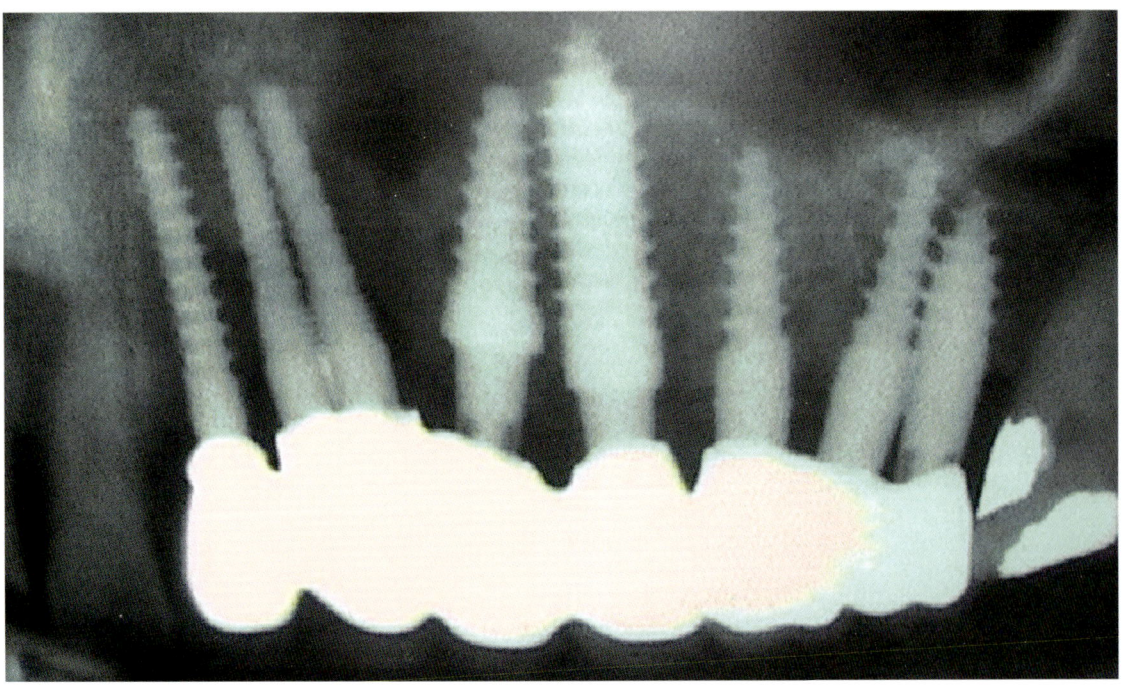

Final cemented splinted crown, lateral view

Panoramic radiographic control, zoomed detail

178

7.4.2/Case 34

Patient: female, 60 years old

11 upper jaw implants performed under general anaesthesia
17-27 three splinted crowns

05/05/2011	18,28	osteotomy
	14,25	extraction, immediate implant placement
	17	Champions® implant Ø 4.5 x 6 mm, 15 Ncm
	16	Champions® implant Ø 3.5 x 6 mm, 30 Ncm
	15	Champions® implant Ø 3.5 x 8 mm, 40 Ncm
	14	Champions® implant Ø 4.5 x 14 mm, 40 Ncm, Prep-Cap
	11	Champions® implant Ø 3.0 x 12 mm, 40 Ncm
	21	Champions® implant Ø 3.0 x 12 mm, 40 Ncm
	24	Champions® implant Ø 3.0 x 14 mm, 30 Ncm
	25	Champions® implant Ø 4.5 x 12 mm, 40 Ncm, Prep-Cap
	26m	Champions® implant Ø 3.5 x 8 mm, 20 Ncm
	26d	Champions® implant Ø 3.5 x 6 mm, 20 Ncm
	27	Champions® implant Ø 3.5 x 8 mm, 15 Ncm
	12, 13, 22, 23	tooth preparation
	17-27	dentist made temporary
06/05/2011		wound control
	17-27	cemented laboratory made temporary
14/07/2011	17-27	impression
21/07/2011		Cemented zirconium dioxide crown
Treatment period:		**2.5 months**
Remarks:		14, 25 immediate implant placement
		Endotracheal anaesthesia
		Immediate loading
		The dental prosthesis was fabricated by the family dentist.

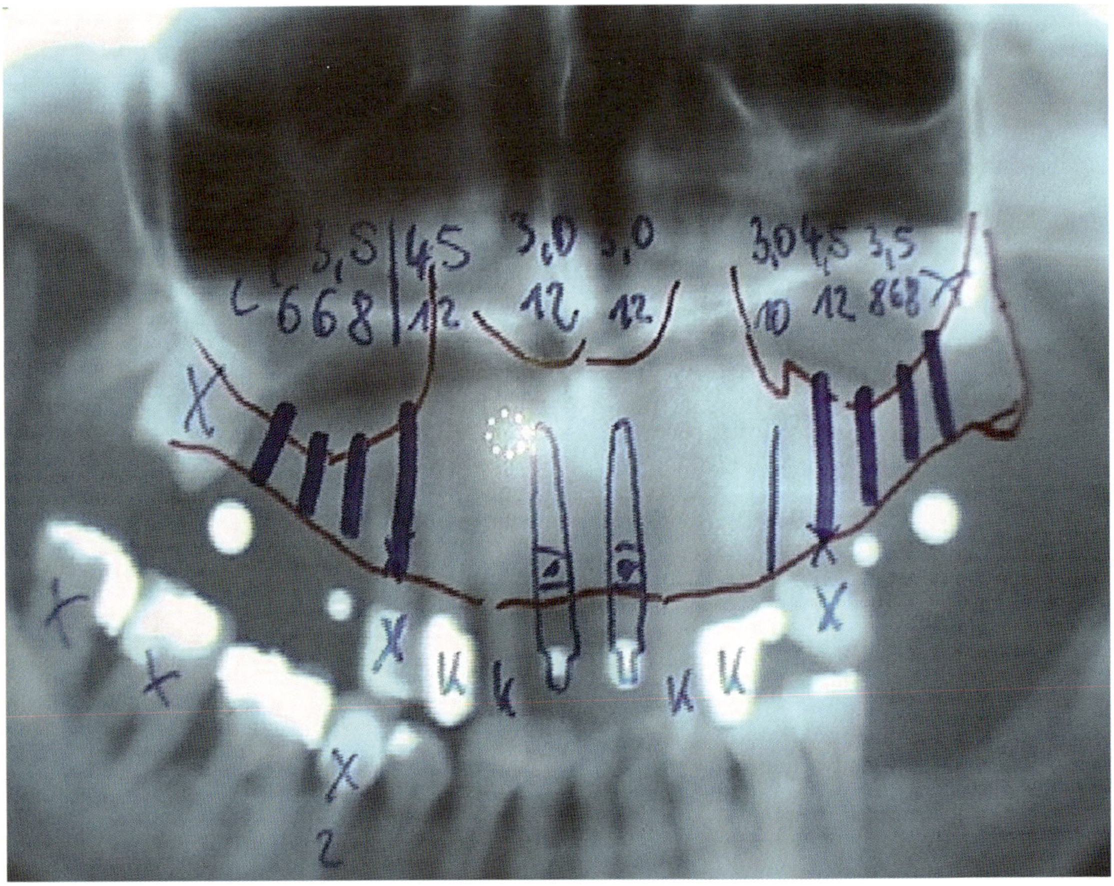

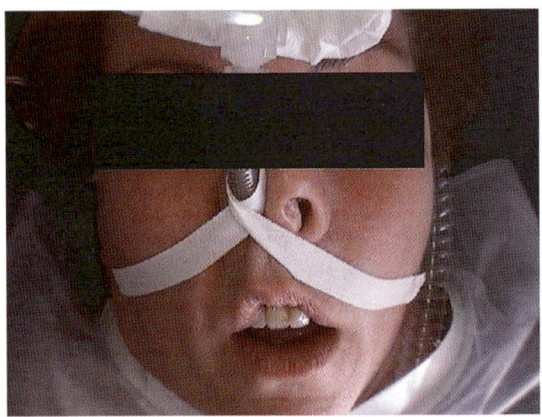

Panoramic radiograph initial findings, planned treatment

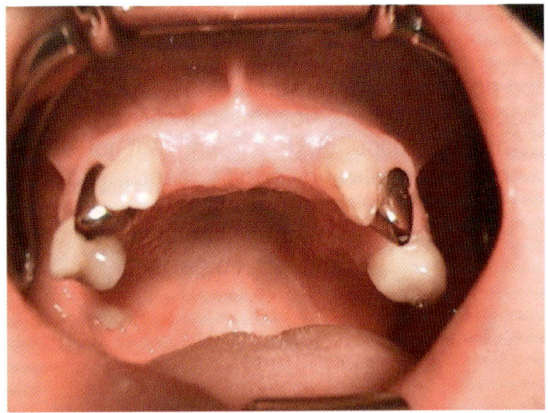

Endotracheal anaesthesia

Clinical initial findings

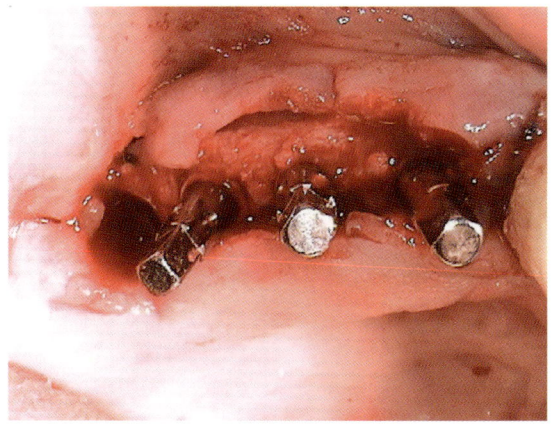

Open implant placement in the right upper jaw

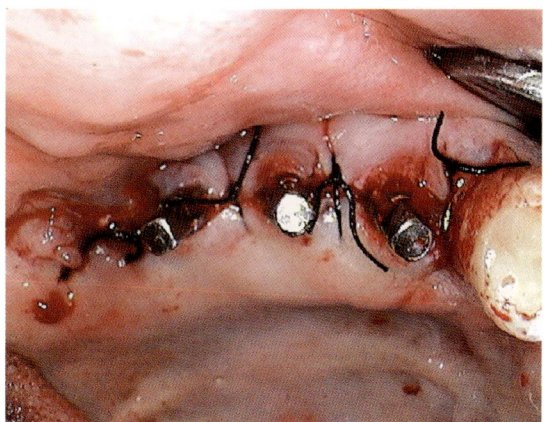

Wound closure

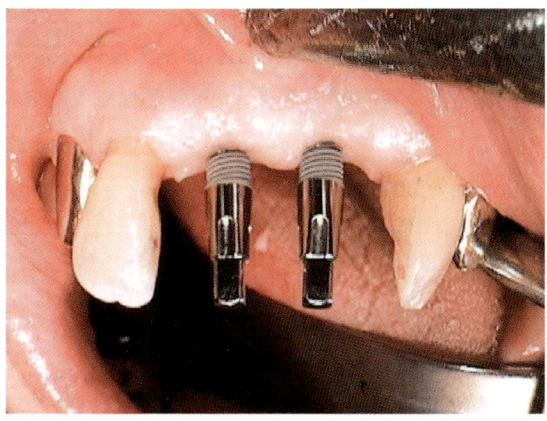

Insertion at the beginning, in the anterior maxillary region

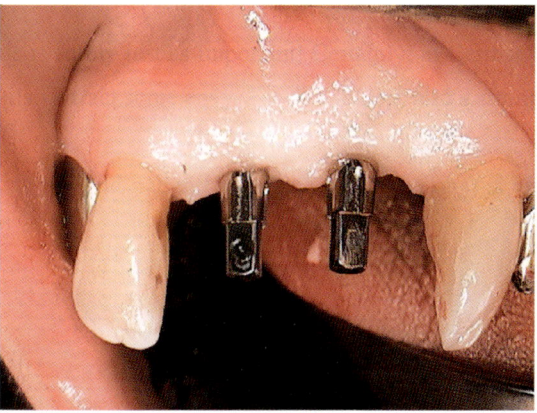

Completed insertion in the anterior maxillary region, anterior view

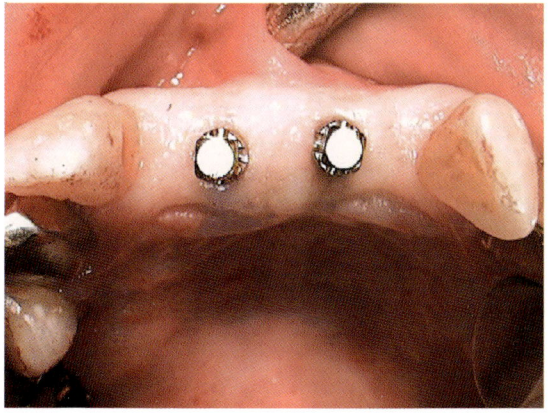

Completed insertion in the anterior maxillary region, occlusal view

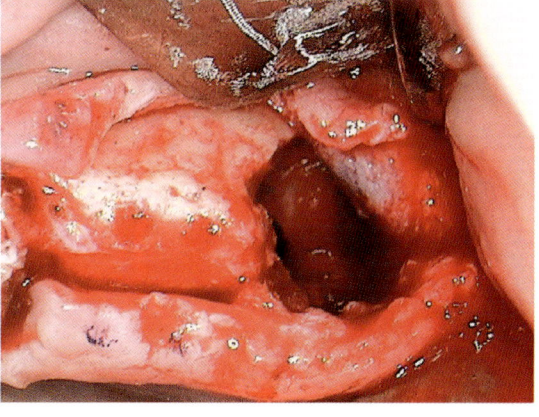

Osteotomy 28

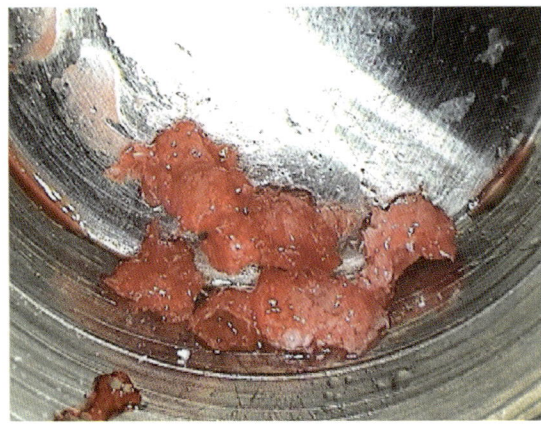

Autologous bone in regio 28

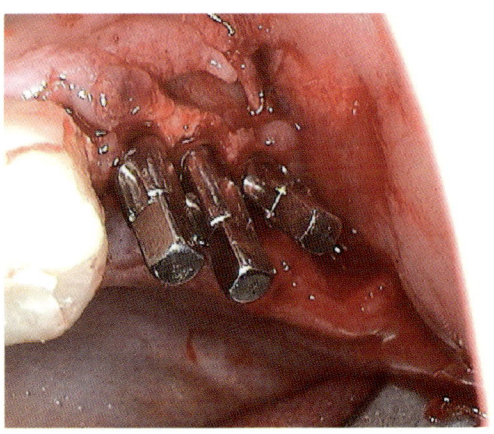

Completed insertion in the left upper jaw

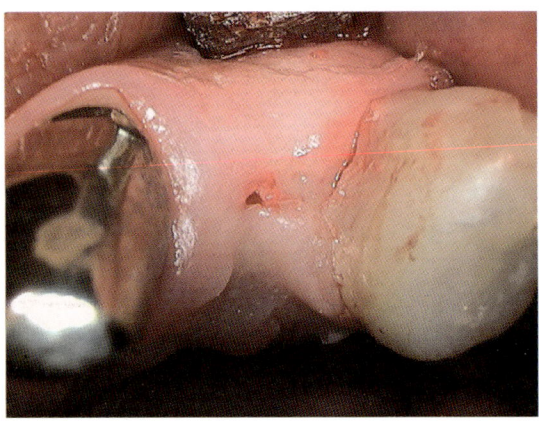

Drilled hole in regio 24

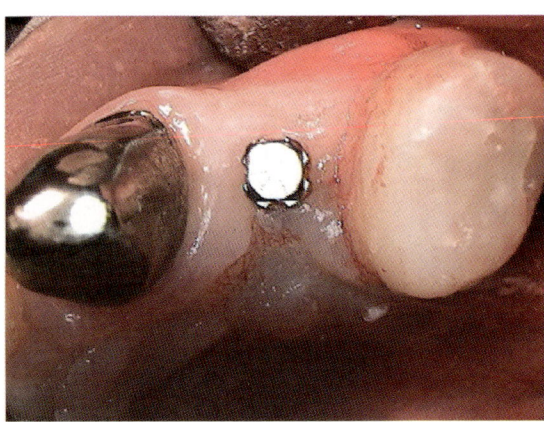

Implant placement in regio 24

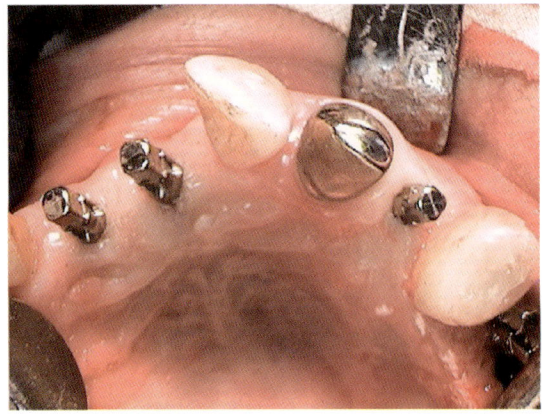

Completed implant placement in the anterior region

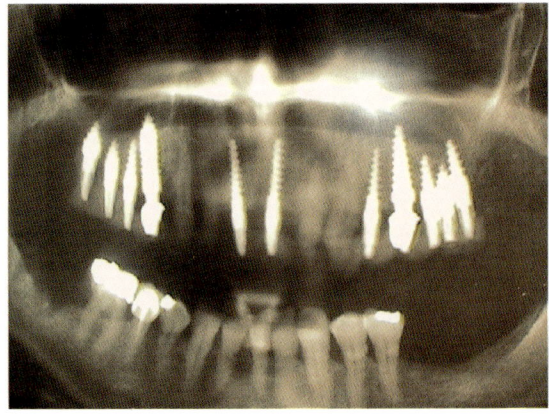

Panoramic radiographic control

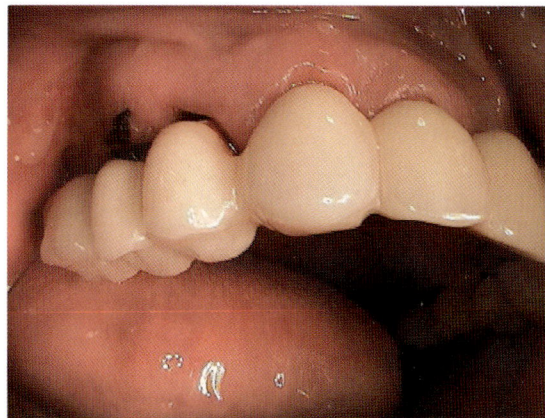

1st postoperative day, laboratory made temporary, upper jaw, right side

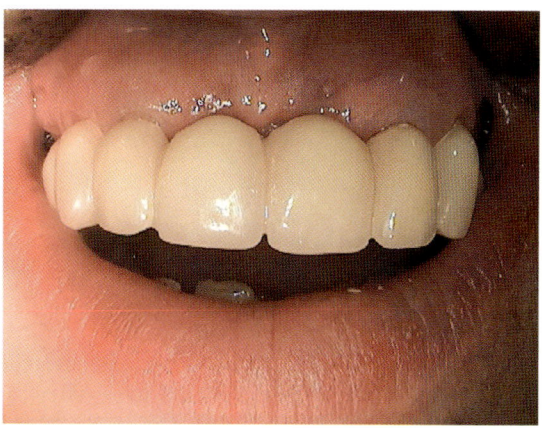

1st postoperative day, laboratory made temporary, upper jaw, anterior region

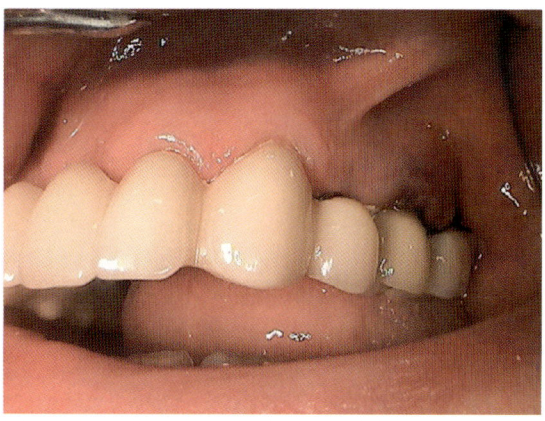

1st postoperative day, laboratory made temporary, upper jaw, left side

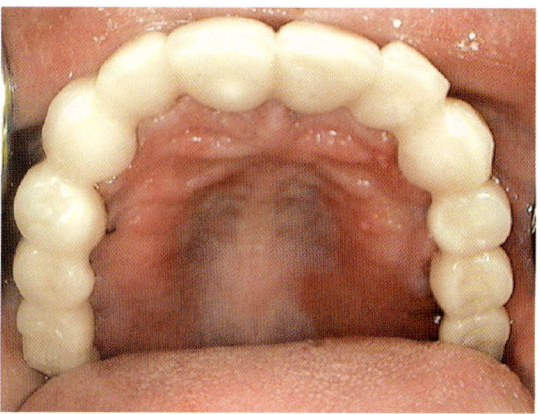

1st postoperative day, laboratory made temporary, occlusal view

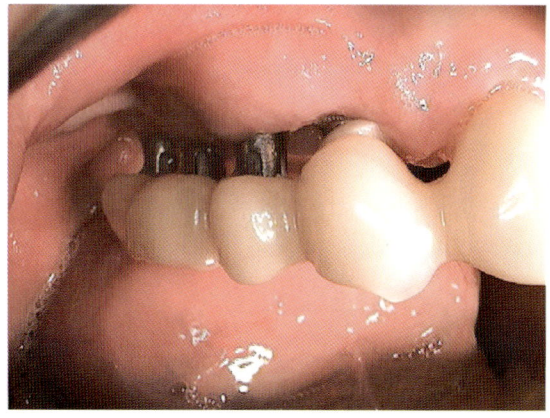

Laboratory made temporary after 9 weeks, right side

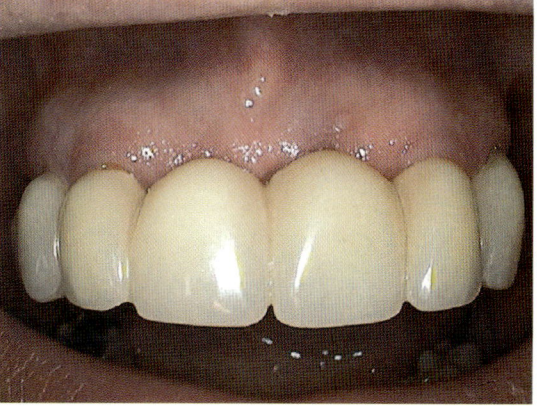

Laboratory made temporary after 9 weeks, anterior region

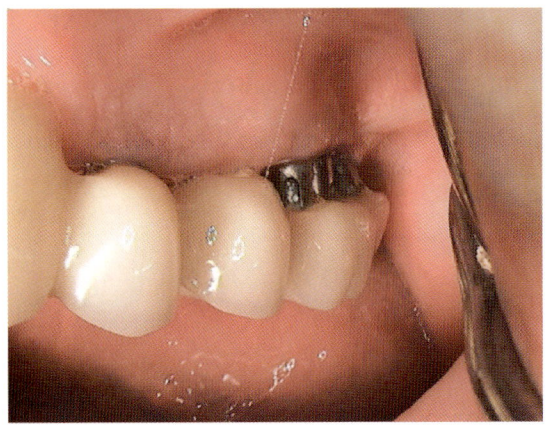

Laboratory made temporary after 9 weeks, left side

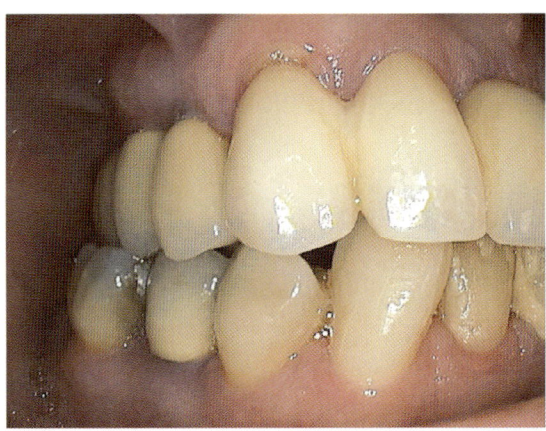

Cemented crown, right side, lateral view

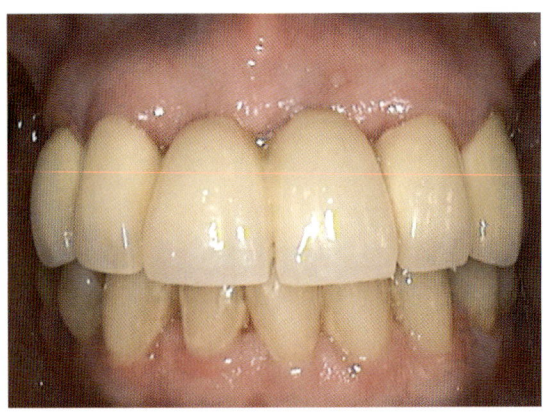

Cemented bridge, anterior view

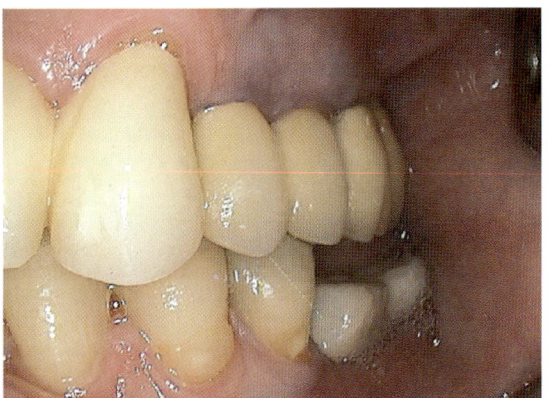

Cemented bridge, left side, lateral view

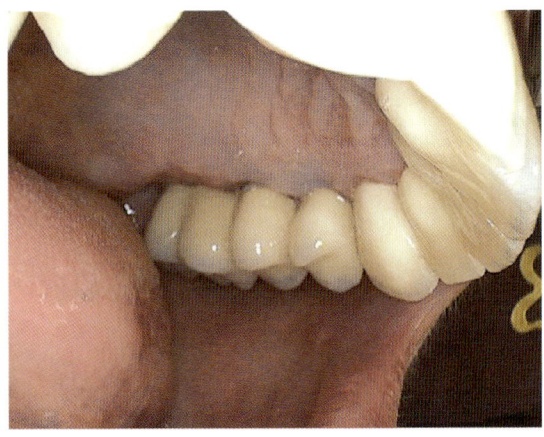

Cemented bridge, left side, palatal view

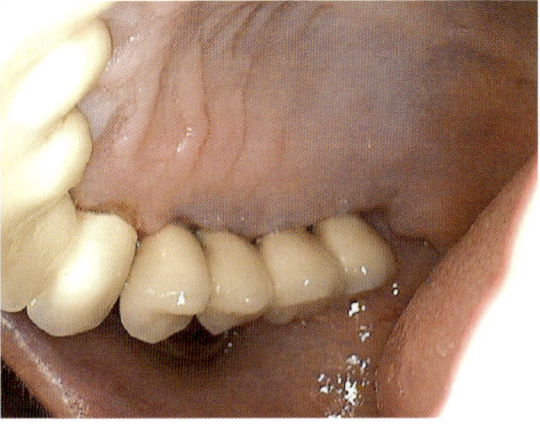

Cemented bridge, right side, palatal view

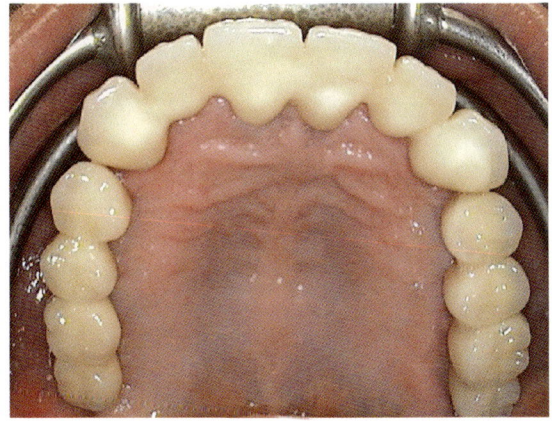

Cemented bridge, occlusal view

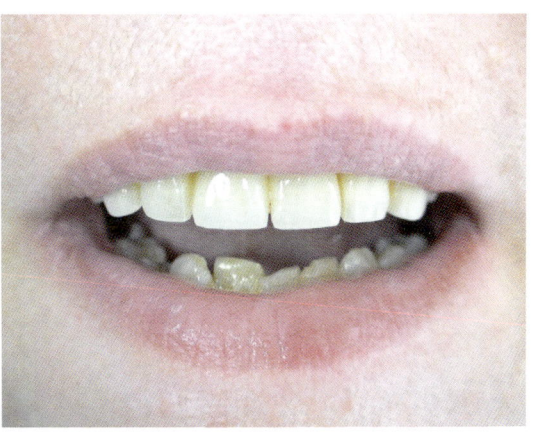

Cemented bridge, labial view

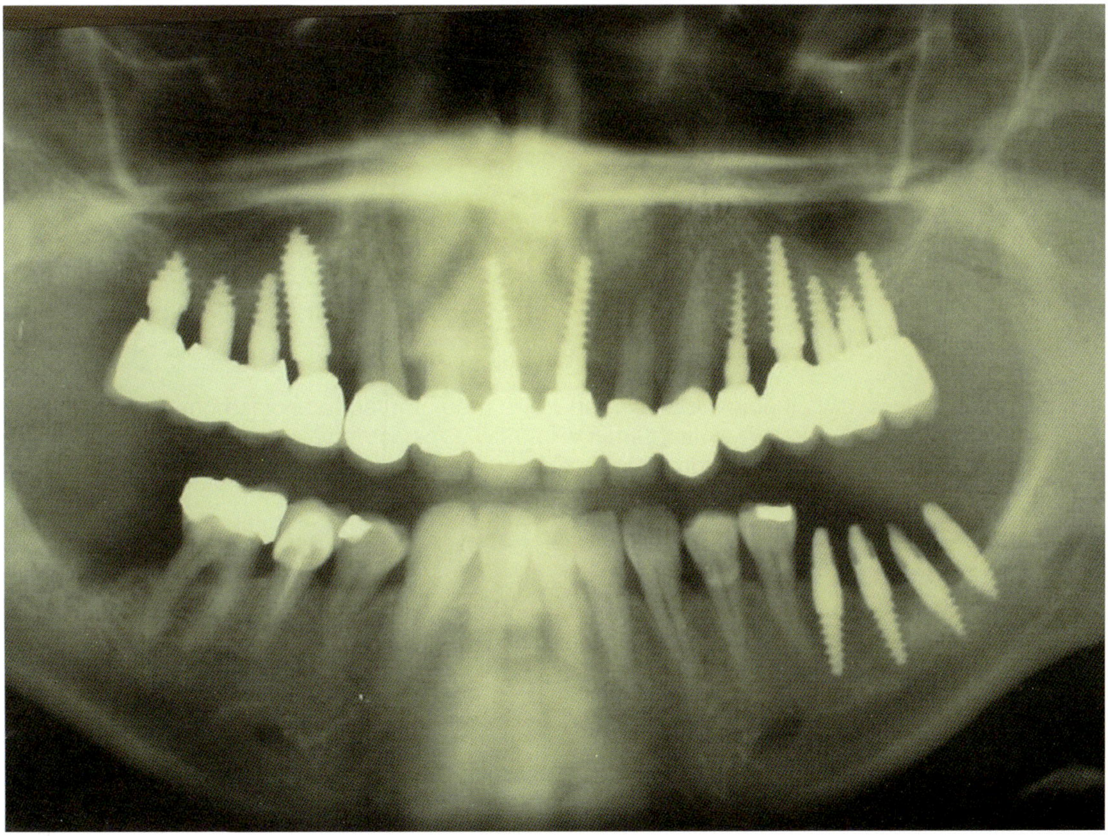

X-ray final control, panoramic radiograph

7.4.3/Case 35

Patient: male, 55 years old

11 implants in the upper jaw, augmentation, 18-28   3 zirconium dioxide splinted crowns

---

06/04/2010	13-24	removed bridge
	22	extraction
	24	abutment definitely screwed (external implant)
	13-24	dentist made temporary
13/04/2010	15	extraction
01/06/2010	11	Champions® implant Ø 3.5 x 12 mm, > 40 Ncm
	21	Champions® implant Ø 3.5 x 14 mm, > 40 Ncm
	22	Champions® implant Ø 3.5 x 16 mm, > 40 Ncm
		cemented zirconium Prep-Cap
		non-reactive beta-tricalcium phosphate, absorbable membrane, suture
	18	Champions® implant Ø 3.5 x 8 mm, 15 Ncm
	17	Champions® implant Ø 3.5 x 8 mm, 15 Ncm
	16	Champions® implant Ø 3.5 x 8 mm, 30 Ncm
	15	Champions® implant Ø 4.5 x 12 mm, 40 Ncm cemented Prep-Cap
	25	Champions® implant Ø 4.5 x 8 mm, 30 Ncm cemented Prep-Cap
	26	Champions® implant Ø 3.5 x 8 mm, 30 Ncm
	27	Champions® implant Ø 3.5 x 8 mm, 20 Ncm
	28	Champions® implant Ø 3.5 x 8 mm, 15 Ncm preparation
		impression for laboratory made temporary
		cemented dentist made temporary
03/06/2010		Cemented laboratory made temporary
03/08/2010		Impression
17/08/2010		Framework try-in, bite registration
24/08/2010	18-13, 12-23 24-28	cemented zirconium dioxide splinted crown
June 2011		Radiographic control

Treatment period: 2.8 months

Remarks:

Integration of an external implant
2 x indirect sinus lift
Augmentation
Avoiding a direct sinus lift
"Highest beer money" that has been ever paid:
a dinner for the entire team

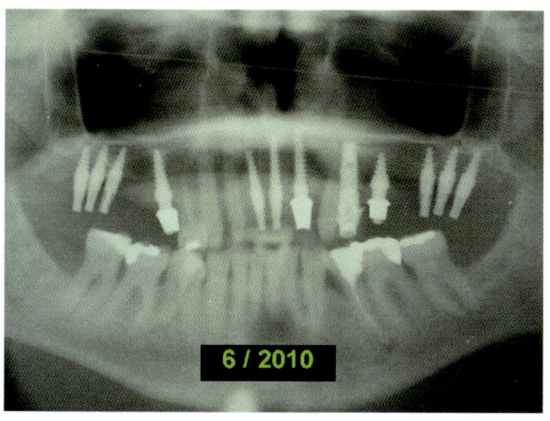

Panoramic radiographic control after implant
placement

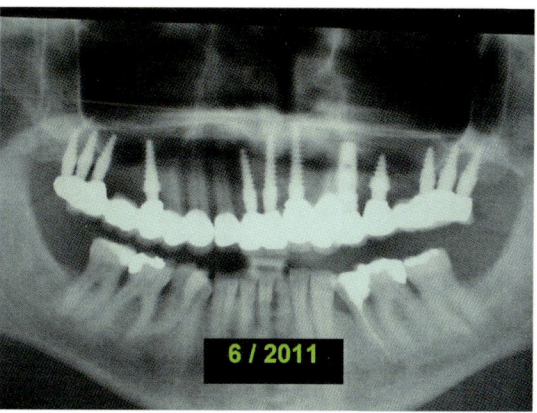

Panoramic radiographic control, 1 year after
implant placement

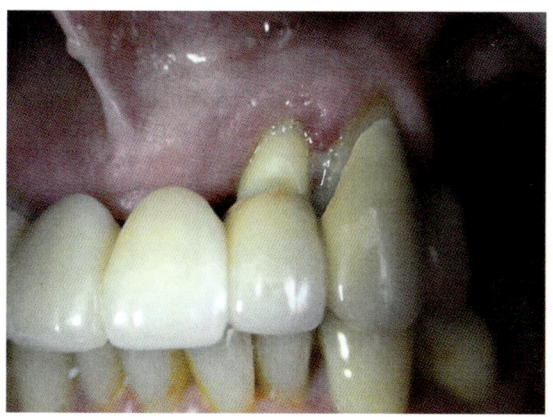

Clinical initial situation

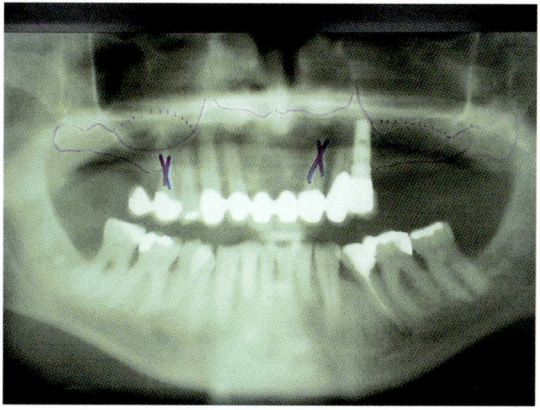

Radiographic illustration of the initial situation

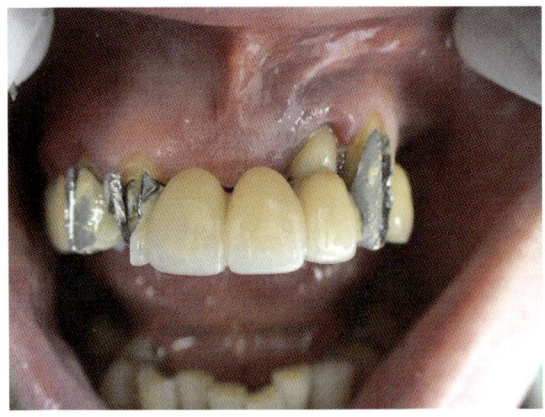

Removal of the existing bridge

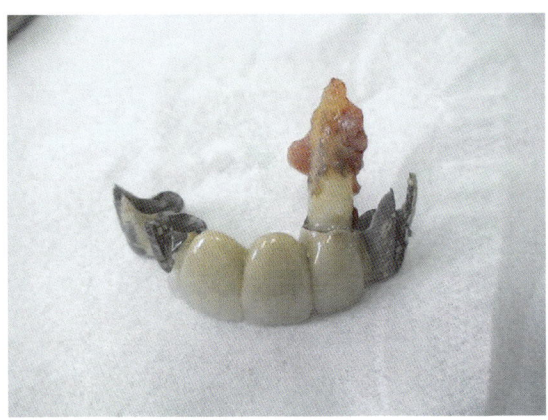

Removed bridge

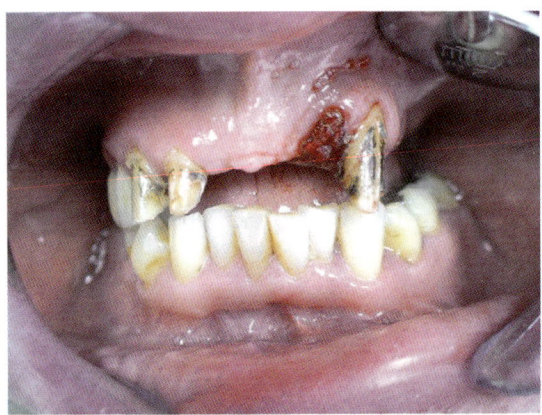

Extraction of tooth 22

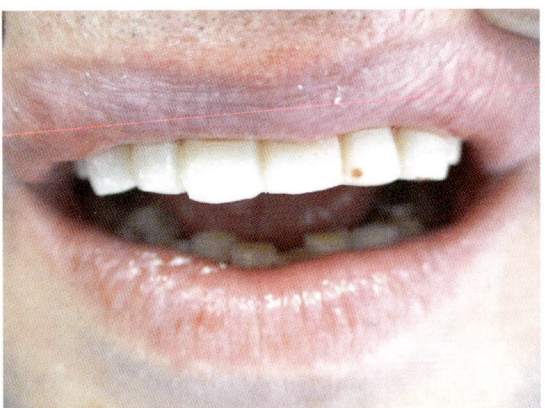

Dentist made temporary 13-24

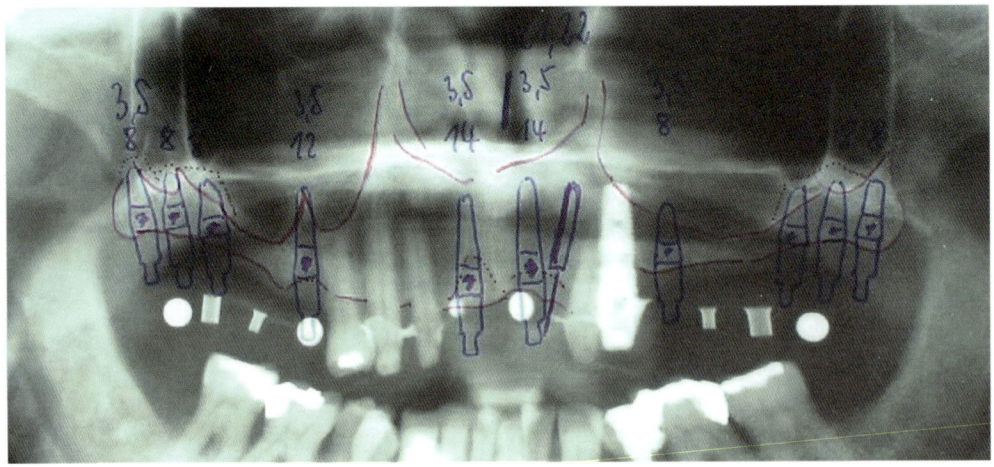

Planned implant treatment, panoramic radiograph

188

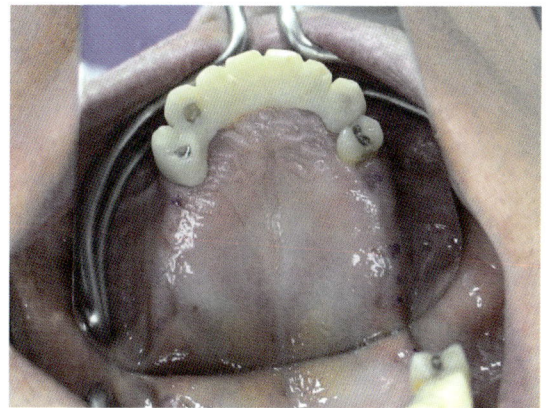

Clinical situation before implant placement

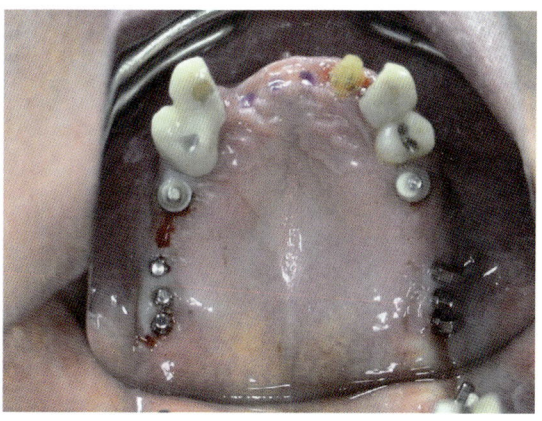

Implant placements in the tuber region, right side, left side

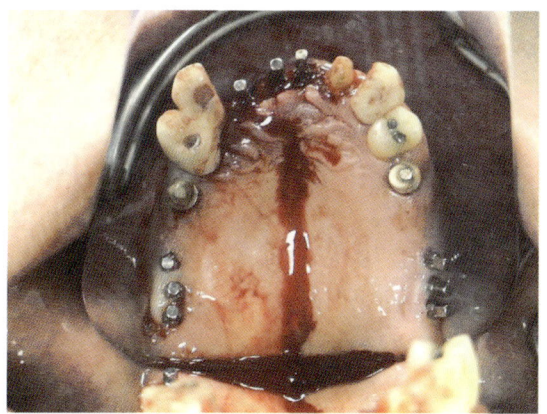

Implant placement in the anterior region

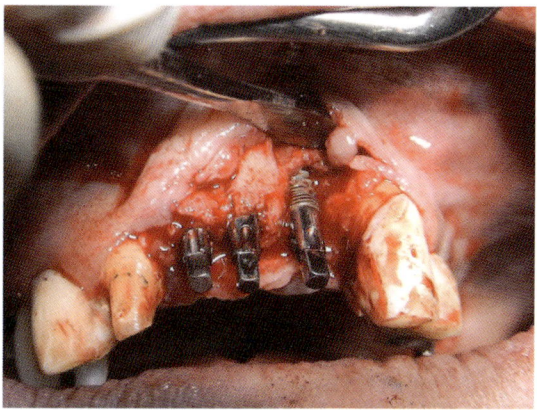

Situation before implant placement...

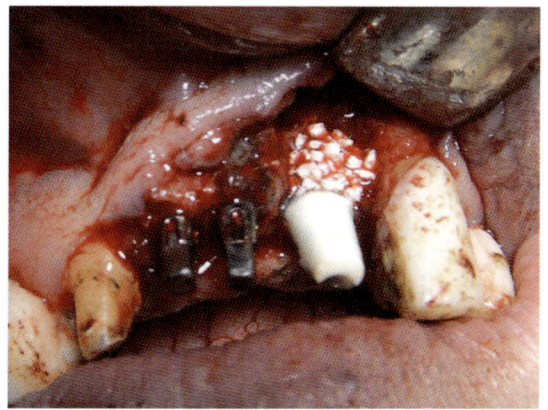

...with non-reactive beta-tricalcium phosphate

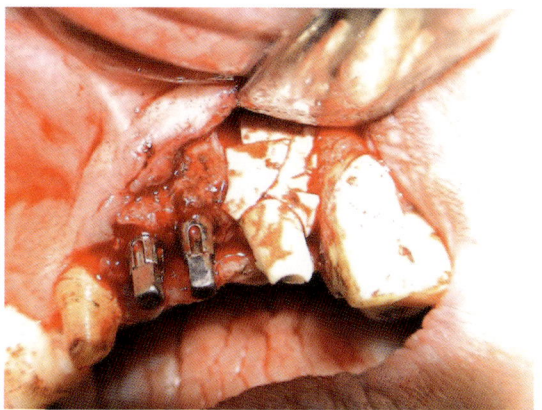

...and of an absorbable membrane

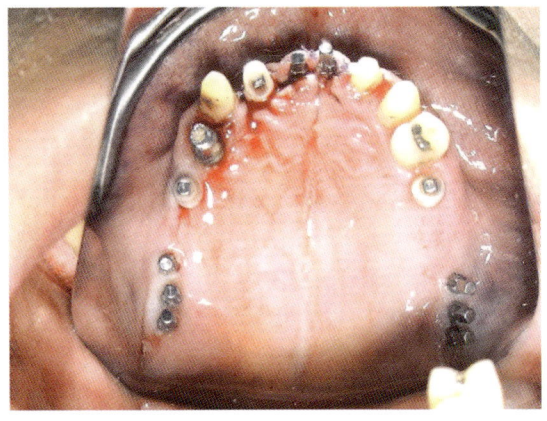

Progressed implant placement, occlusal view

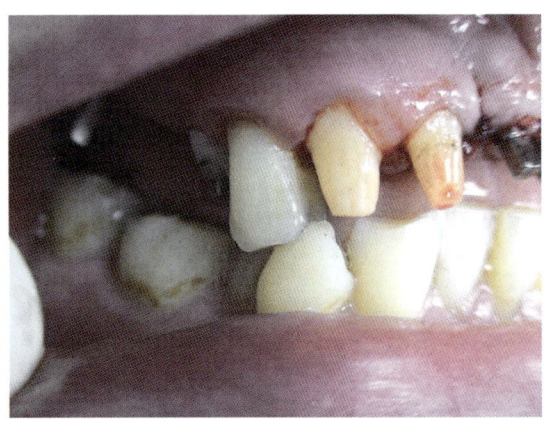

All abutments are prepared, apart from 14...

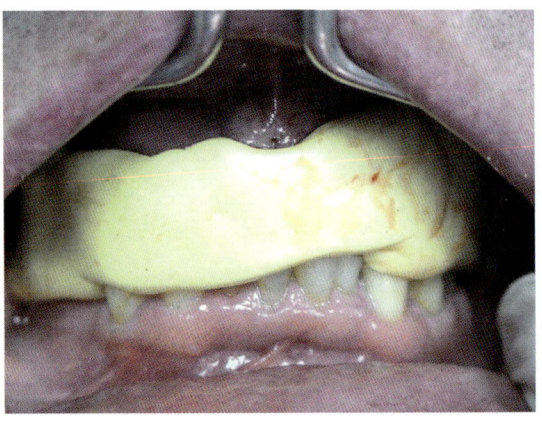

...in order to realise a proper bite registration

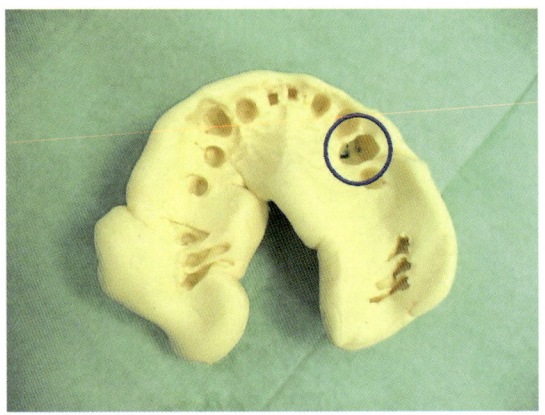

Bite registration with non-prepared tooth 14

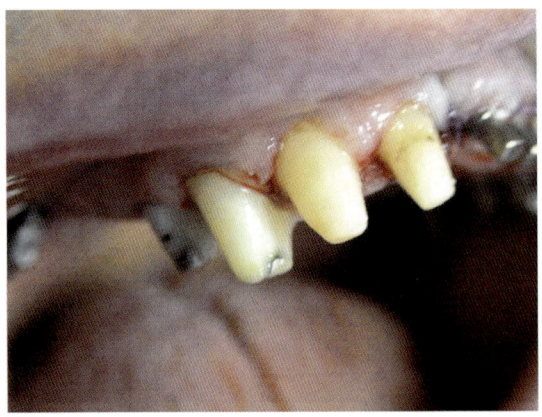

Preparation of tooth 14, lateral view

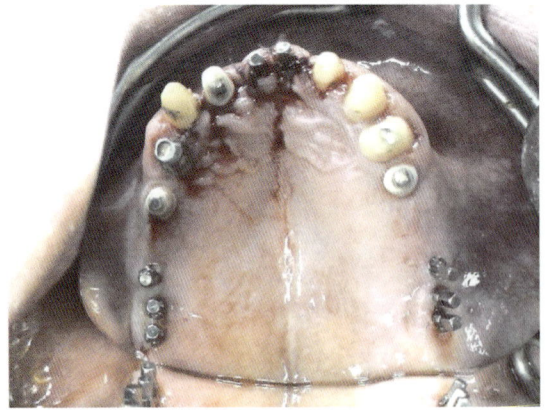

Preparation of all abutments, occlusal view

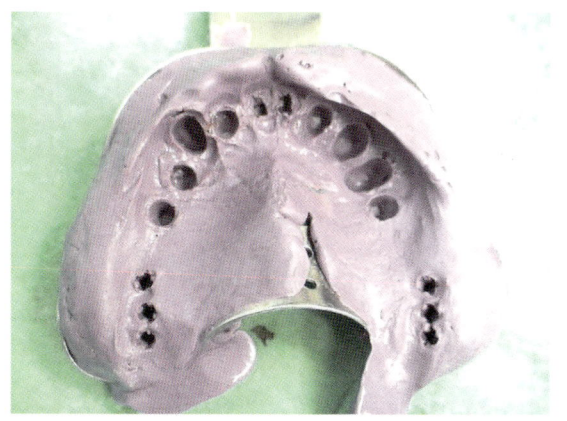

Impression for the laboratory made temporary

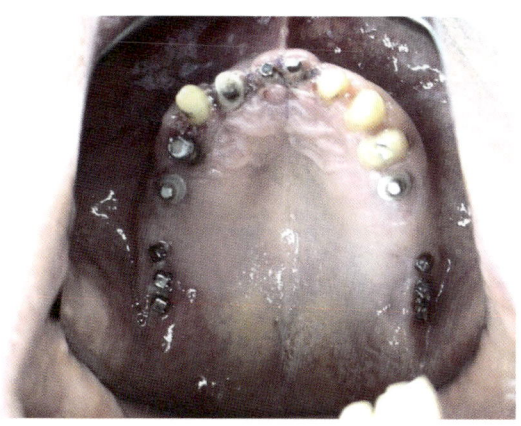

1st postoperative day

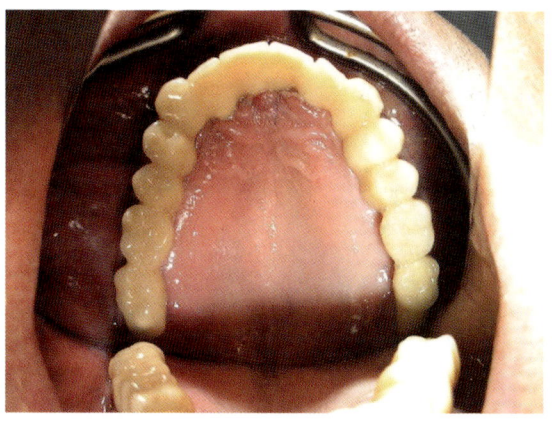

Cemented laboratory made temporary,
1st postoperative day, occlusal view

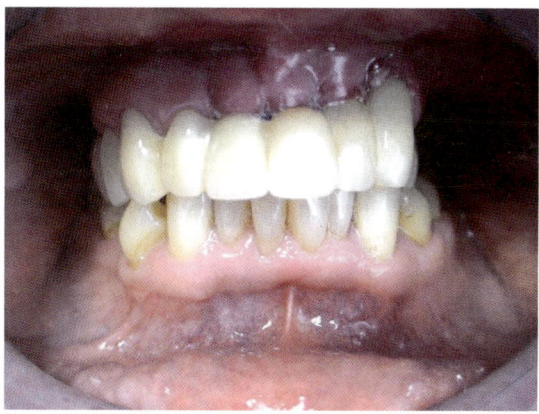

Cemented laboratory made temporary,
1st postoperative day, anterior view

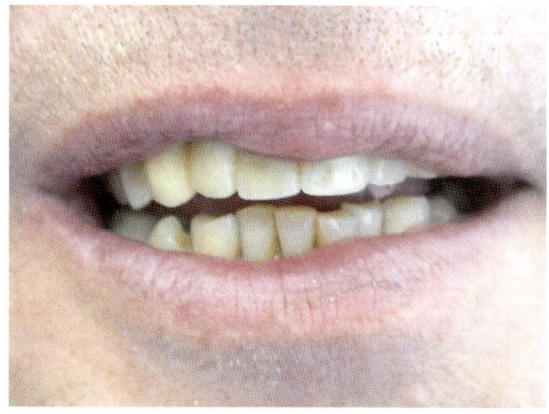

Cemented laboratory made temporary,
1st postoperative day, view of the lip region

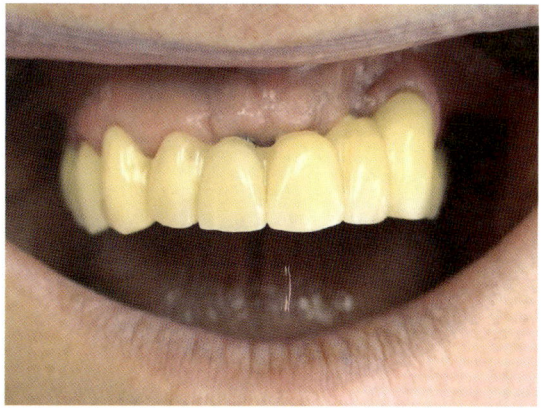

After osseointegration, before impression taking

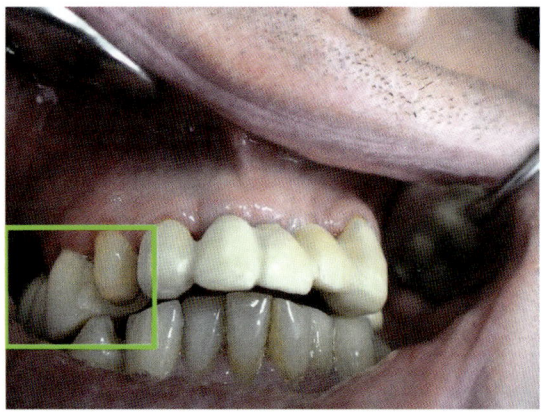

Framework try-in, parts of the laboratory made temporary protect the bite position

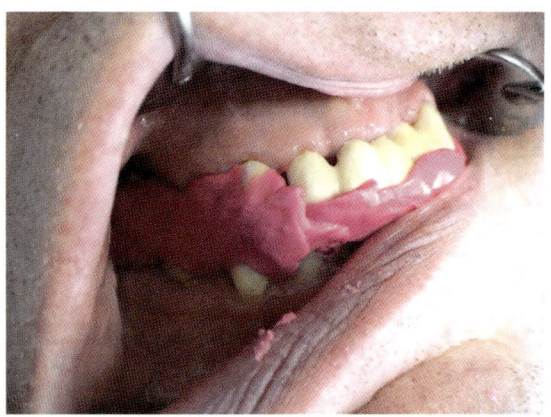

Registration of the habitual occlusion

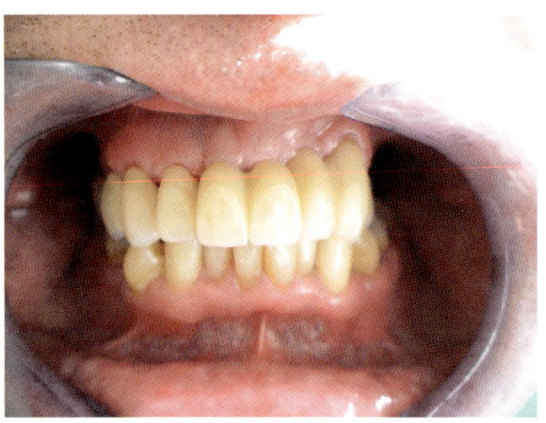

Cemented bridge, anterior view

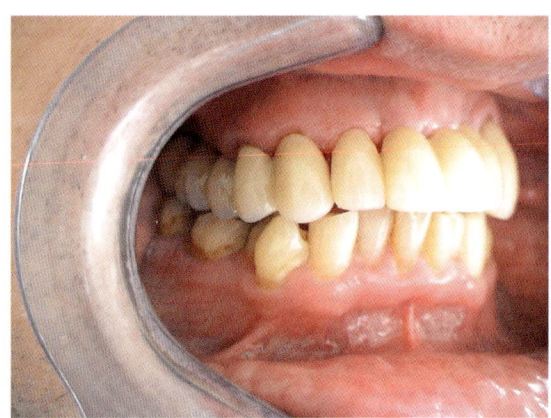

Cemented bridge, lateral view

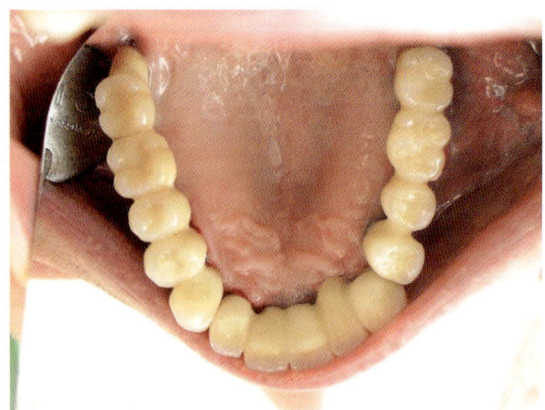

General occlusal view

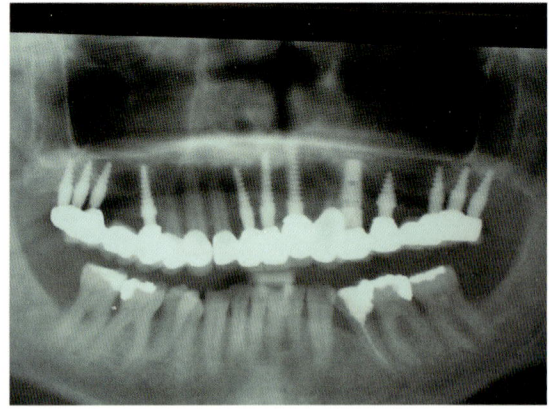

Radiograph final control

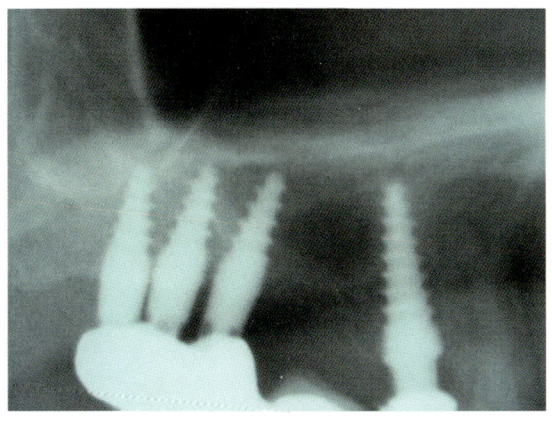

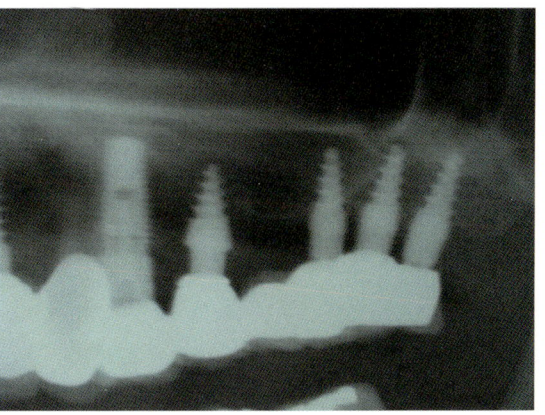

X-ray final control, macro image, right side...   X-ray final control, macro image, left side...

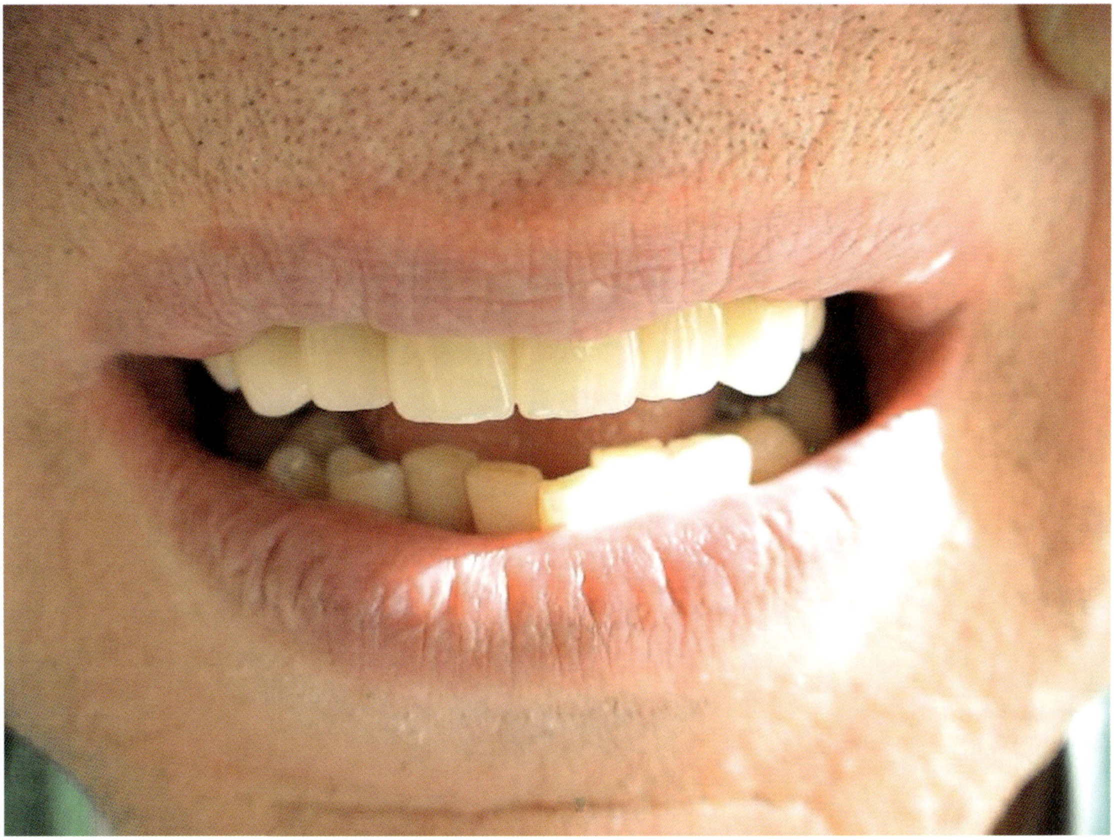

...a smile!

7.4.4/Case 36

Patient: male, 56 years old

12 lower jaw implants
36 additional implant placement,
bridge

02/07/2009	32	Champions® implant Ø 3.5 x 14 mm, 40 Ncm
	33	Champions® implant Ø 3.5 x 14 mm, 40 Ncm
	34	Champions® implant Ø 3.5 x 10 mm, 35 Ncm
	35	Champions® implant Ø 3.5 x 12 mm, 35 Ncm
	36	Champions® implant Ø 3.5 x 12 mm, 35 Ncm
	37	Champions® implant Ø 3.5 x 10 mm, 30 Ncm
	42	Champions® implant Ø 3.5 x 14 mm, 30 Ncm
	43	Champions® implant Ø 3.5 x 14 mm, 30 Ncm
	44	Champions® implant Ø 3.5 x 10 mm, 40 Ncm
	45	Champions® implant Ø 3.5 x 12 mm, 35 Ncm
	46	Champions® implant Ø 3.5 x 12 mm, 35 Ncm
	47	Champions® implant Ø 3.5 x 12 mm, 35 Ncm
		Impression taking with Impregnum and prepared ground overdenture
		The dentist made temporary has been manufactured by means of of a deep drawn splint and has then been cemented.
17/07/2009		Cemented laboratory made temporary
14/09/2009	36	explantation
26/10/2009	36	additional implant placement impression
13/11/2009	37-47	inserted non-precious metal ceramic bridge
22/08/2011		Panoramic radiographic control, images
Treatment period:		**3.2 months**
Remarks:		Today,we do not longer manufacture non-precious metal ceramic bridges: The gingiva only "loves" ceramic and titanium! 35, 36, 37 stump preparation by means of plastic caps More than 2 years after implant placement no bone loss!

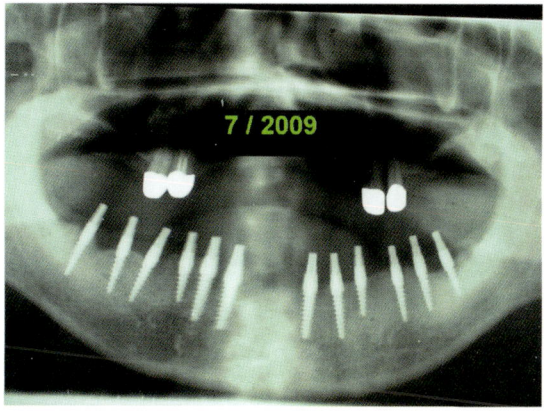

Panoramic radiograph after implant placement

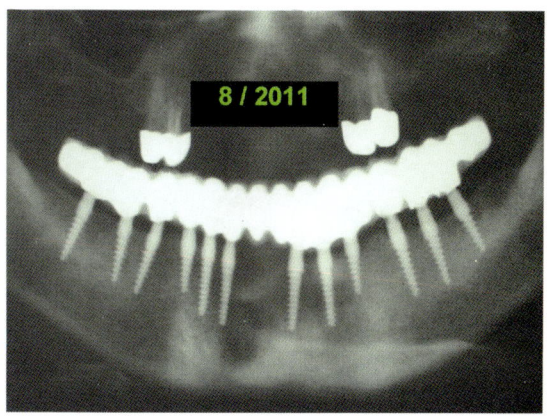

Panoramic radiograph after more than 2 years

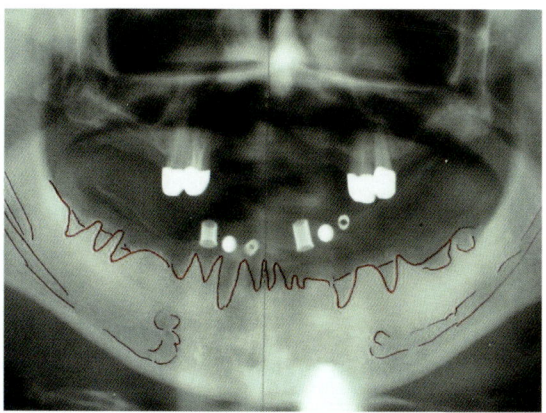

Radiological initial situation, panoramic radiograph

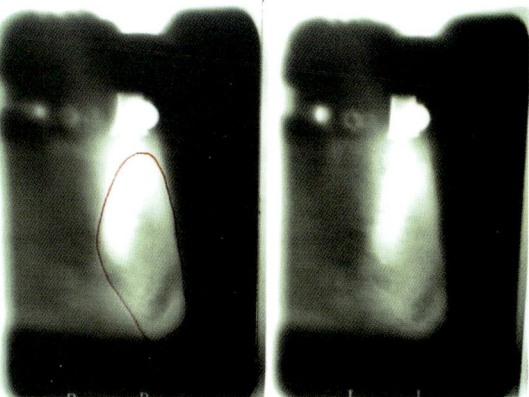

Cross-sectional images, left side

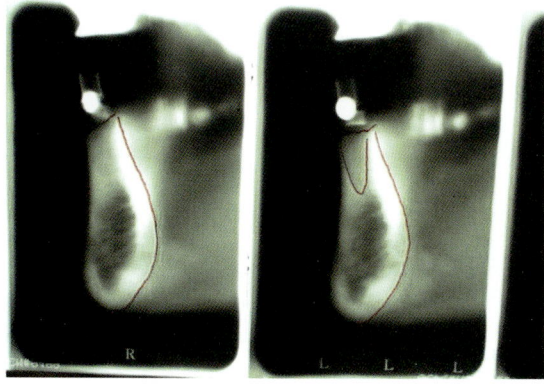

Cross-sectional images, right side

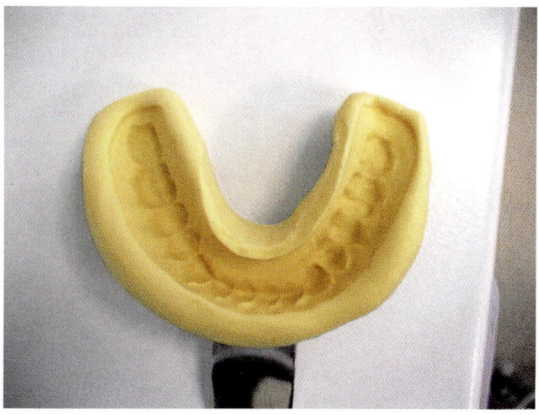

Impression of an overdenture...

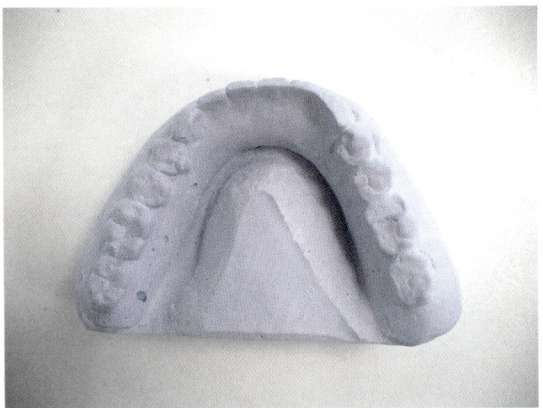

...to create the cast

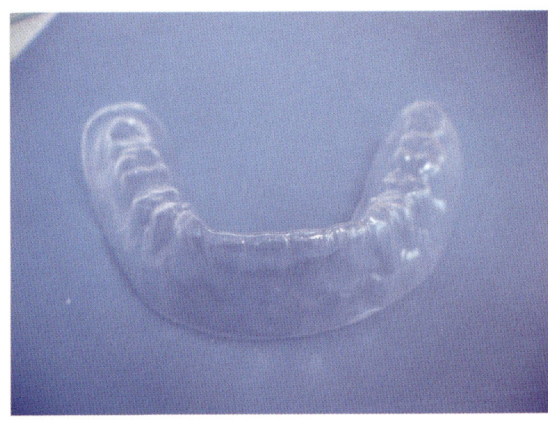

...and to create the splint for the dentist made temporary

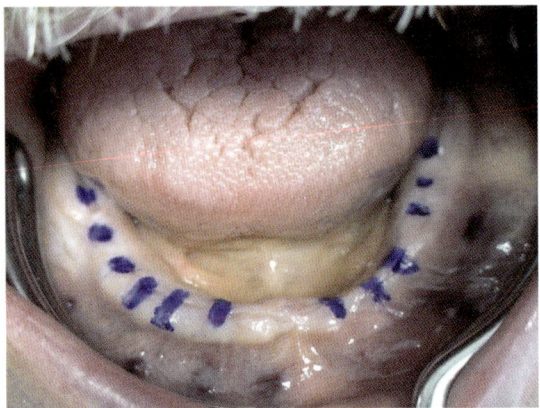

Marked points for planned initial holes

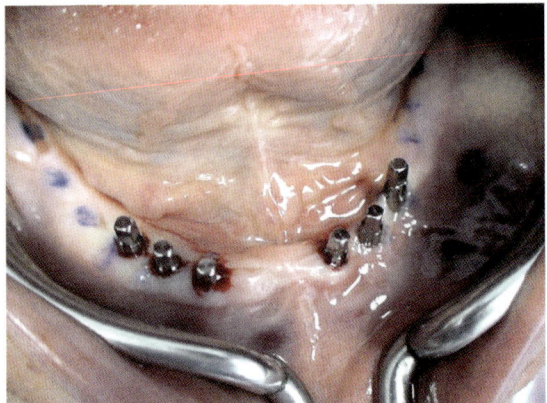

Implant placement in the anterior region

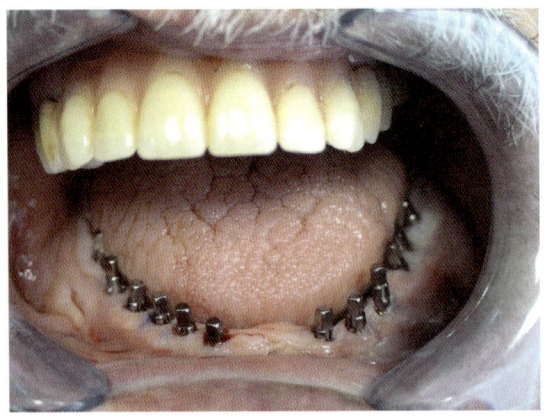

Completed implant placement

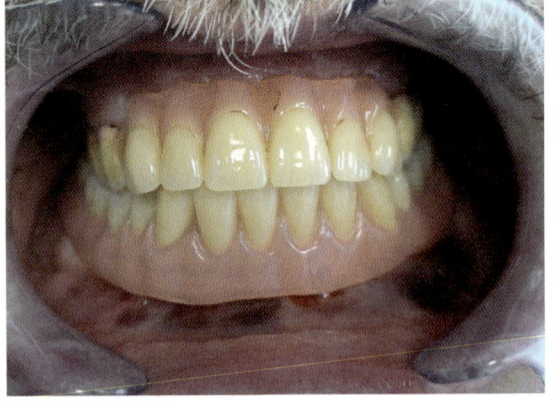

Try-in of the ground overdenture to take an impression for the laboratory made temporary

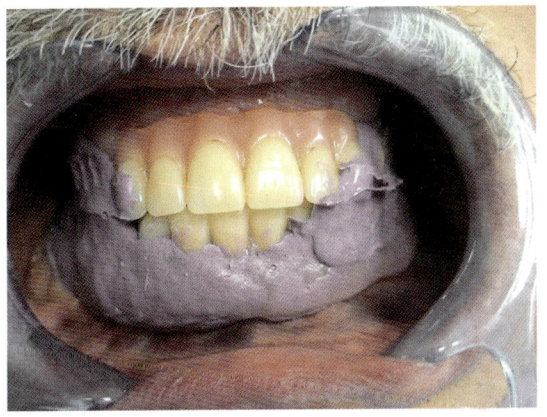

Impression taking for the laboratory made temporary...

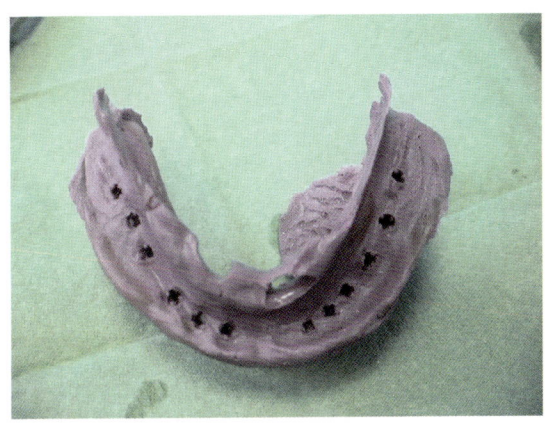

...basal view

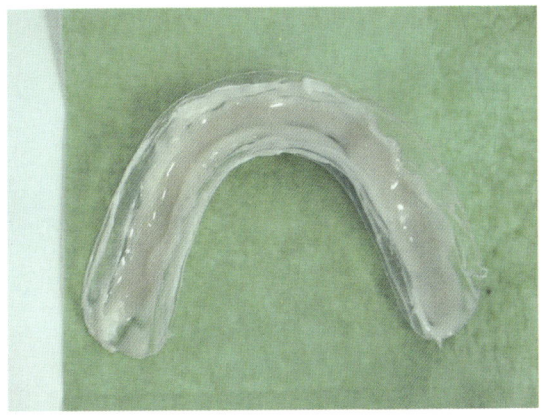

Splint for the dentist made temporary

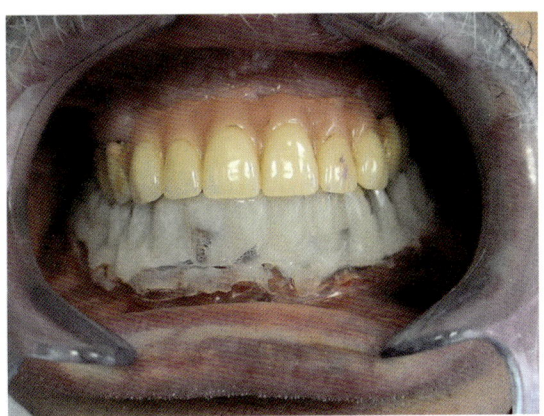

Splint in situ

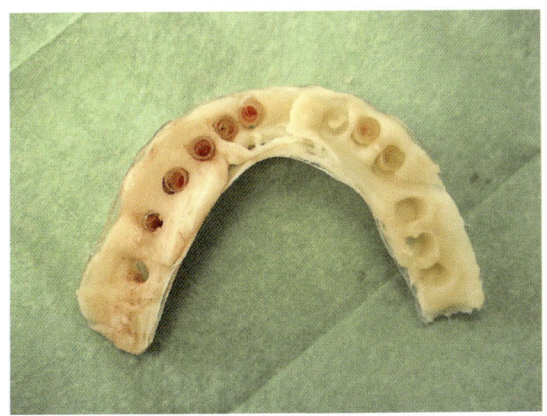

Non-ground dentist made temporary

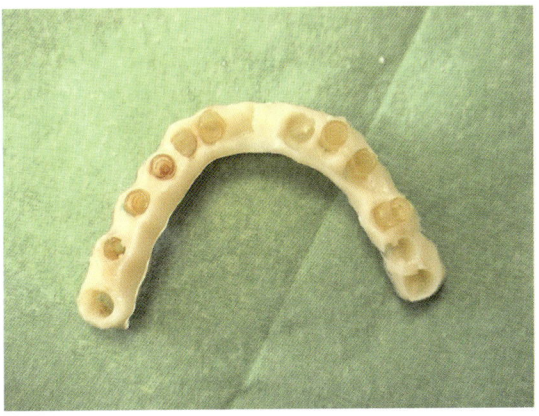

Ground dentist made temporary

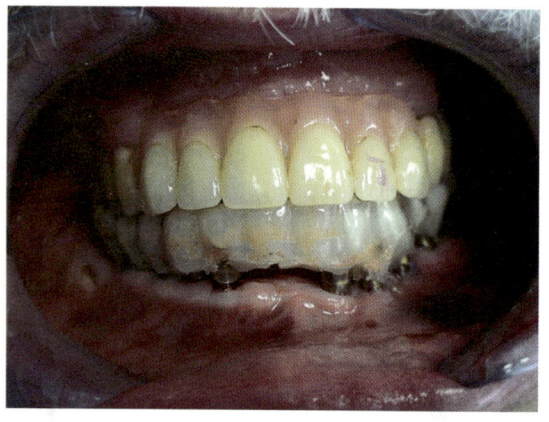

Cemented dentist made temporary

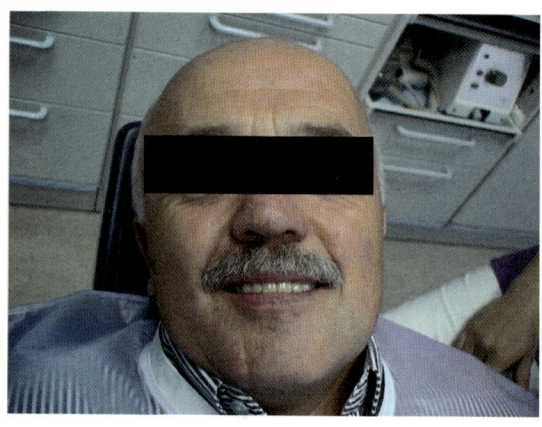

1st postoperative day, no swellings!

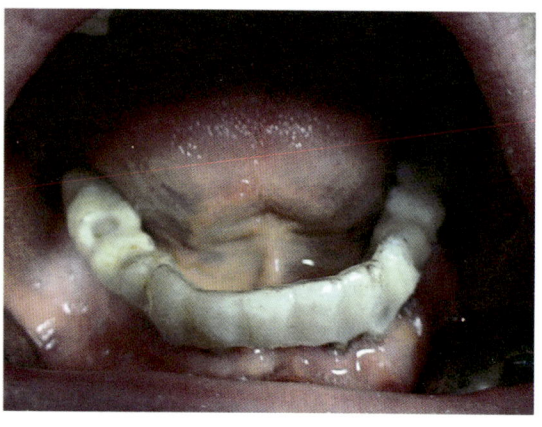

Before the insertion of the laboratory made temporary

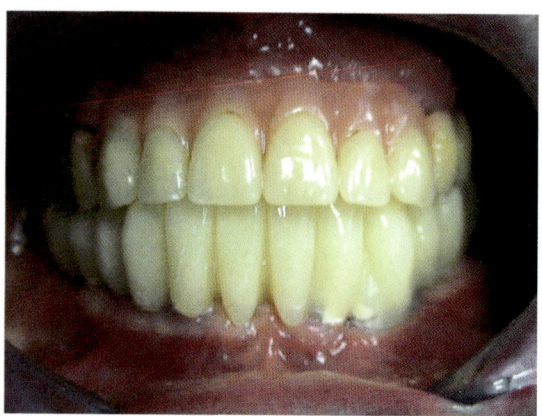

Cemented laboratory made temporary...

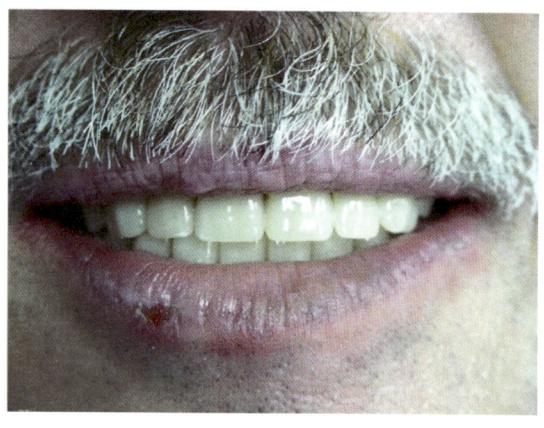

...with a smile

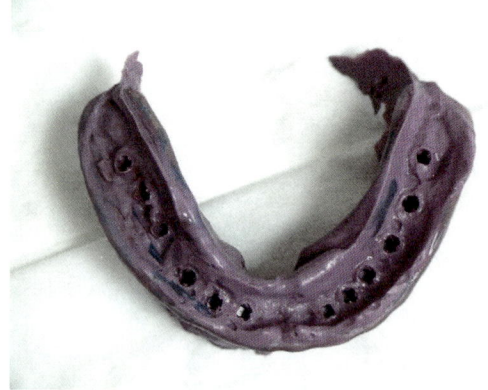

Additional implant placement 36 and impression

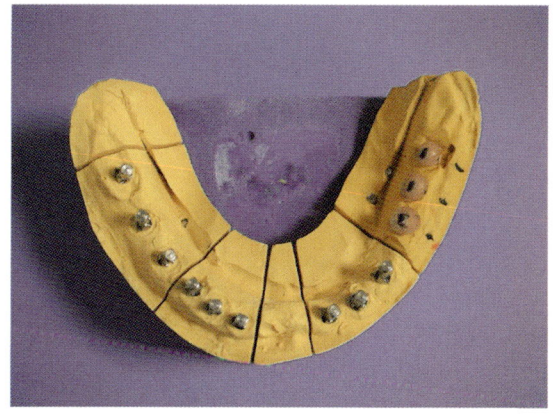

Cast

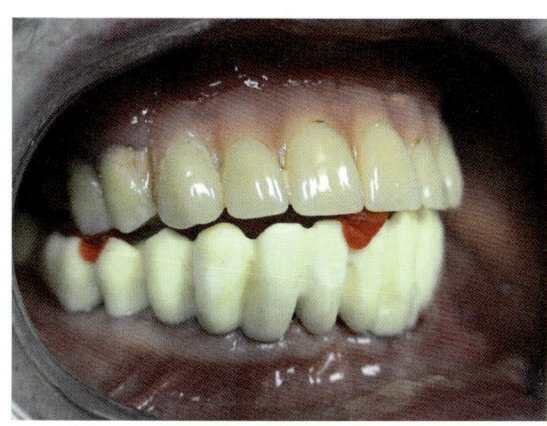

Try-in of the framework...

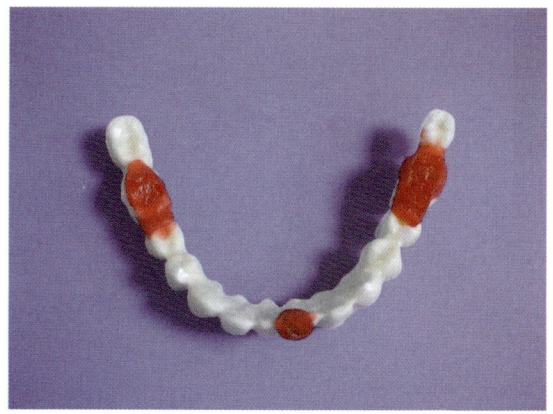

...bite registration

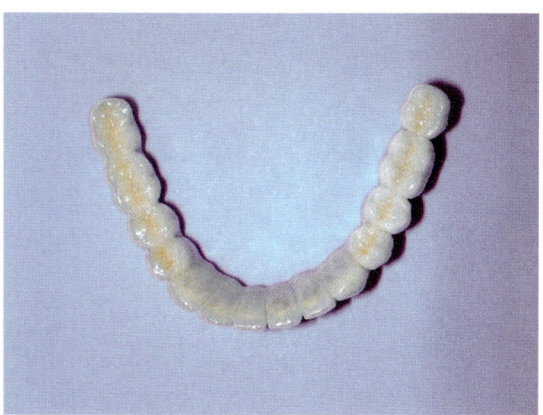

Circular bridge...

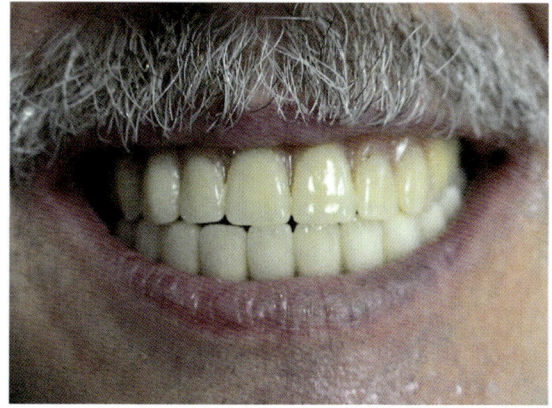

...in situ

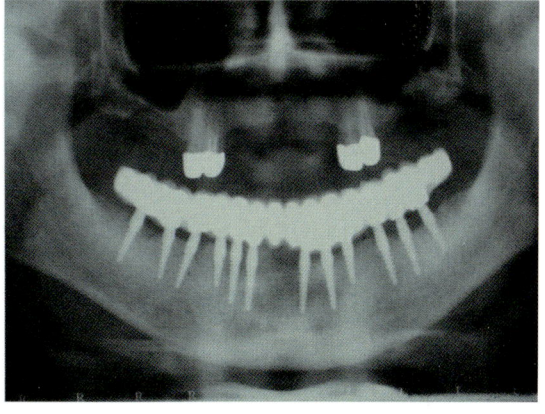

Panoramic radiographic control after more than 2 years

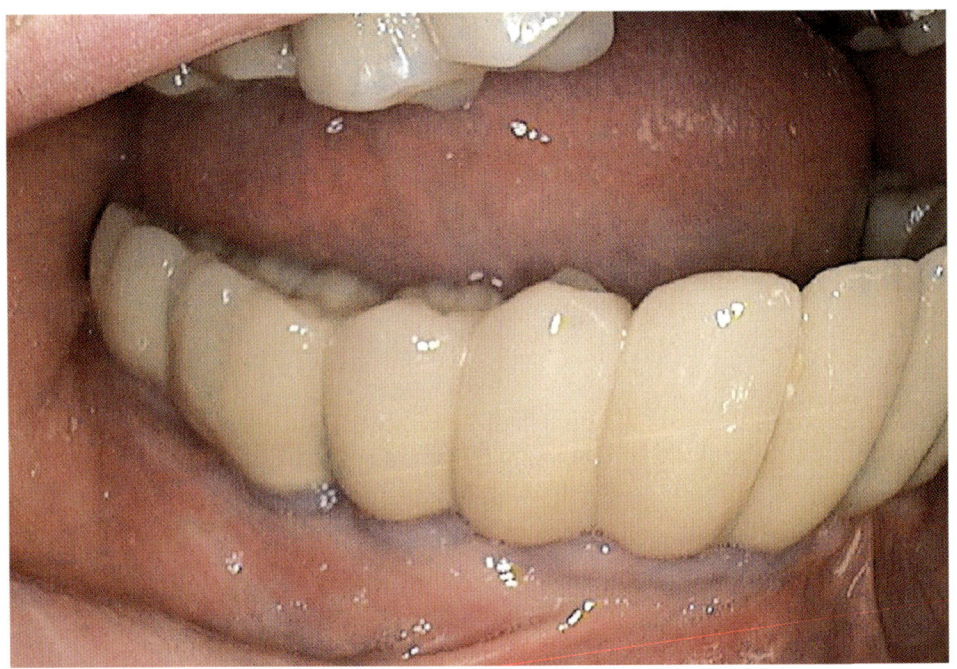

Lateral detailed view after more than 2 years

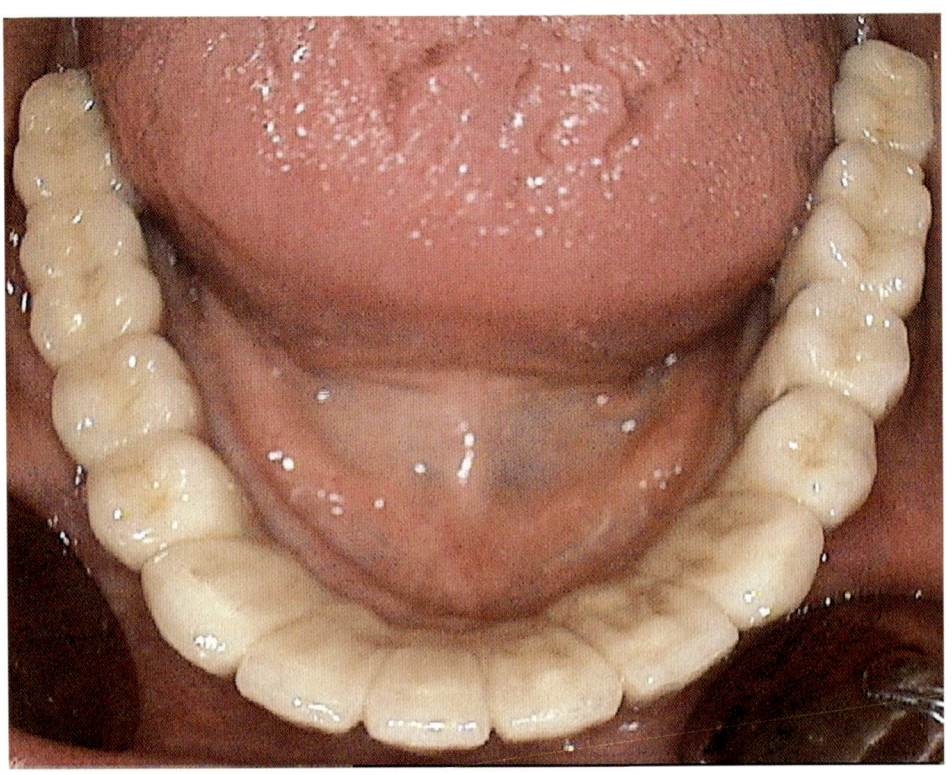

Occlusal view after more than 2 years

7.4.5/Case 37

Patient: male, 57 years old

8 x extraction, 15 lower jaw implants, 43 explantation
33-37/32-47 zirconium dioxide bridges

28/09/2010	37	extraction
02/11/2010	43-32,34	extraction
	44	osteotomy
	47	Champions® implant Ø 3.5 x 8 mm, 40 Ncm, cemented Prep-Cap
	46 d	Champions® implant Ø 3.5 x 10 mm, 60 Ncm
	46 m	Champions® implant Ø 3.5 x 10 mm, 60 Ncm
	45	Champions® implant Ø 3.5 x 10 mm, 40 Ncm, cemented Prep-Cap
	44	Champions® implant Ø 3.5 x 14 mm, 60 Ncm, cemented Prep-Cap
	43	Champions® implant Ø 3.5 x 18 mm, 40 Ncm
	42	Champions® implant Ø 3.0 x 14 mm, 40 Ncm
	31	Champions® implant Ø 3.0 x 14 mm, 30 Ncm
	32	Champions® implant Ø 3.0 x 12 mm, 30 Ncm
	34	Champions® implant Ø 3.5 x 16 mm, 60 Ncm, cemented Prep-Cap
	35	Champions® implant Ø 3.5 x 8 mm, 40 Ncm, cemented Prep-Cap
	36 m	Champions® implant Ø 3.5 x 10 mm, 60 Ncm
	36 d	Champions® implant Ø 3.5 x 10 mm, 60 Ncm
	37	Champions® implant Ø 3.5 x 10 mm, 60 Ncm, cemented Prep-Cap
		bite registration
		impression taking for laboratory made temporary
		cemented dentist made temporary
03/11/2010		Cemented laboratory made temporary
05/01/2011		Removed laboratory made temporary
	43	loosened implant → explantation
		impression
19/01/2011	33-37	cemented zirconium dioxide crown
	32-47	cemented zirconium dioxide crown
Treatment period:		**2.5 months**
Remarks:		43 no additional implant placement because enough osseointegrated implants were available.

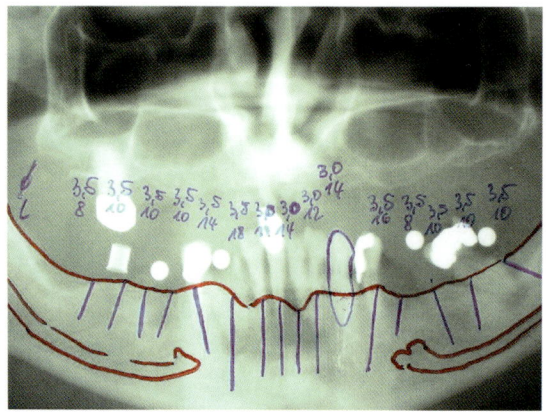

Panoramic radiograph for planned treatment

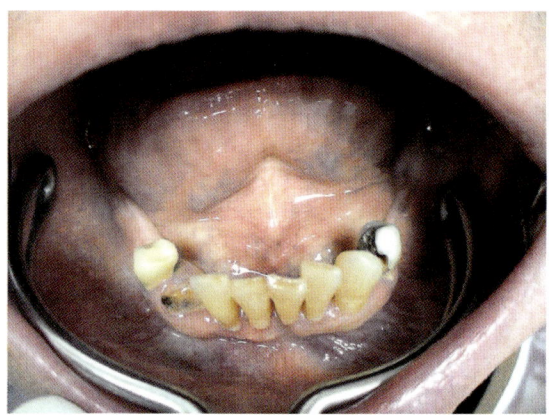

Clinical initial situation

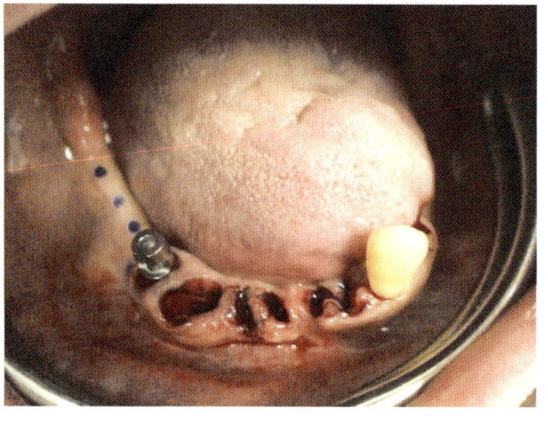

Alveoli after extraction,
for the bite registration tooth 33 has not been
removed

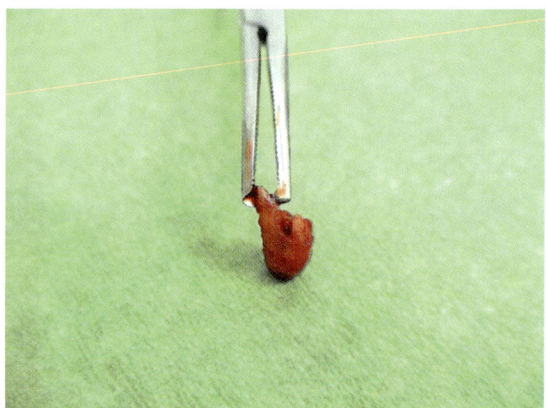

Residual root after osteotomy 44

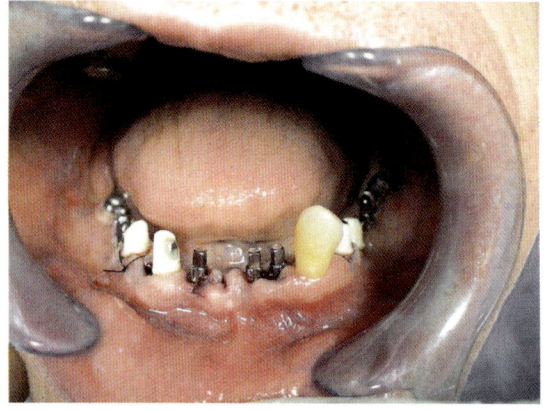

Completed implant placement, apart from tooth 33

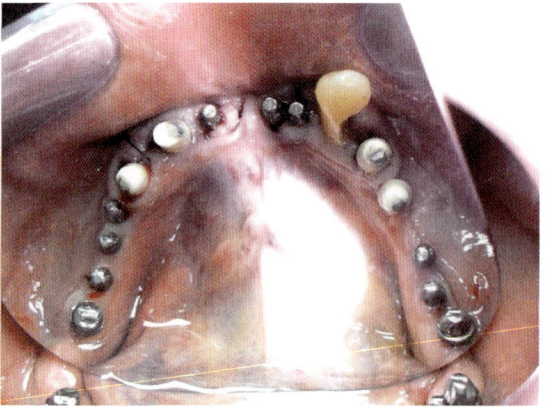

Occlusal view, mirror image

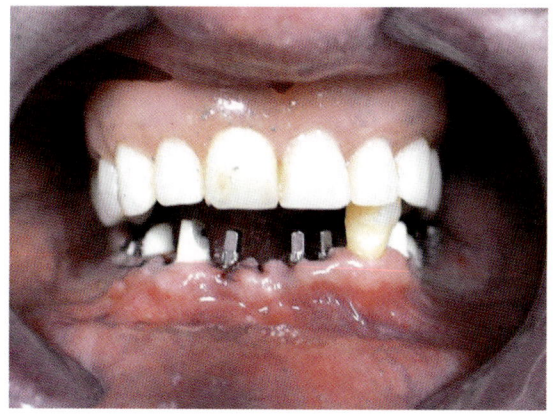

Verification of the habitual occlusion...

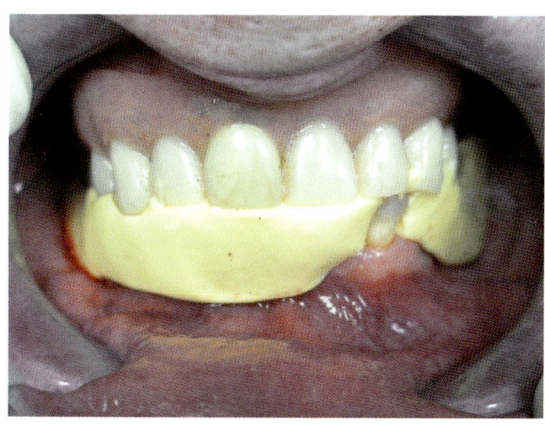

...and bite registration

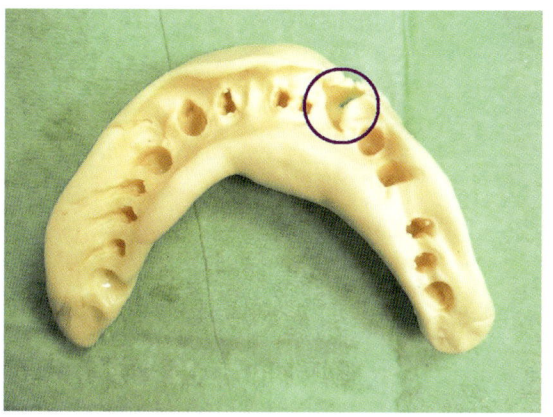

Bite registration, own tooth 33 is not prepared

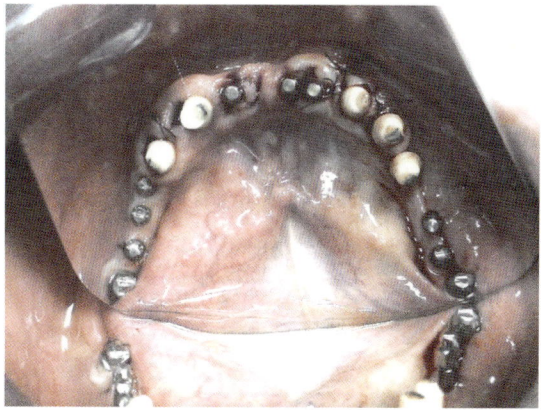

33 immediate implant placement, all implants are prepared

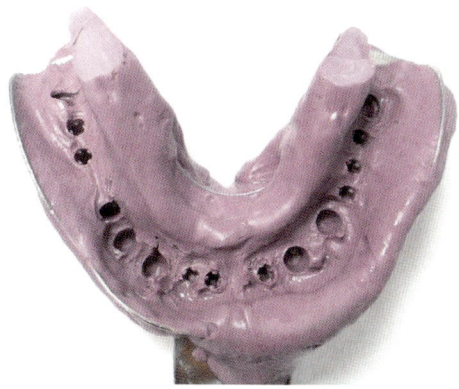

Impression for laboratory made temporary

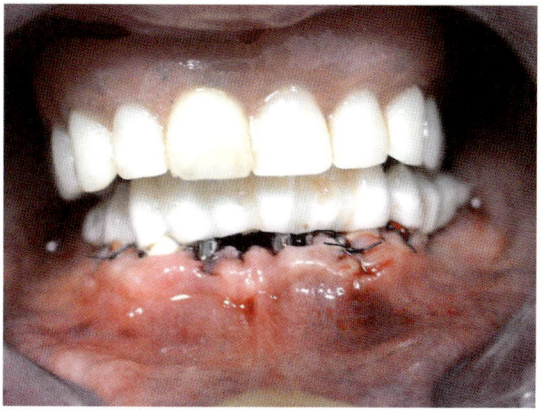

Dentist made temporary for the 1st day

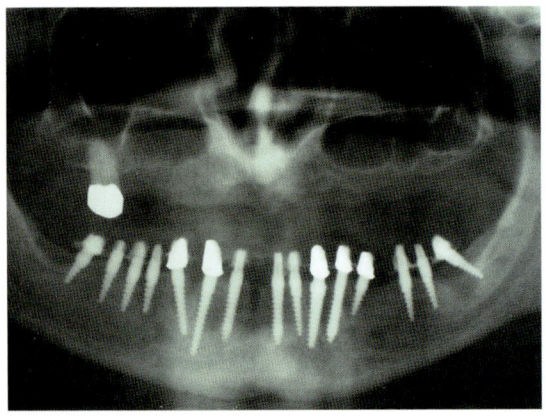

Radiographic control, panoramic radiograph

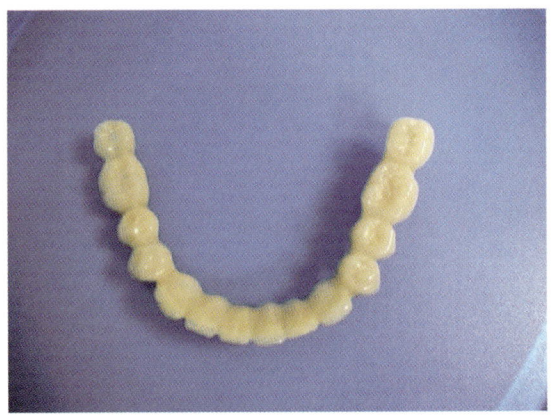

Laboratory made temporary...

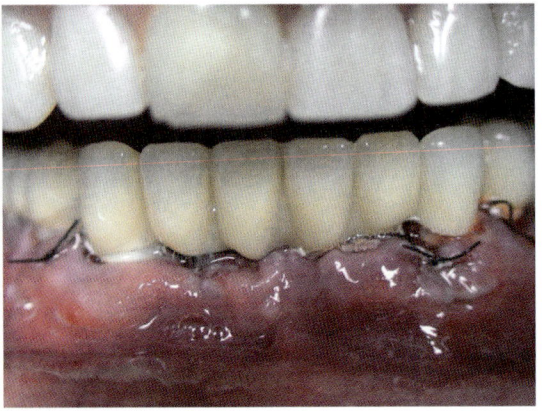

...cemented

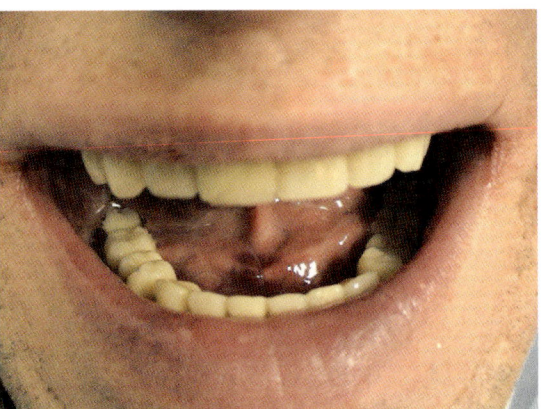

Laboratory made temporary, speaking view

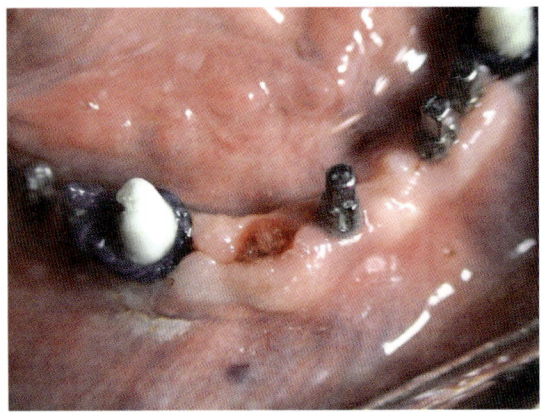

Explantation of tooth 43 without additional implant placement and new impression taking

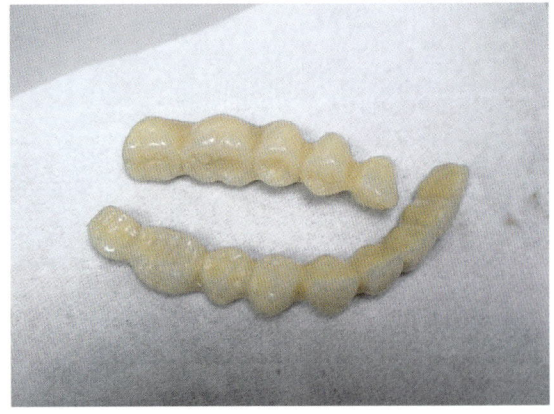

Final zirconium dioxide bridge

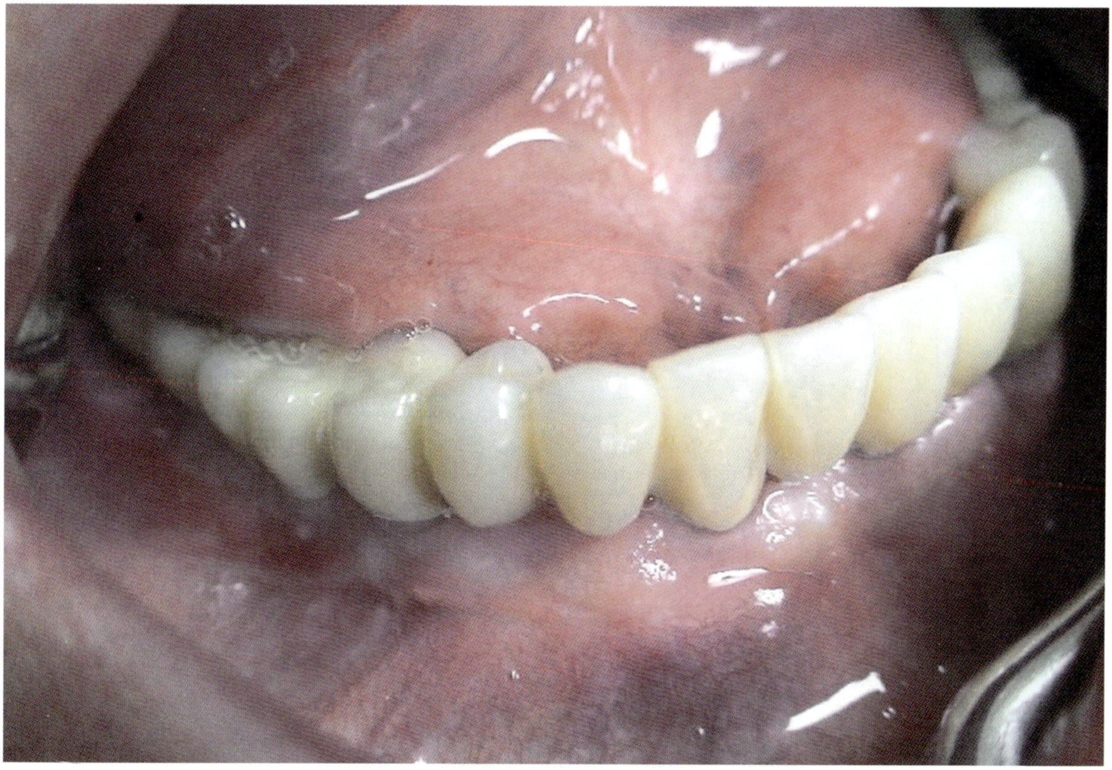

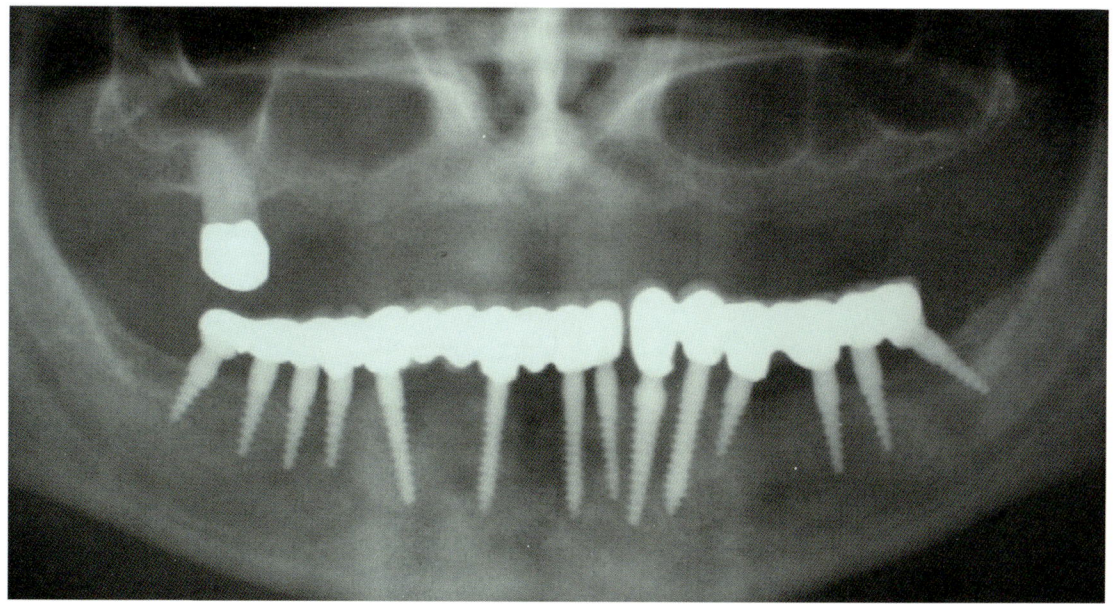

Final cemented bridges in situ

Final radiographic control, panoramic radiograph

7.4.6/Case 38

Patient: female, 55 years old

38-48 16 implants, 3 zirconium dioxide splinted crowns

15/06/2010	34,44	extraction
	48	Champions® implant Ø 3.5 x 10 mm, 25 Ncm
	47	Champions® implant Ø 3.5 x 12 mm, 30 Ncm
	46	Champions® implant Ø 3.5 x 14 mm, 50 Ncm
	45	Champions® implant Ø 3.5 x 10 mm, 60 Ncm
	44	Champions® implant Ø 3.5 x 16 mm, 60 Ncm
	34	Champions® implant Ø 3.5 x 16 mm, 60 Ncm
	35	Champions® implant Ø 3.5 x 10 mm, 60 Ncm
	36	Champions® implant Ø 3.5 x 12 mm, 60 Ncm
	37	Champions® implant Ø 3.5 x 12 mm, 60 Ncm
	38	Champions® implant Ø 3.5 x 12 mm, 60 Ncm
	42	Champions® implant Ø 3.5 x 18 mm, 60 Ncm
	41	Champions® implant Ø 3.0 x 14 mm, 50 Ncm
	31	Champions® implant Ø 3.0 x 14 mm, 30 Ncm
	32	Champions® implant Ø 3.5 x 18 mm, 60 Ncm
	44,43,33,43	cemented Prep-Cap
		preparation
		impression for the laboratory made temporary
		cemented dentist made temporary

| 16/06/2010 | 38-48 | cemented laboratory made temporary |

| 06/09/2010 | | Impression |

| 13/09/2010 | 48-44,43-33 | cemented zirconium dioxide splinted crown |
| | 34-38 | |

| 07/06/2011 | | Radiographic control |

Treatment period: **3 months**

Remarks:
Immediate implant placement
Immediate loading
33 and 43 has been extracted after bite registration.
Post-control without bone loss!
(Almost) no swellings, as usual!
Upper low restoration at a German university took more than 1 year.

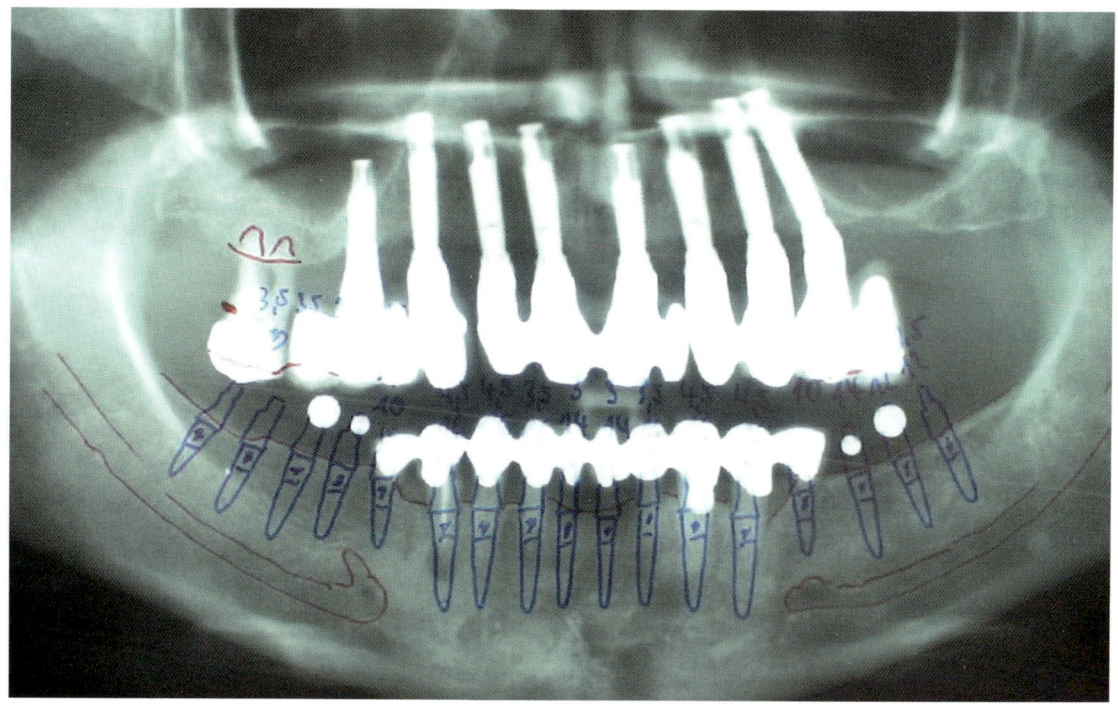

Panoramic radiograph for planned treatment

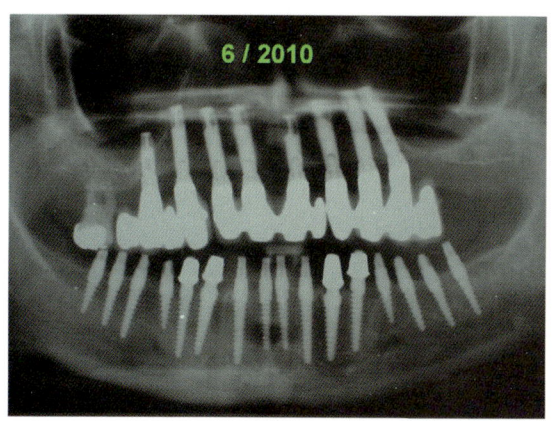

Panoramic radiograph after implant placement

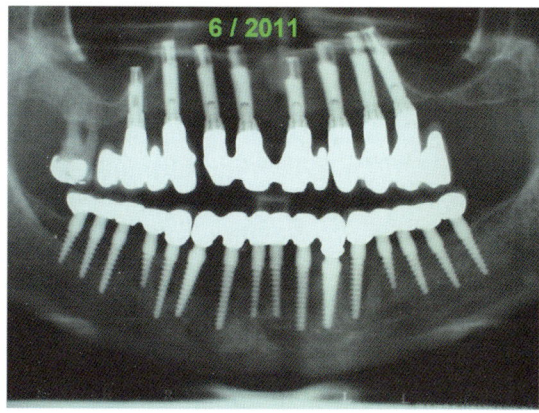

Panoramic radiograph after 1 year

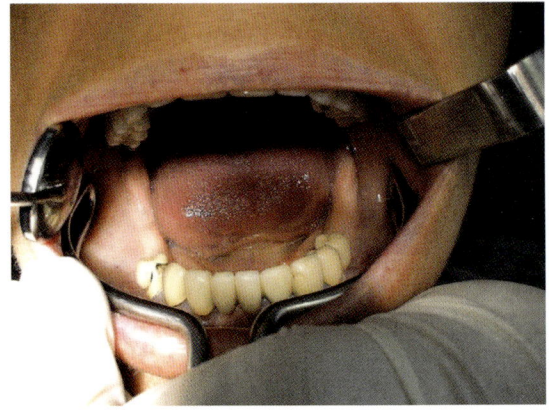

Clinical initial situation

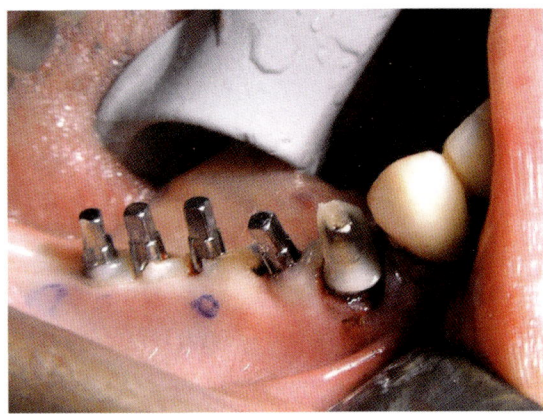

Implant placement, right side

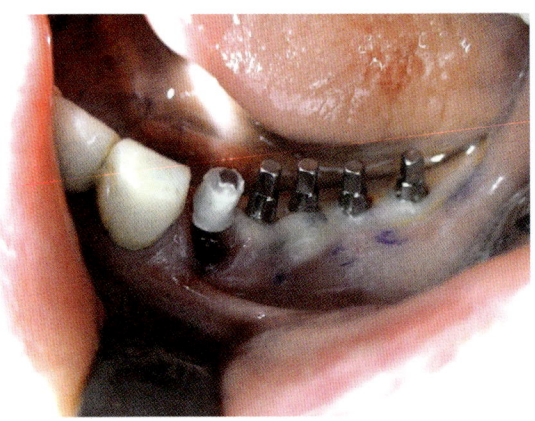

Implant placement, left side

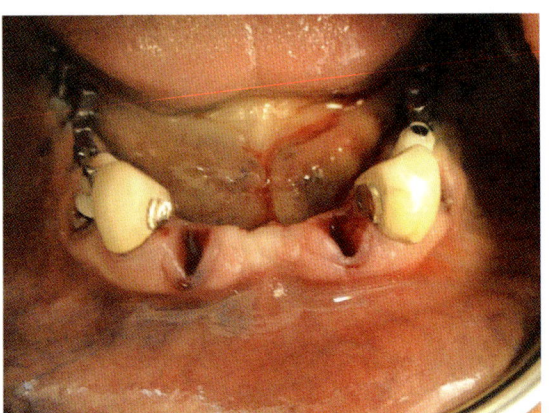

Anterior tooth extraction

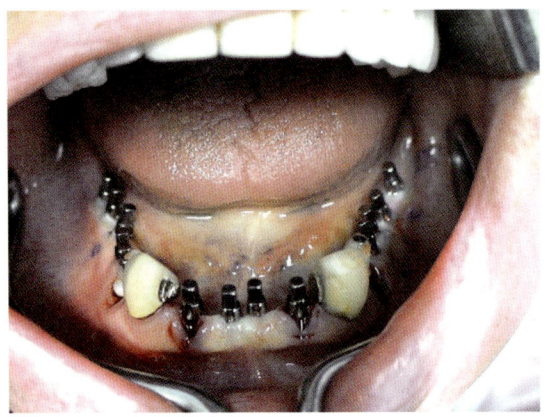

Implant placement of the anterior tooth

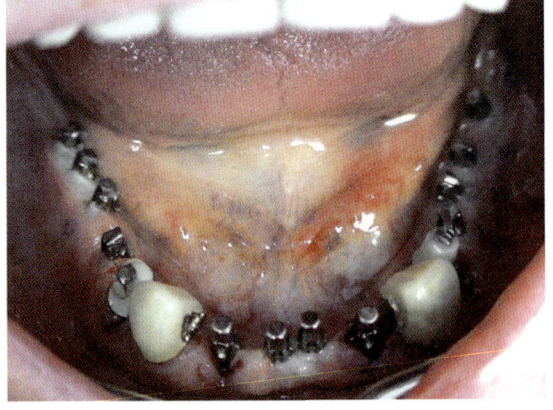

Preparation of the implant head with following bite registration

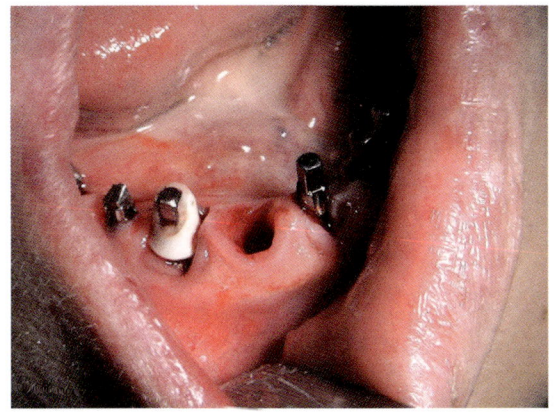

Extraction 43 (33)...

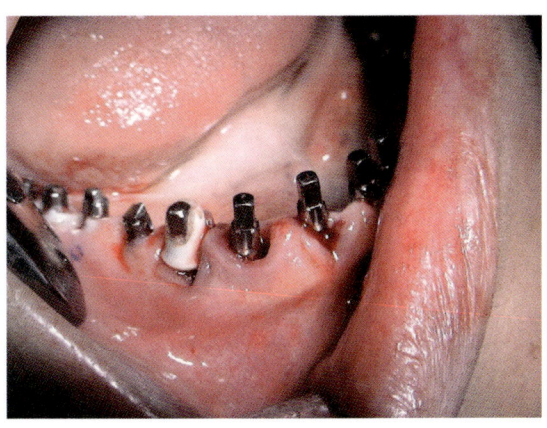

.,,implant placement...

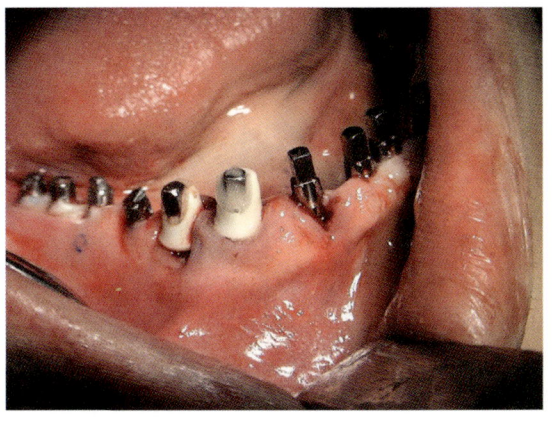

...Prep-Cap cementing...

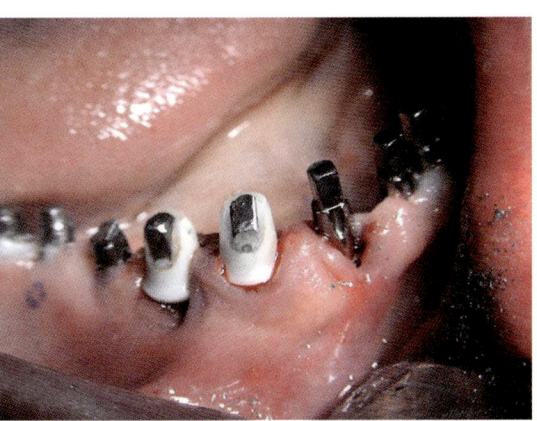

...and preparation

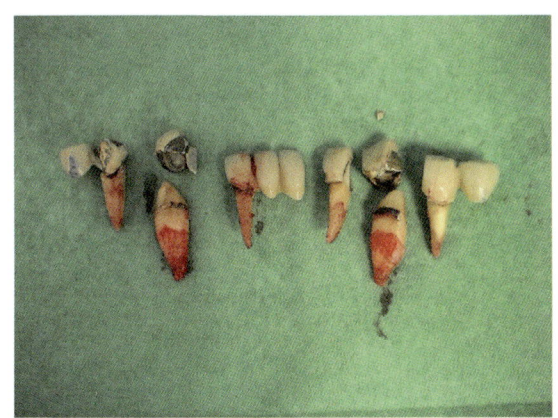

Extracted teeth

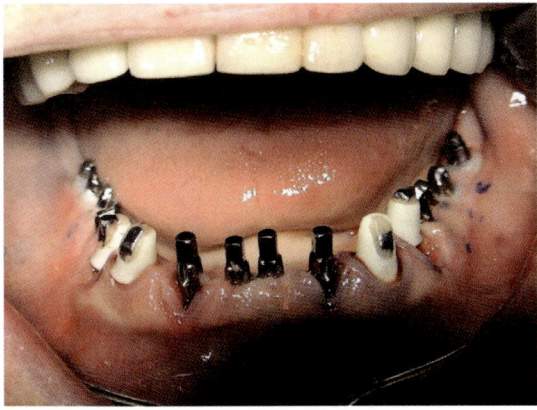

Completed preparations

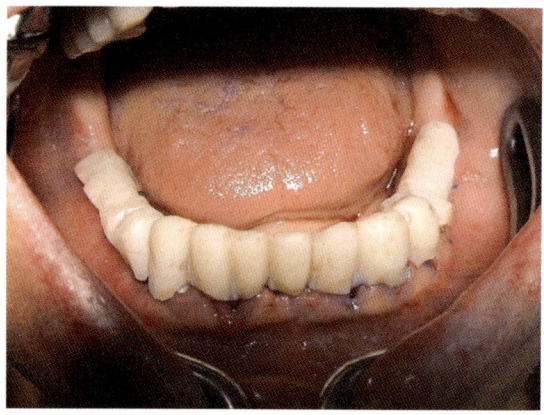

Cemented dentist made temporary

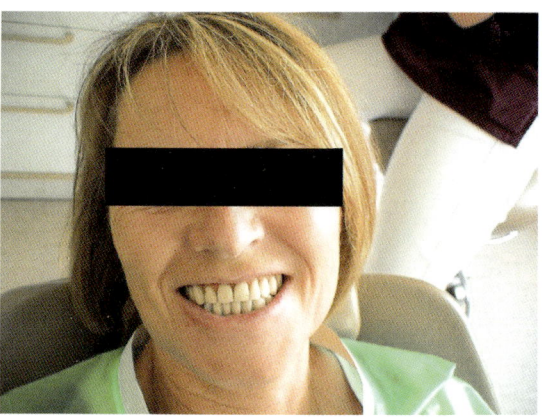

1st postoperative day

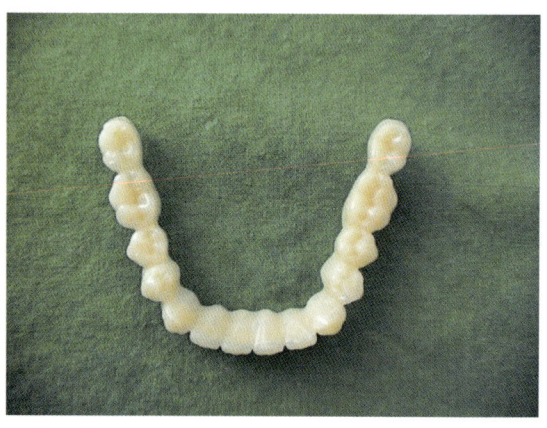

Laboratory made temporary, occlusal view

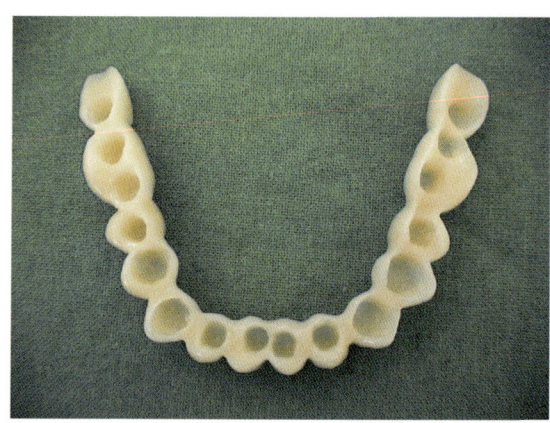

...basal view...

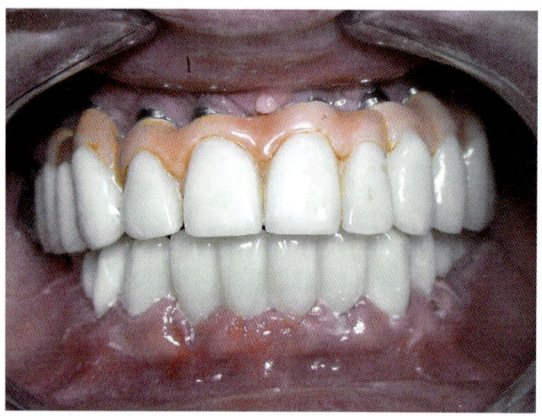

...anterior view...

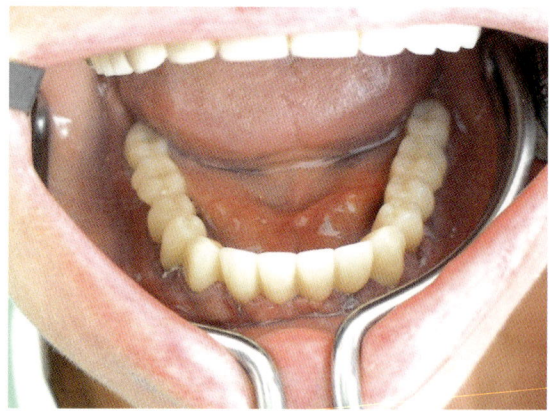

...as well as occlusal view in situ

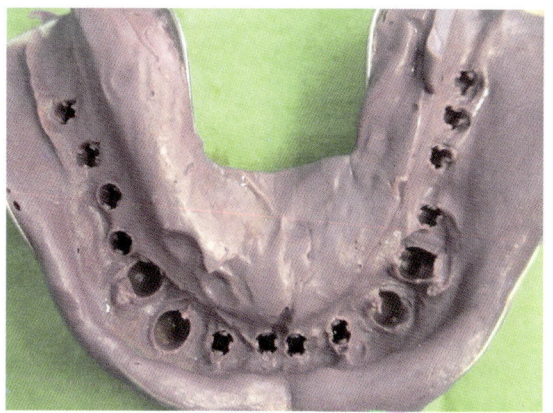

Impression

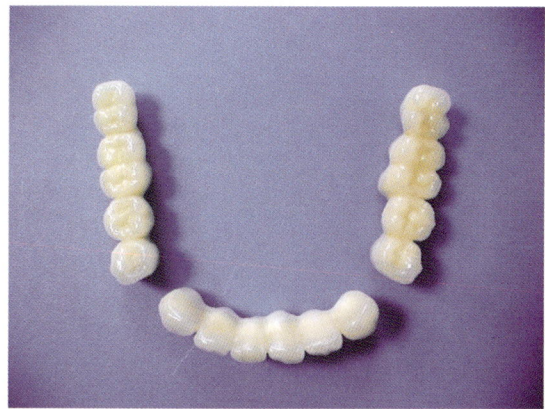

Final zirconium dioxide splinted crowns, occlusal view

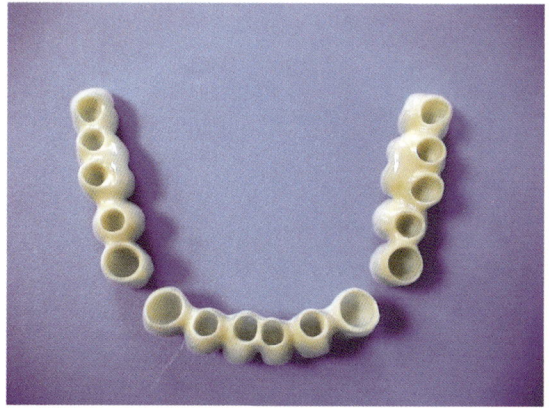

Final zirconium dioxide splinted crowns, basal view

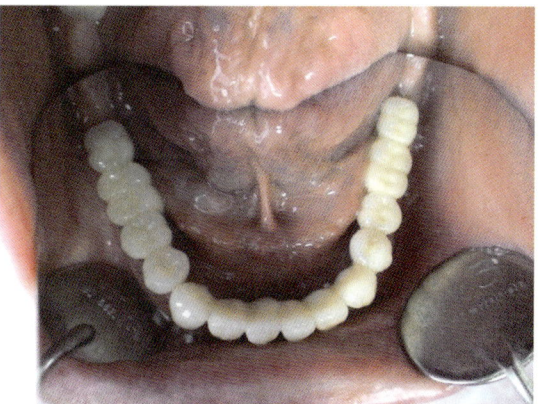

Final zirconium dioxide splinted crowns, occlusal view

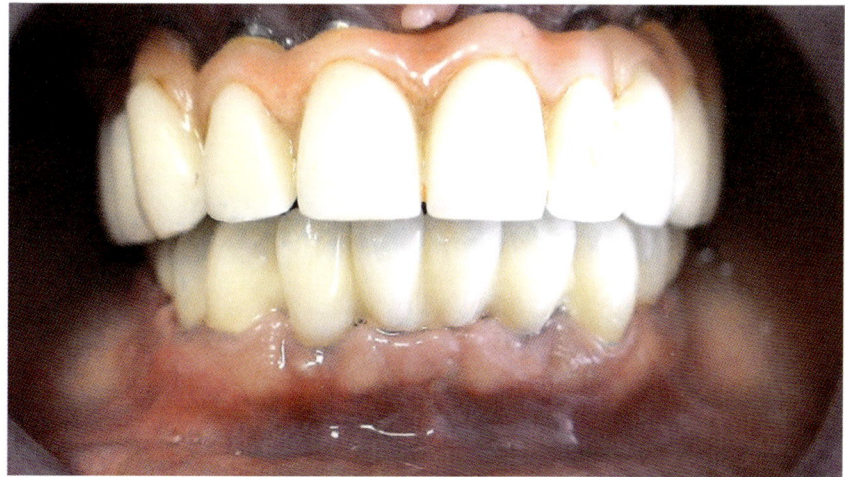

Final zirconium dioxide splinted crowns, anterior view

Overdentures

7.5.1/Case 39

Patient: male, 74 years old

6 lower jaw implants with direct matrix integration

11/07/2011	Lower jaw	Repair acceptance, reworking to a lower jaw overdenture without metal
12/07/2011	33	Champions® implant Ø 3.0 x 8 mm, >60 Ncm, Periotest -2
	32	Champions® implant Ø 3.0 x 10 mm, >40 Ncm, Periotest +5
	31	Champions® implant Ø 3.0 x 12 mm, >60 Ncm, Periotest +4
	41	Champions® implant Ø 3.0 x 12 mm, >60 Ncm, Periotest -1
	42	Champions® implant Ø 3.0 x 10 mm, 30 Ncm, Periotest +2
	43	Champions® implant Ø 3.0 x 10 mm, >40 Ncm, Periotest +3
		6 matrices cured into denture resin
13/07/2011		Wound control
Treatment period:		**90 minutes**
Remarks:		Late implant placement, immediate loading

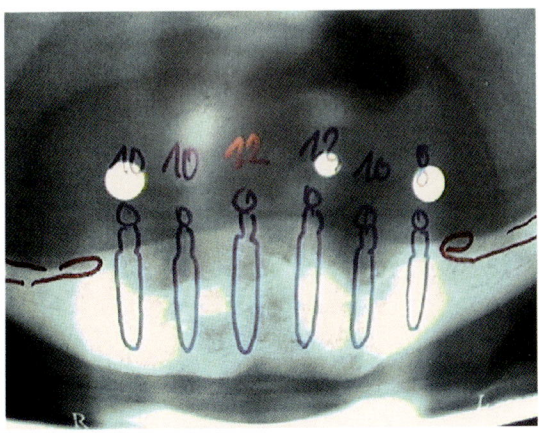

Panoramic radiograph for planned treatment

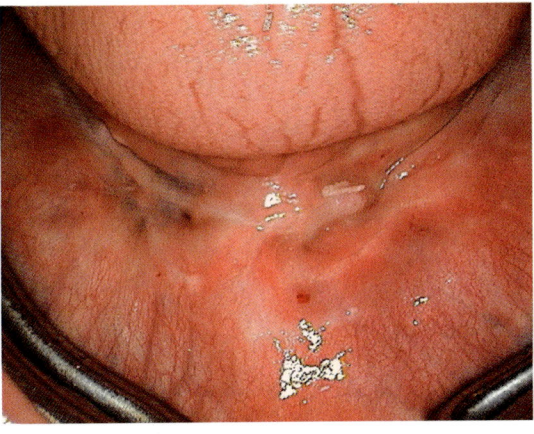

Clinical initial situation

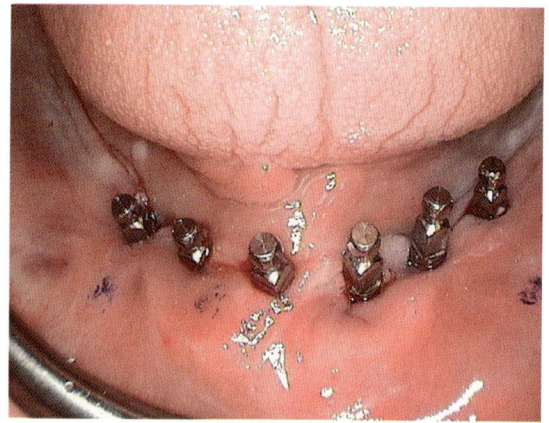

Performed implant placement

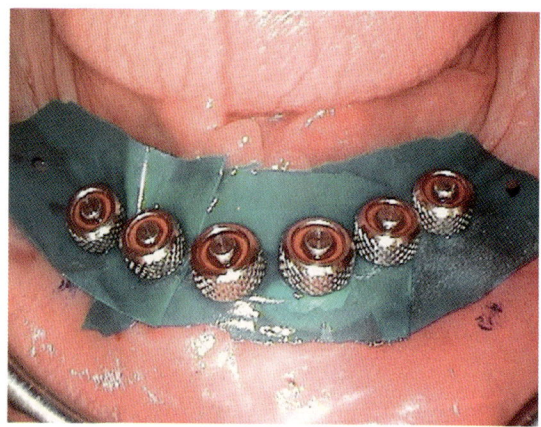

Preparation for the polymerisation process, rubber dam to protect the gingiva

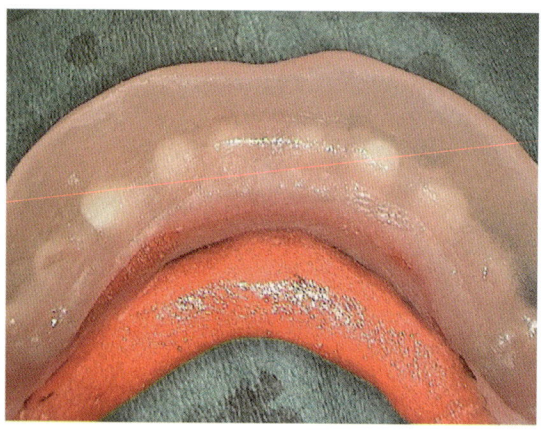

Ground and reinforced prosthesis

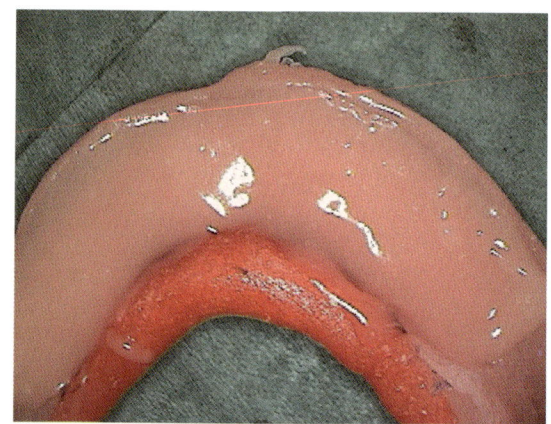

Inserted polymer

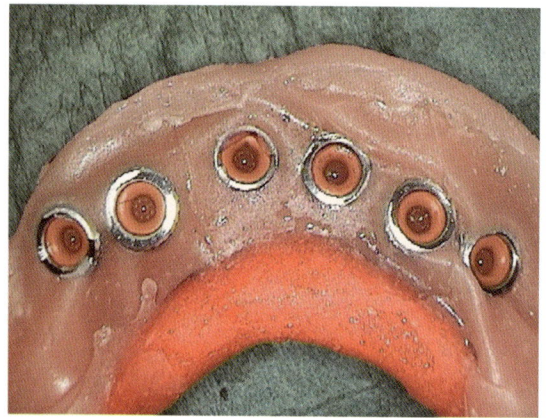

Cured matrices, before prosthesis preparation

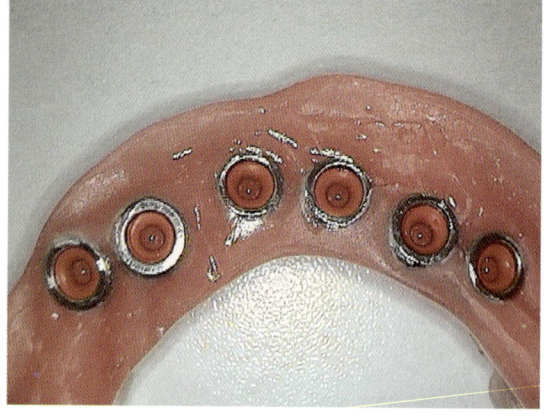

Inserted matrices, after prosthesis preparation

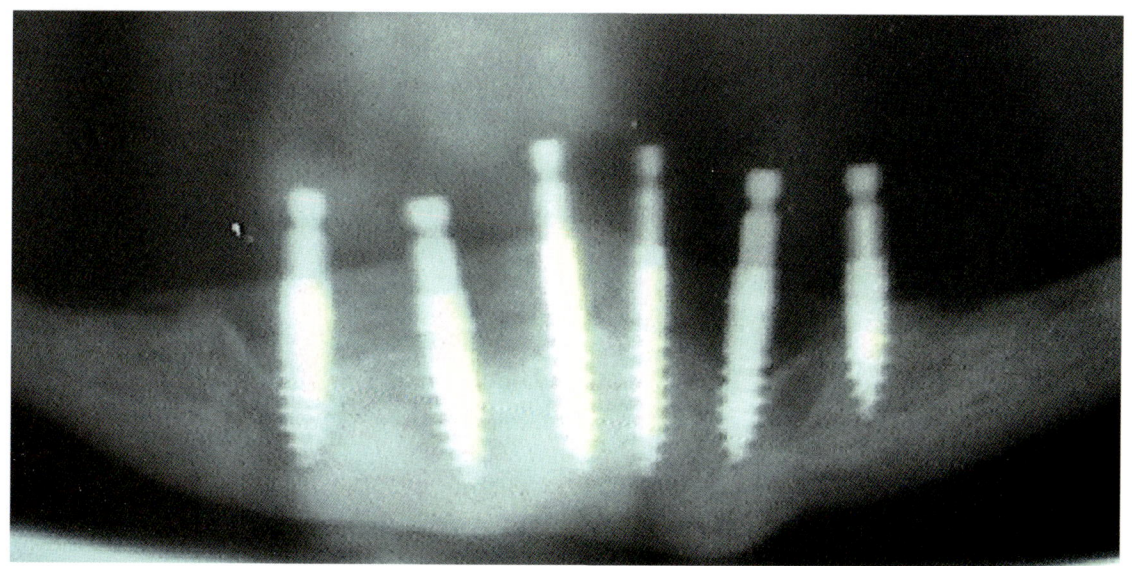

Radiographic control, panoramic radiograph

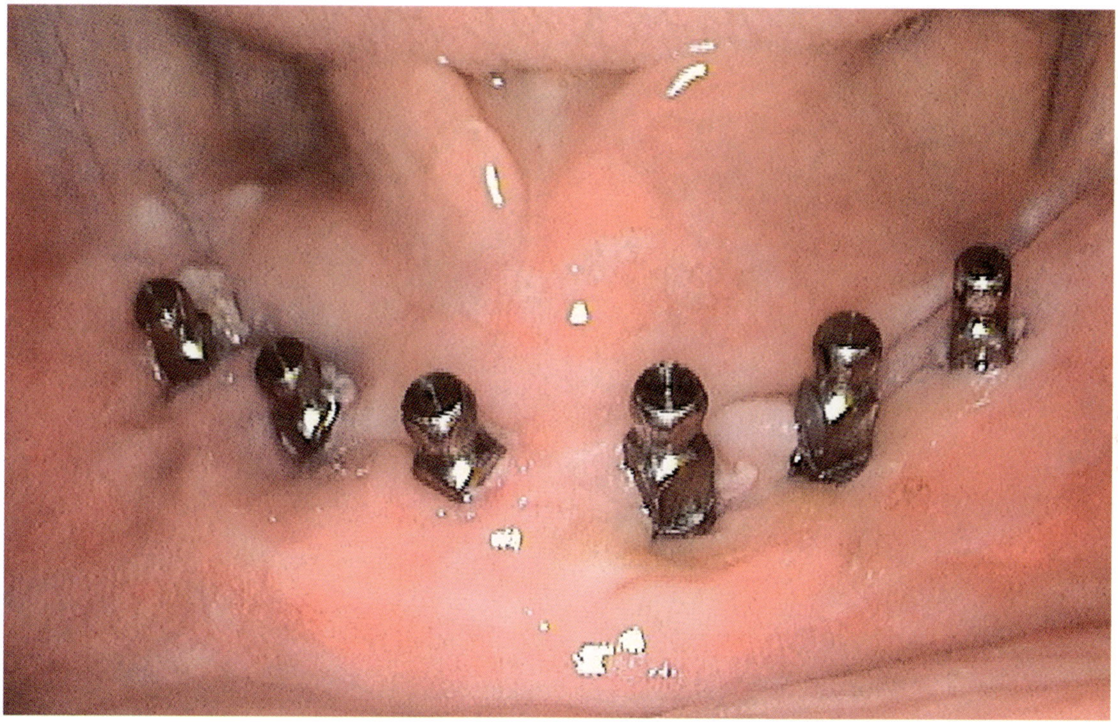

1st postoperative day

7.5.2/Case 40

Patient: female, 88 years old

43-33 6 tulip head implants with early loading

16/03/2010	43-33	6 Champions® ball head implants (Ø 3.0 x 12 mm, >60 Ncm), so-called "tulips", inserted with appropriate metal matrices for tulips cured into denture resin
May 2011	Upper jaw Lower jaw	Overdenture Implant prosthesis Control images
Treatment period:		**90 minutes**
Remarks:		Late implant placement, immediate loading Reinforcement of the prosthesis with resinous material in order to avoid fractures during grinding procedures

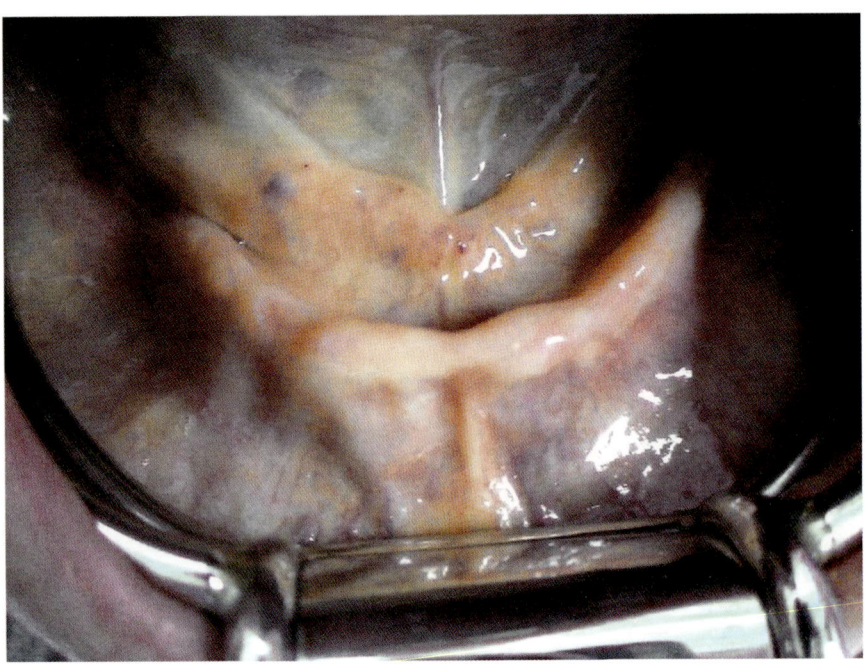

Clinical initial situation

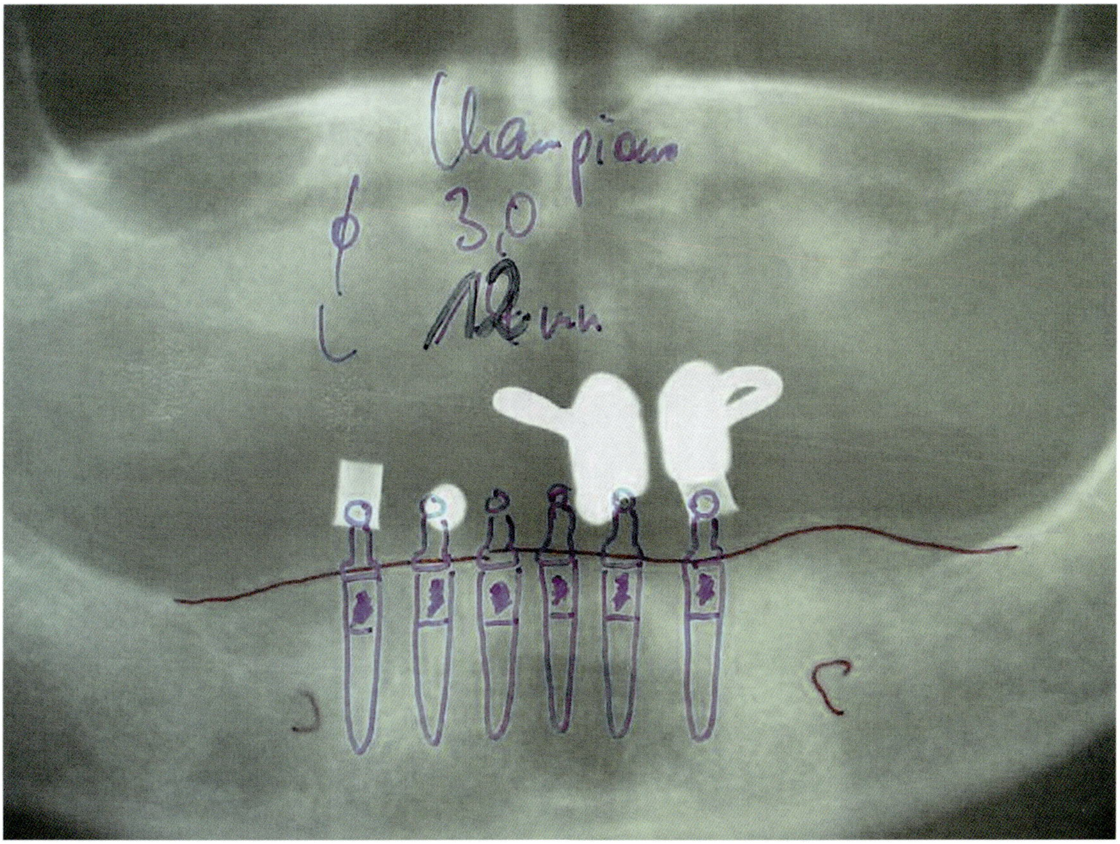

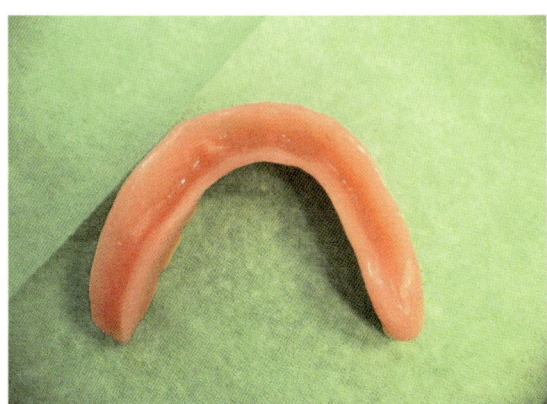

Planned implant placement, panoramic radiograph

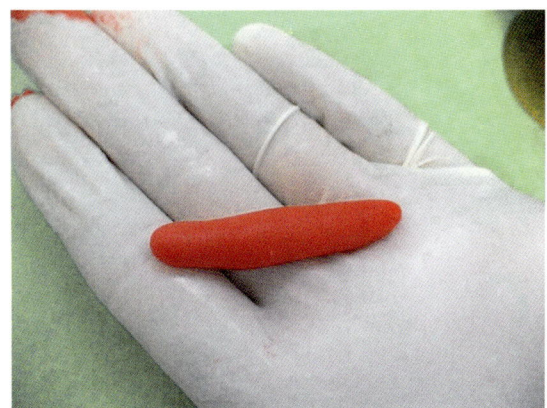

Available prosthesis, bottom side

Resin serves as...

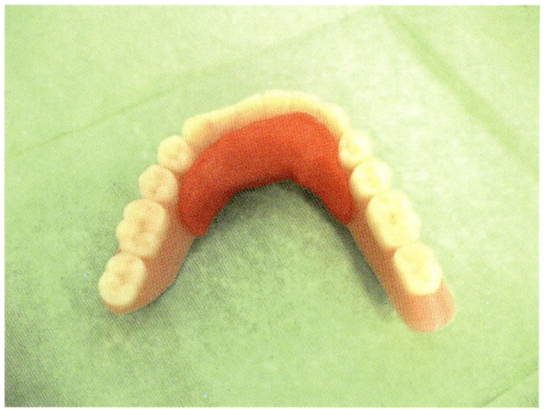

...lingual reinforcement

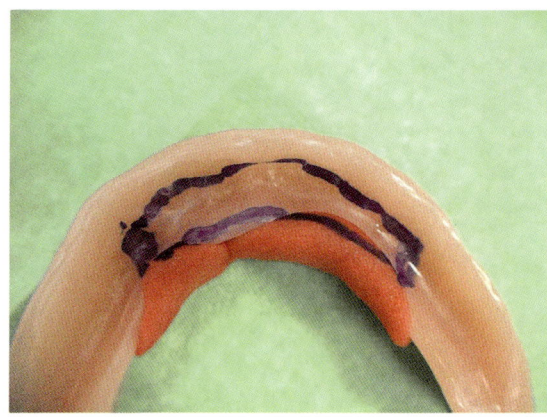

The marked section will be ground

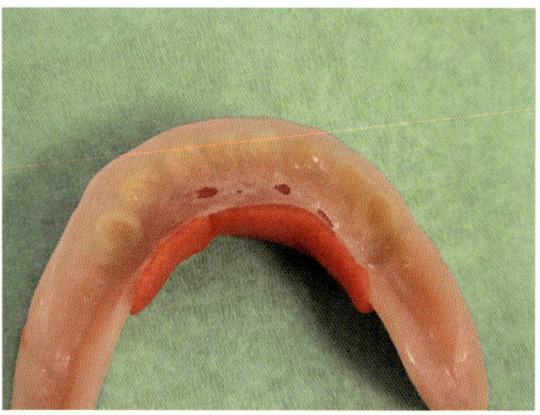

The ground section is now prepared for the insertion of the matrices

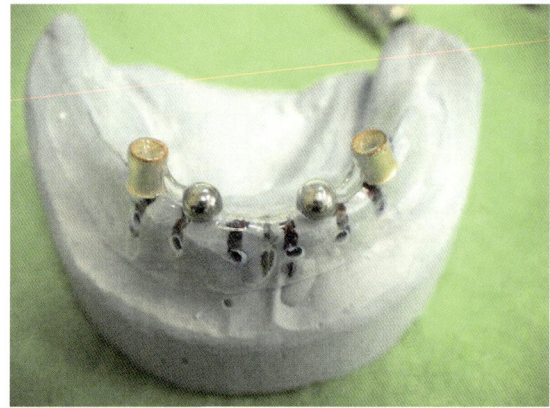

X-ray template onto the cast

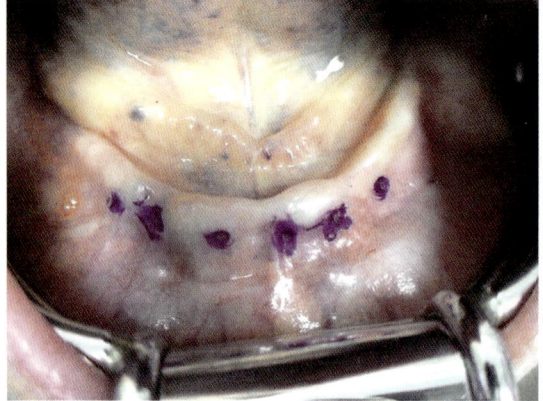

From the X-ray template onto the mucosa transferred marks

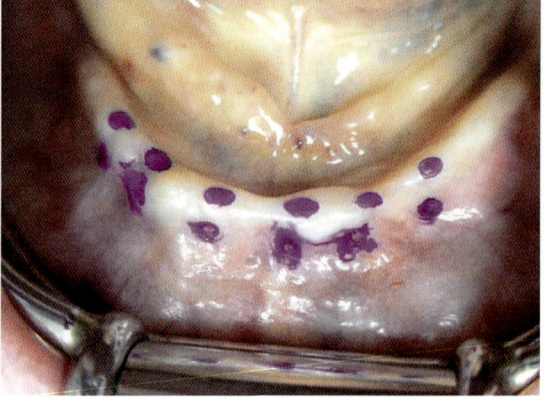

Transferred marks for initial pilot hole preparation

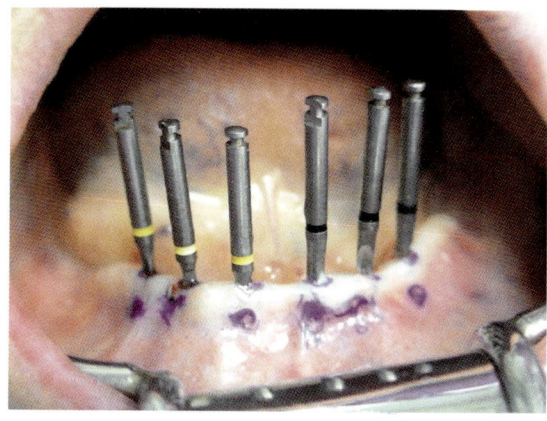

Control of the performed pilot hole preparation

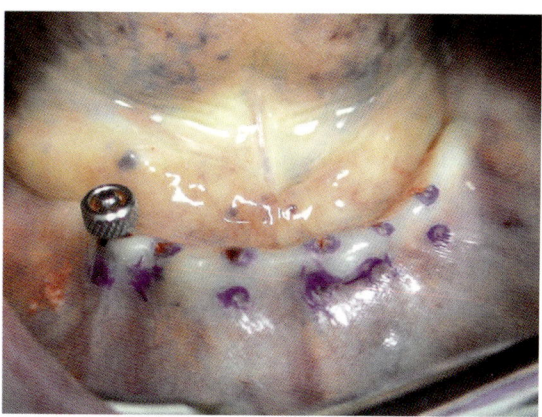

Implant placement at the beginning

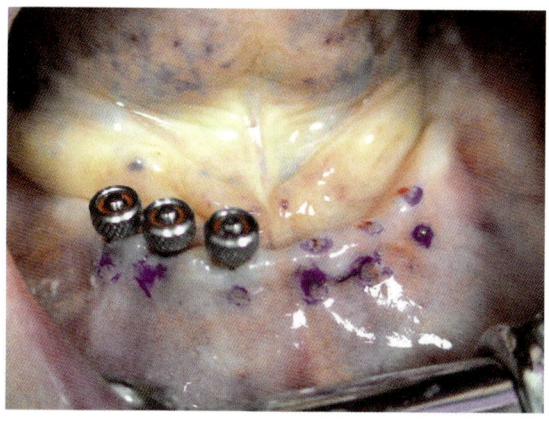

Distance control due to attached matrices

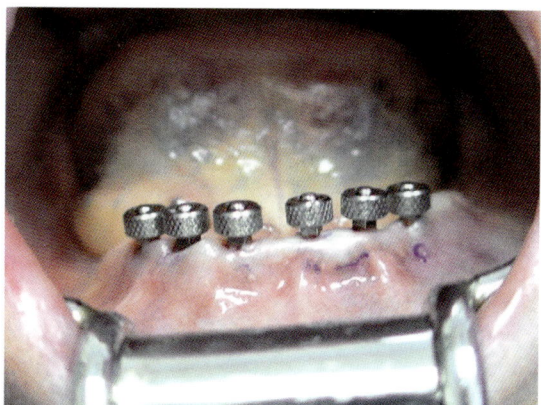

Implant placement at the end

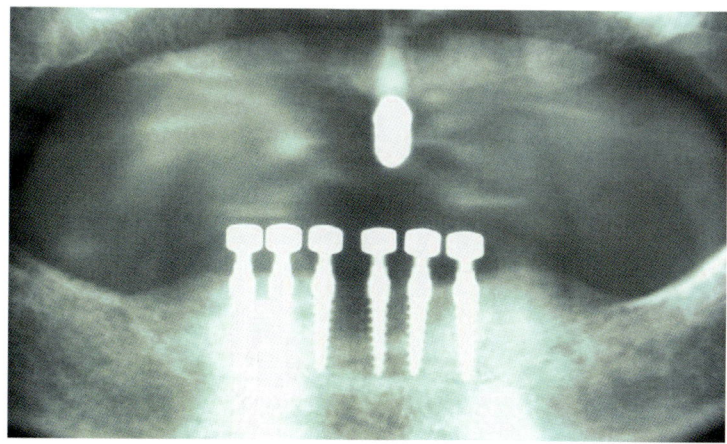

Final control, panoramic radiograph

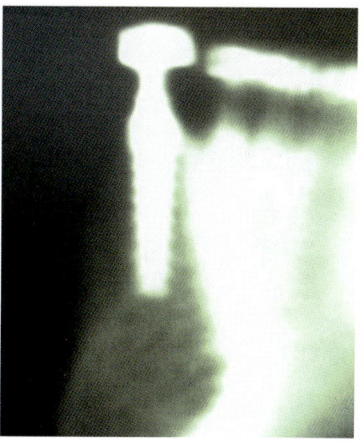

Radiographic control, cross-sectional image

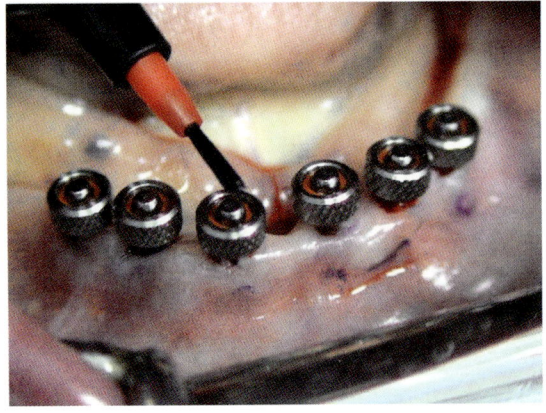

Matrix isolation

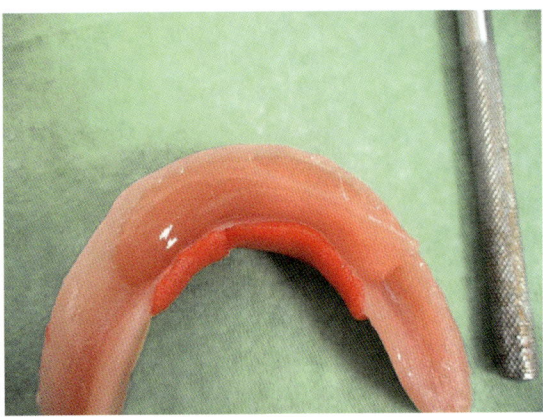

Injected cold-cured polymer

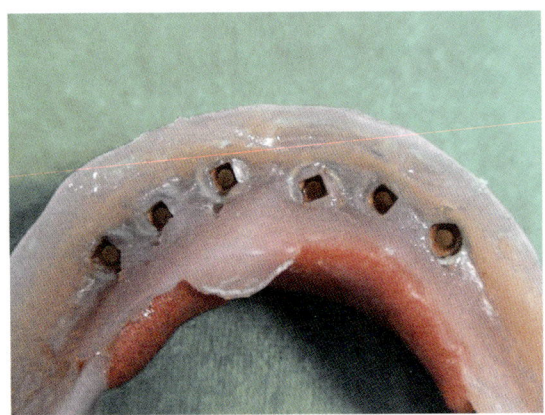

Cured cold-cured polymer

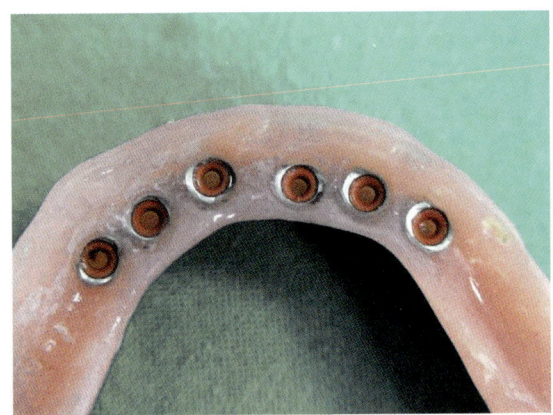

Prepared prosthesis

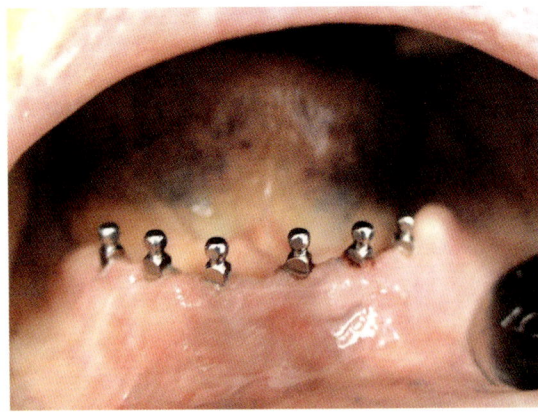

Clinical situation, more than one year after implant placement

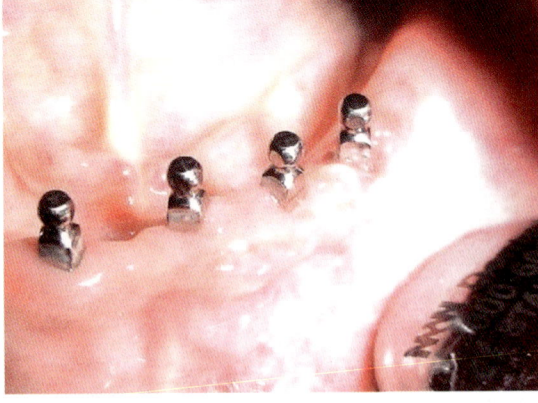

Clinical situation, more than one year after implant placement, macro view

7.5.3/ Fall 41

Patient: männlich, 57 Jahre alt

6   UK-Implantate mit direkter Matrizeneinarbeitung

11/10/2010	33	Champions® implant Ø 3.5 x 10 mm, 60 Ncm, Periotest -2
	32	Champions® implant Ø 3.5 x 12 mm, 60 Ncm, Periotest -1
	31	Champions® implant Ø 3.5 x 12 mm, 60 Ncm, Periotest -3
	41	Champions® implant Ø 3.5 x 12 mm, 40 Ncm, Periotest -1
	42	Champions® implant Ø 3.5 x 12 mm, 40 Ncm, Periotest -1
	43	Champions® implant Ø 3.5 x 10 mm, 40 Ncm, Periotest -1
		6 matrices cured into denture resin

17/05/2011   Post-control

Treatment period: **90 minutes**

Remarks: Matrices are cemented into the former prosthesis
later onwards: a) relining
                        b) new lower jaw prosthesis

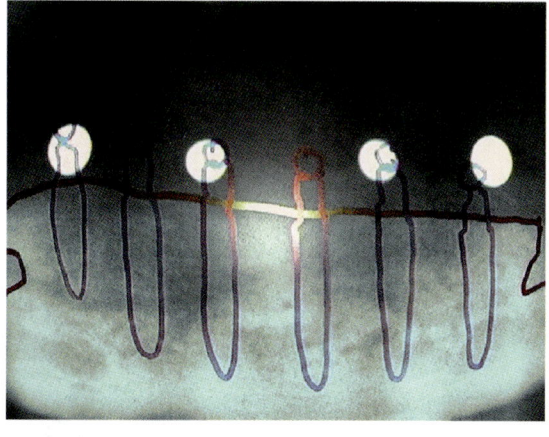

Radiographic planning, panoramic radiograph,
detail

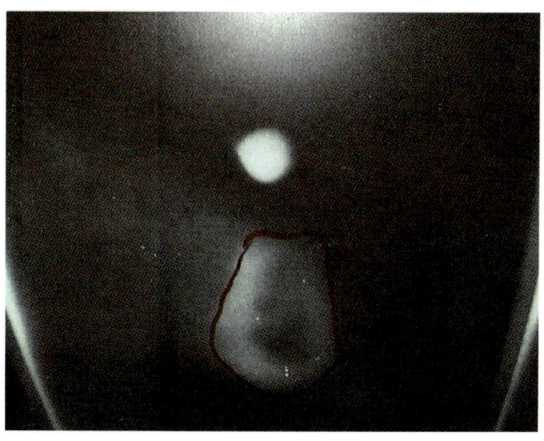

Radiographic planning, cross-sectional image

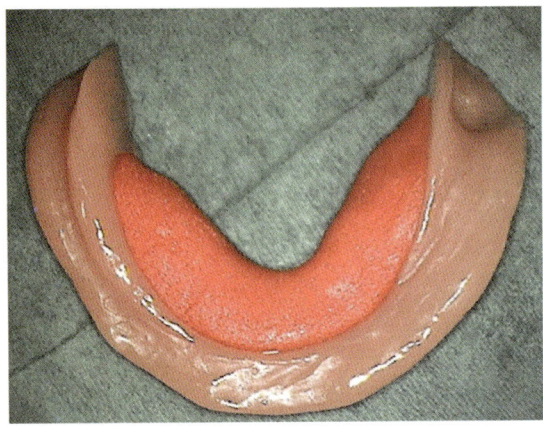

With resin reinforced prosthesis due to danger of fractures

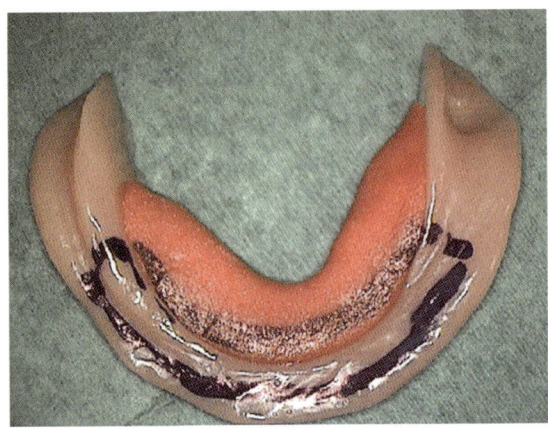

Former prosthesis with marking of the section which has to be ground

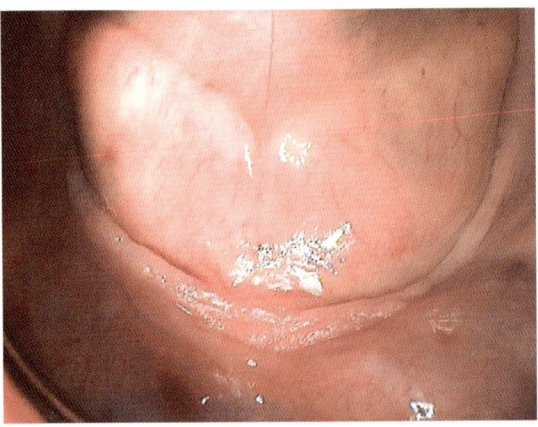

Clinical initial findings

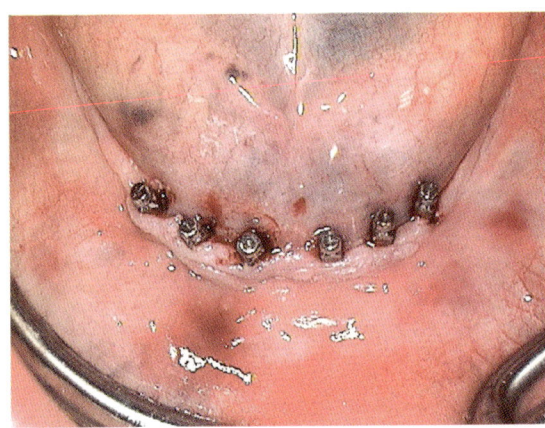

Properly lingually placed implants

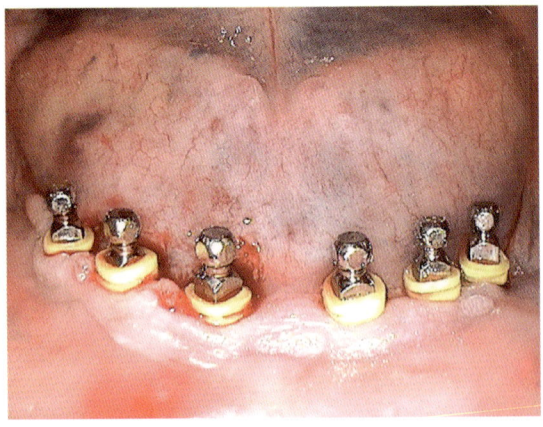

Block-out of the square below the ball by means of placed rubber rings

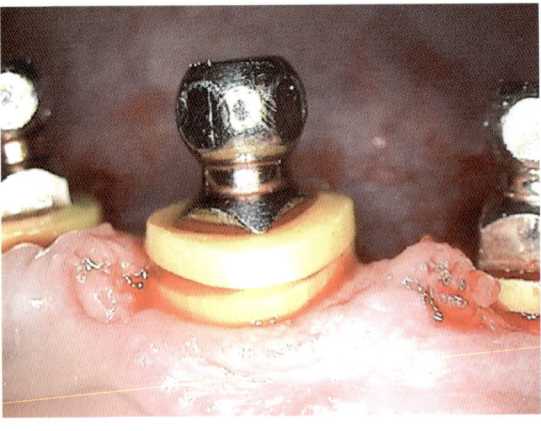

Placed rubber ring, macro view

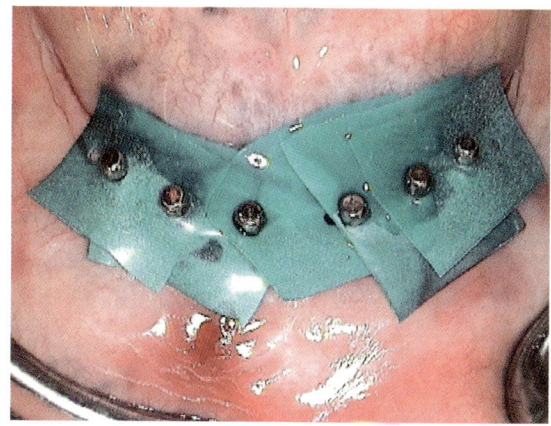

Rubber dam to protect the gingiva from resin...

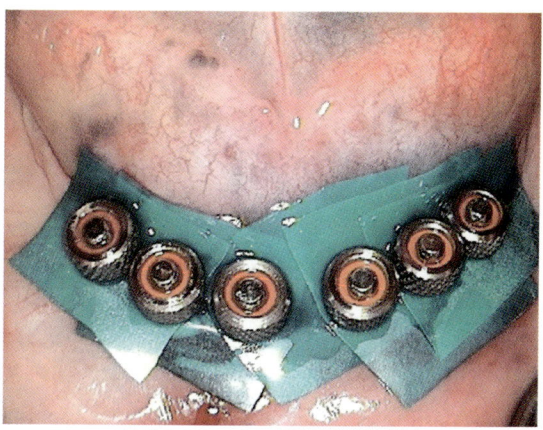

...with attached matrices

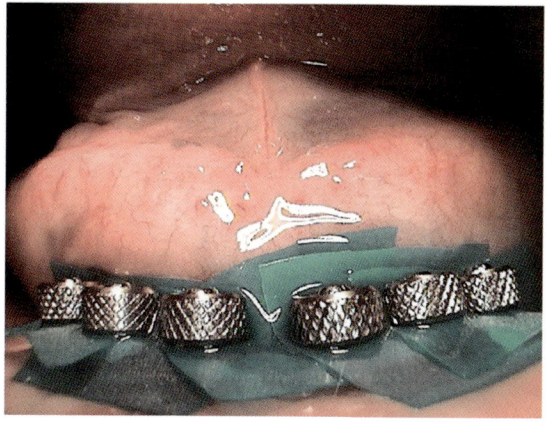

Anterior view

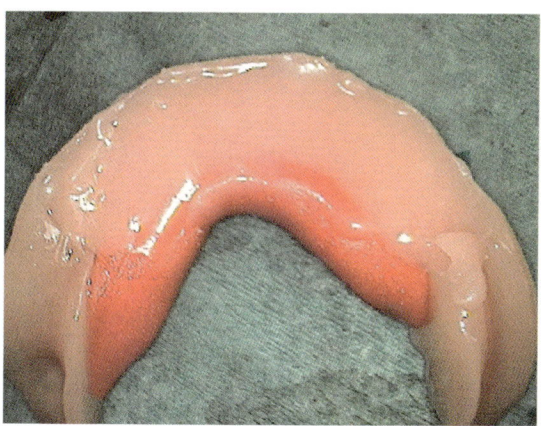

Injected cold-cured polymer

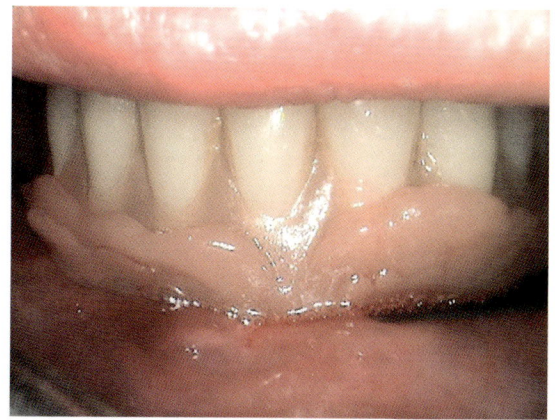

Mouth-closed taken impression, polymerisation process...

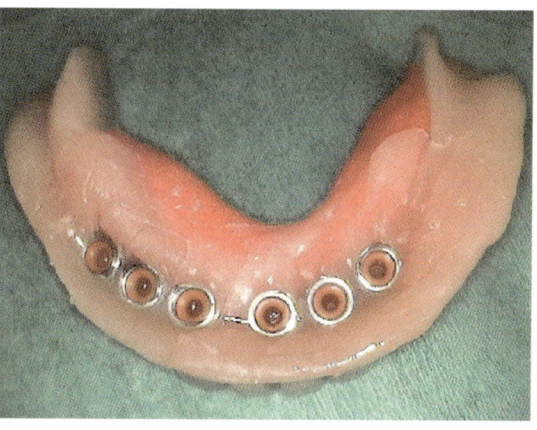

...and situation after removal of the prosthesis

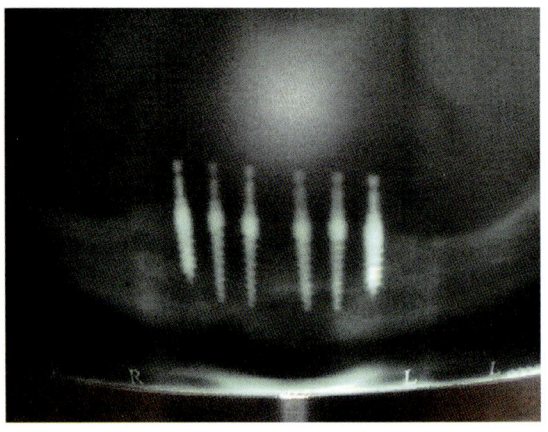

Radiographic control, panoramic radiograph

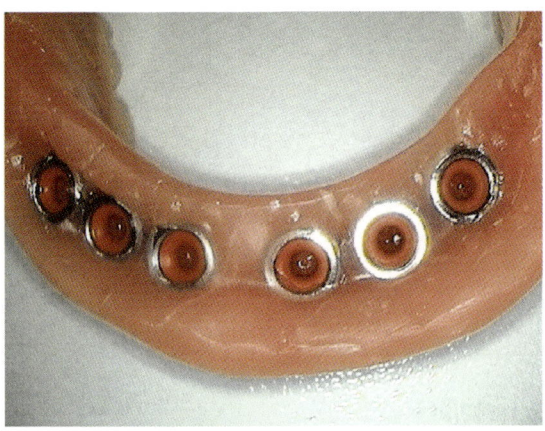

Situation after prosthesis preparation

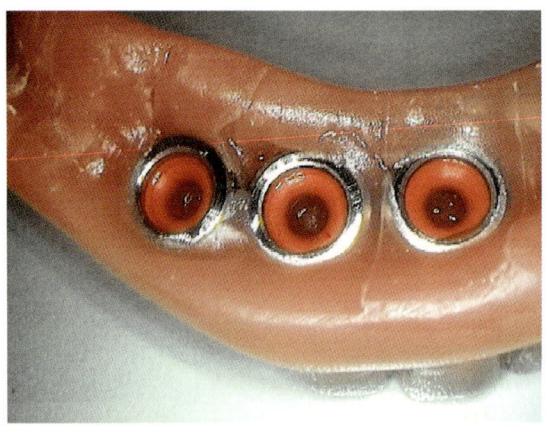

Small failures are subsequently levelled with resin!

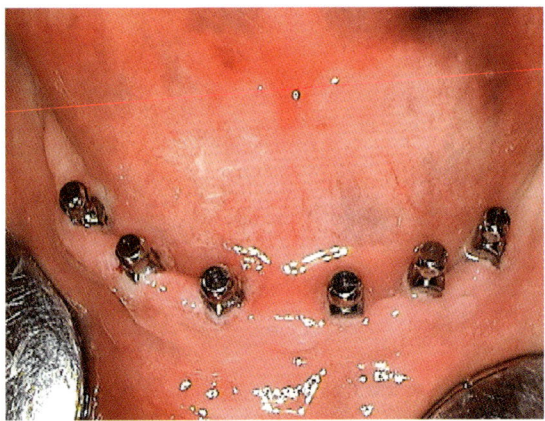

7 months post-surgery

7.5.4/Case 42

Patient: male, 56 years old

6 lower jaw implants with direct matrix integration

10/12/2009	43-34	extraction impression taking for the reworking to an overdenture
15/12/2009	34	
	33	Champions® implant Ø 4.0 x 20 mm,>60 Ncm
	32	Champions® implant Ø 4.0 x 20 mm,>60 Ncm
	41	Champions® implant Ø 4.0 x 16 mm,>50 Ncm
	42	Champions® implant Ø 4.0 x 16 mm, 30 Ncm
	43	Champions® implant Ø 4.0 x 16 mm, >40 Ncm
		Champions® implant Ø 4.0 x 20 mm, 60 Ncm
		6 matrices directly cemented into the prosthesis
16/12/2009		Wound control, image
08/02/2010		Final image
Treatment period:		**2 hours**
Remarks:		Early implant placement, immediate loading Vestibular bone loss 33 Due to space limits one implant had been spared

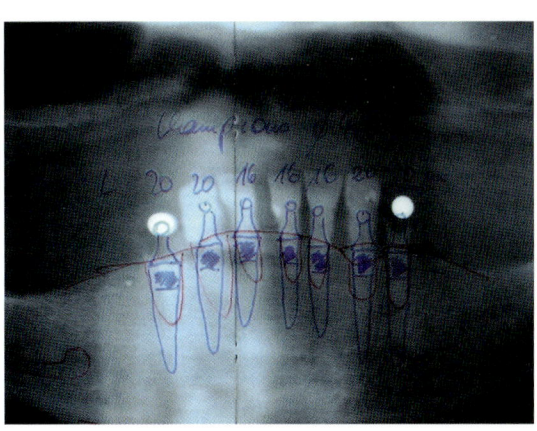

Panoramic radiograph for planned treatment

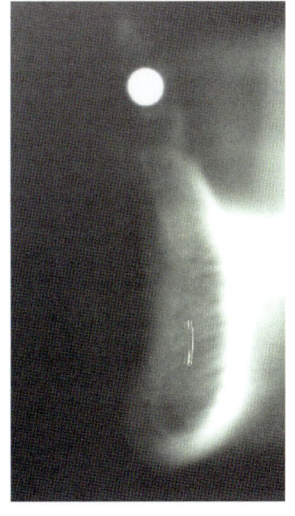

Cross-sectional

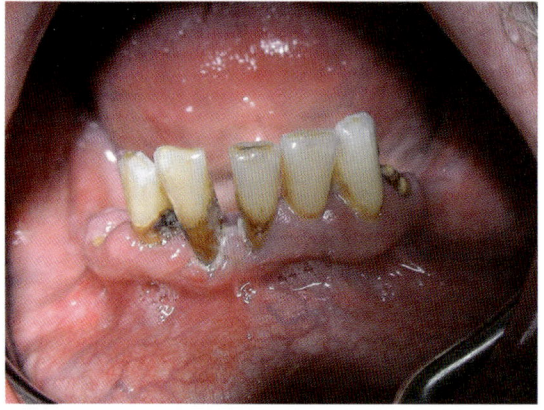

Clinical initial findings

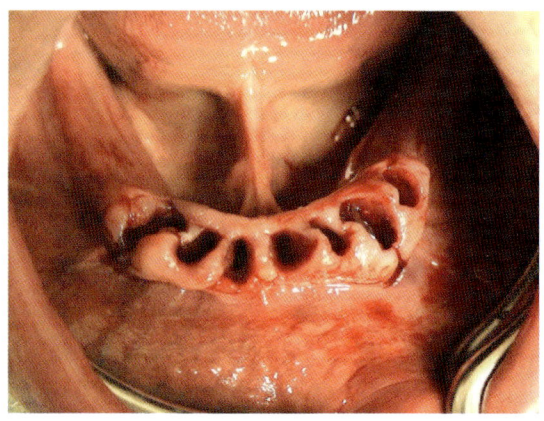

Situation after extraction

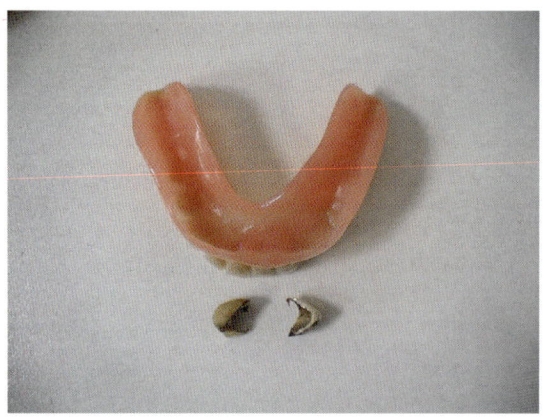

Reworked prosthesis

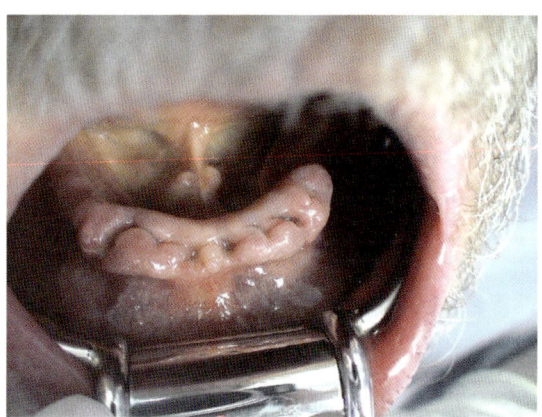

5 days after extraction...

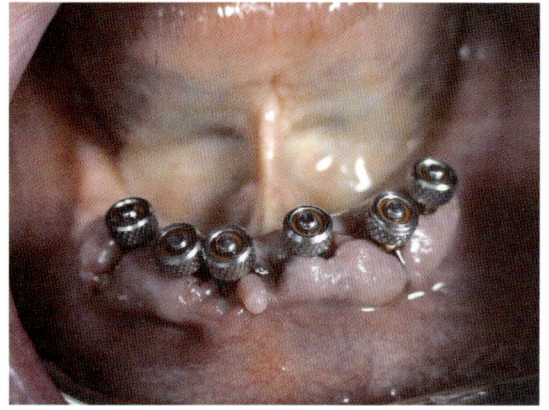

...completed implant placement, with attached metal matrices for tulips

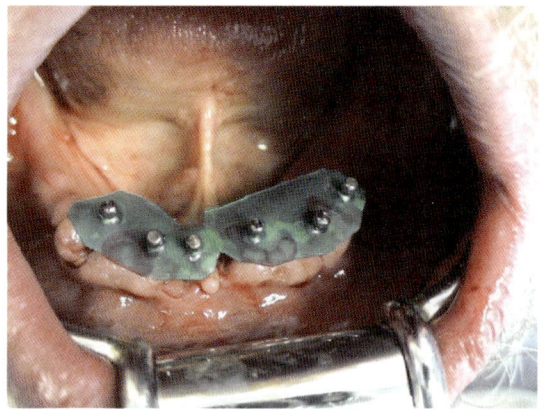

Preparation for the polymerisation process

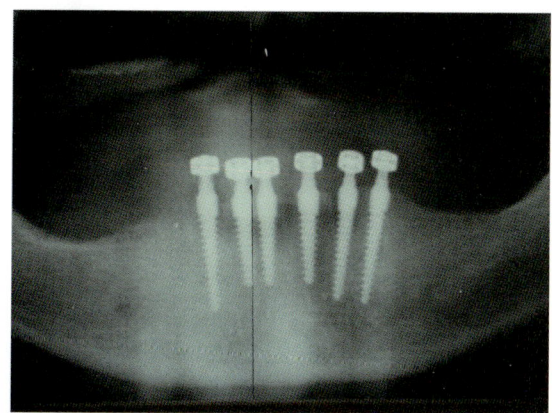

Radiographic control, panoramic radiograph

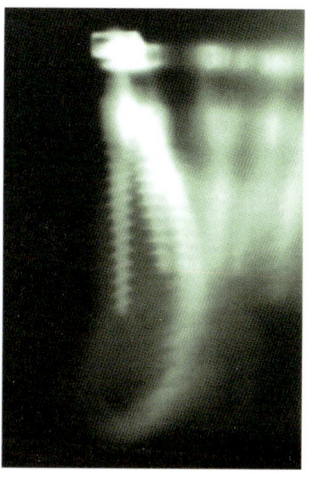

Radiographic control, cross-sectional image

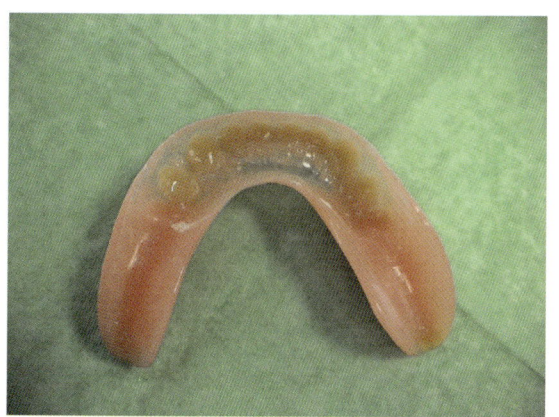

Ground prosthesis

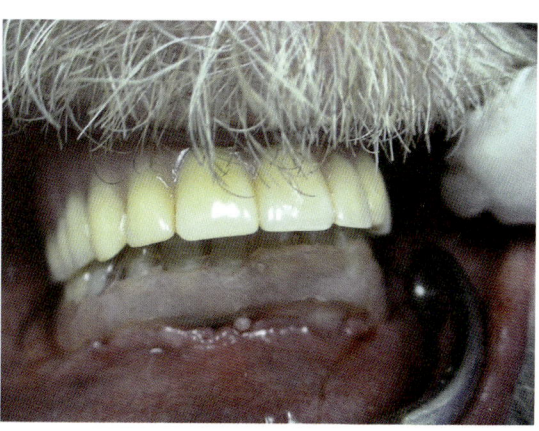

Mouth-closed polymerisation process

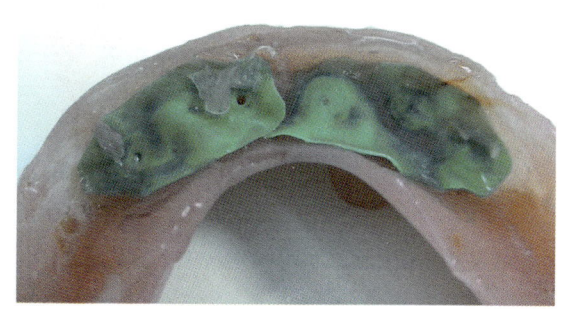

Completed polymerisation process, basal view

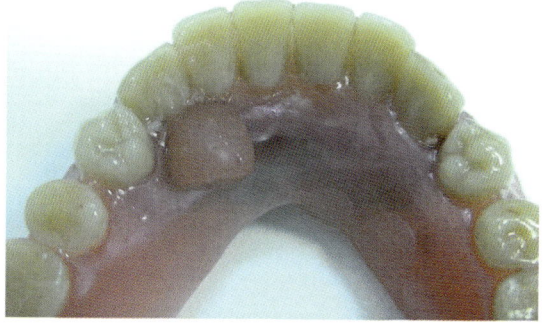

Completed polymerisation process, occlusal view

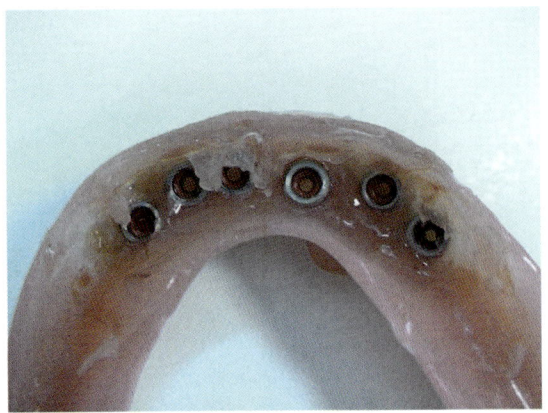

Prosthesis before preparation

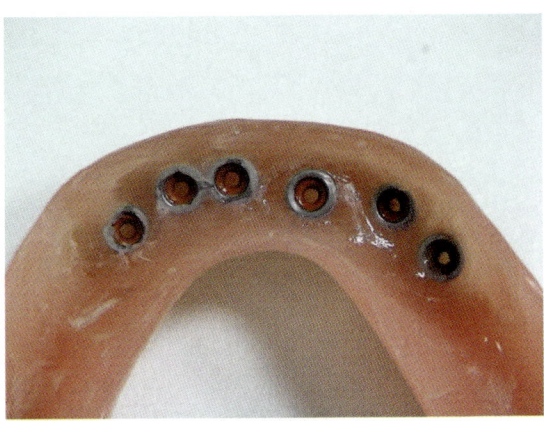

Prosthesis after preparation

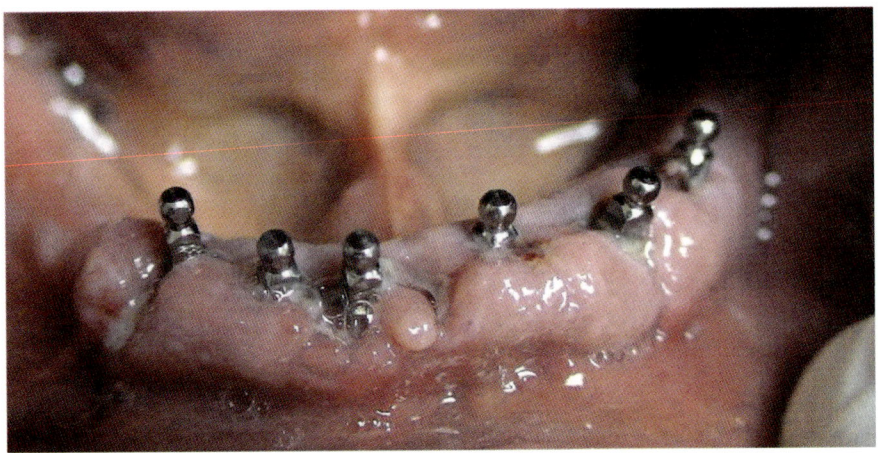

1st postoperative day

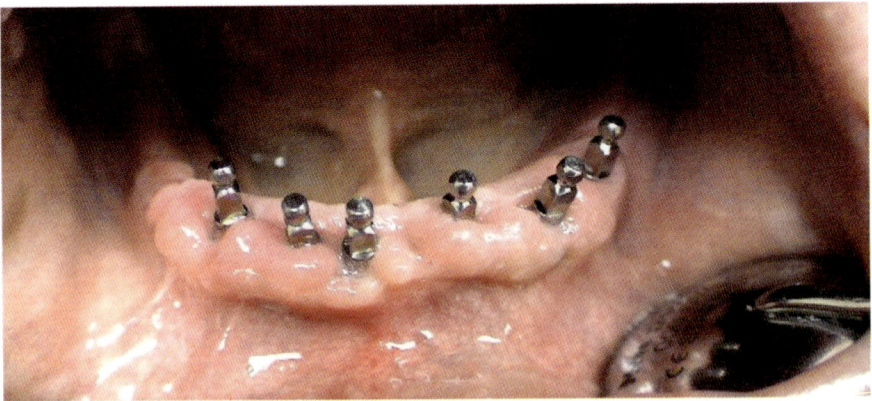

7 weeks after surgery

7.5.5/Case 43

Patient: female, 75 years old

6 lower jaw implants with direct matrix integration
43 immediate implant placement

10/01/2011	44,47	extraction
21/03/2011	Lower jaw	alginate impression taking for the reworking to an overdenture
22/03/2011	43	extraction
	33	Champions® implant Ø 3.0 x 14 mm, >60 Ncm
	32	Champions® implant Ø 3.0 x 14 mm, >30 Ncm
	31	Champions® implant Ø 3.0 x 14 mm, >40 Ncm
	41	Champions® implant Ø 3.0 x 14 mm, >60 Ncm
	42	Champions® implant Ø 3.0 x 14 mm, >60 Ncm
	43	Champions® implant Ø 4.0 x 20 mm, >60 Ncm
		6 matrices (metal matrices for tulips) cured into denture resin
11/10/2011		Post-control, images
Treatment period:		**90 minutes**
Remarks:	43	immediate implant placement
	43-33	immediate loading

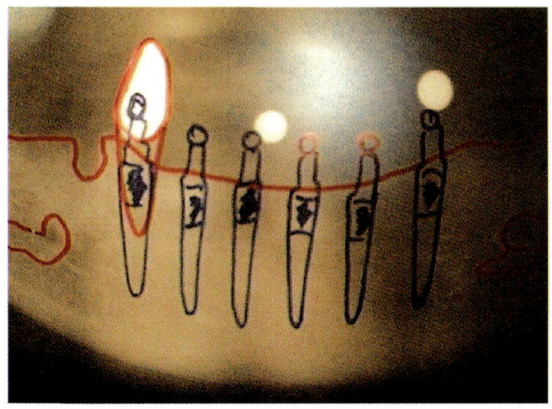

Panoramic radiograph for planned treatment

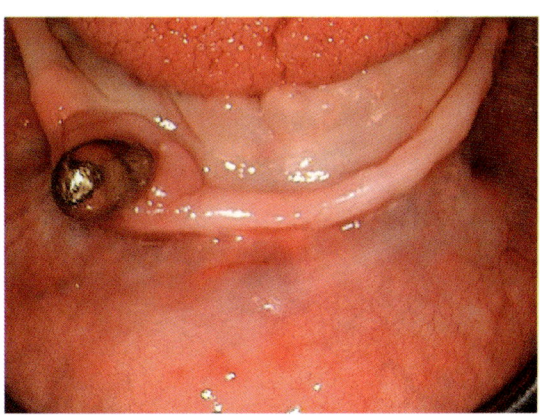

Clinical initial situation

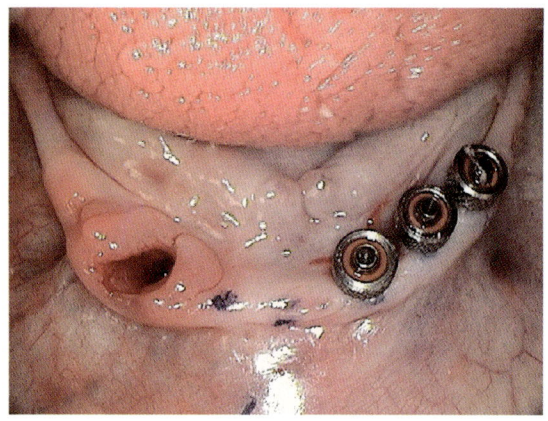

Extraction of tooth 43, implant placement at the beginning

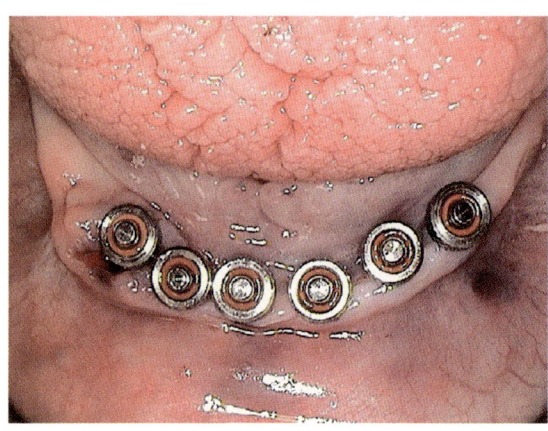

Completed implant placement

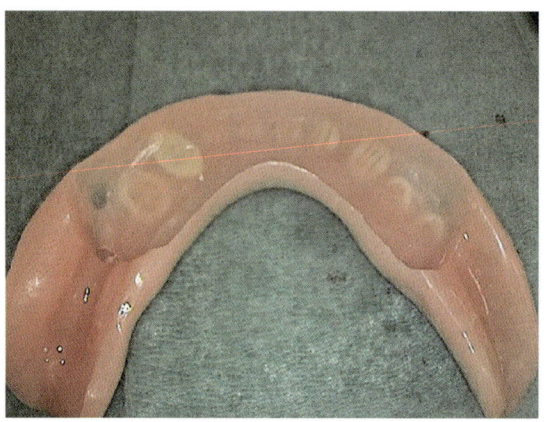

Ground prosthesis

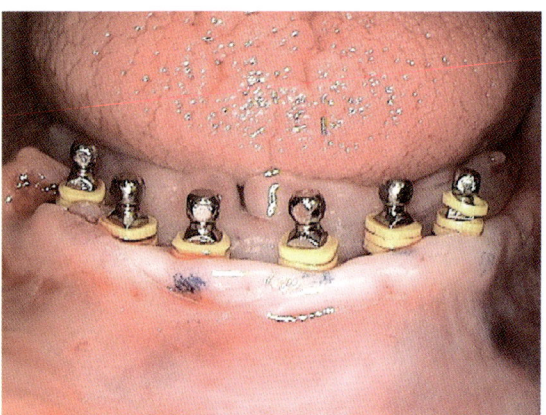

Block-out of the square below the ball by means of placed rubber rings, anterior view

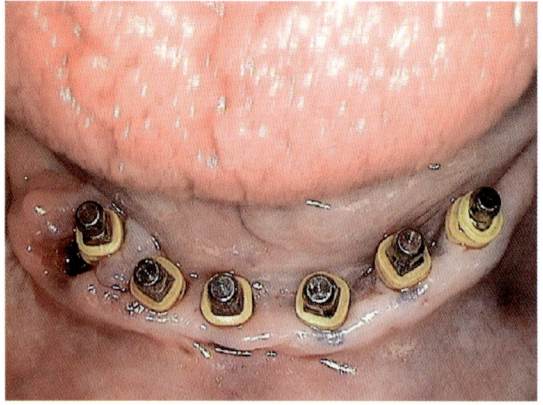

Block-out of the square below the ball due to placed rubber rings, occlusal view

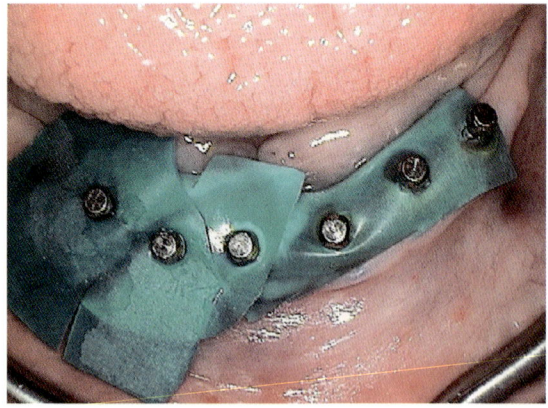

Rubber dam to protect the gingiva of resin...

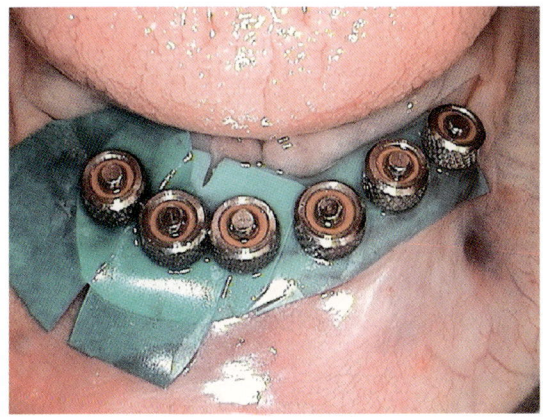

...with attached matrices, occlusal view

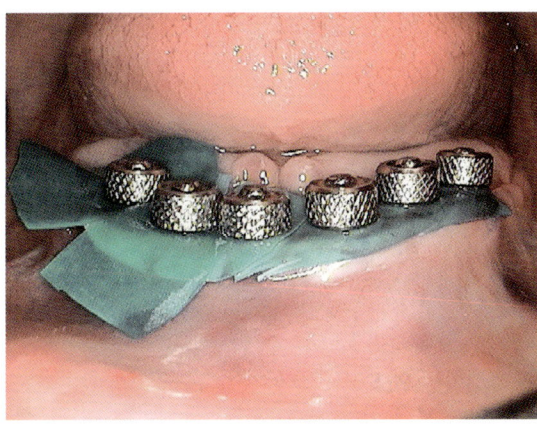

Attached matrices, anterior view

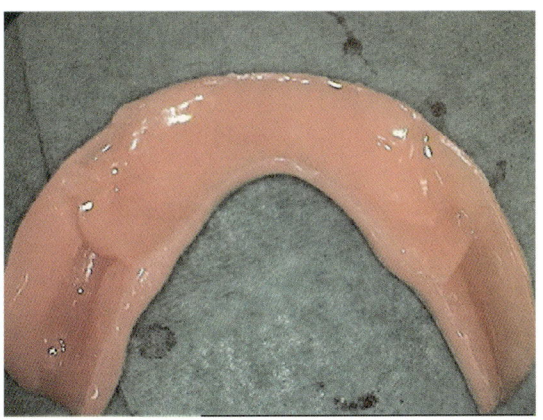

Painted cold-cured polymer

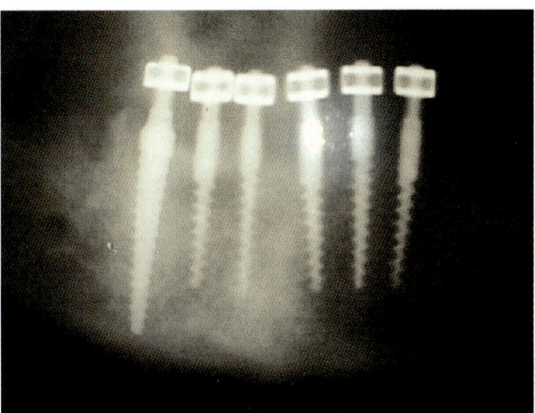

Panoramic radiographic control

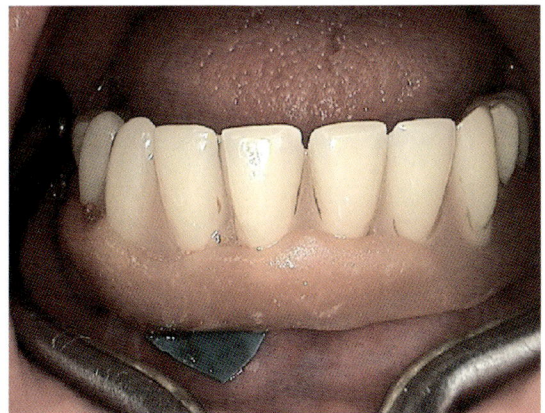

Polymerisation process with mound-closed impression taking

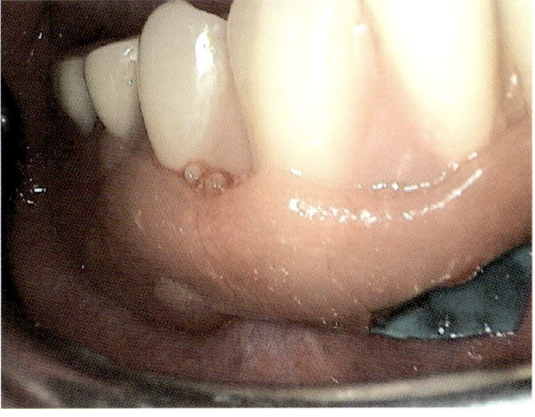

Detailed image

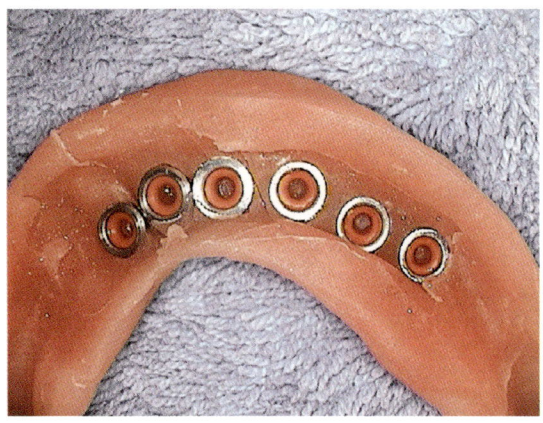

Before the preparation of the prosthesis, basal view

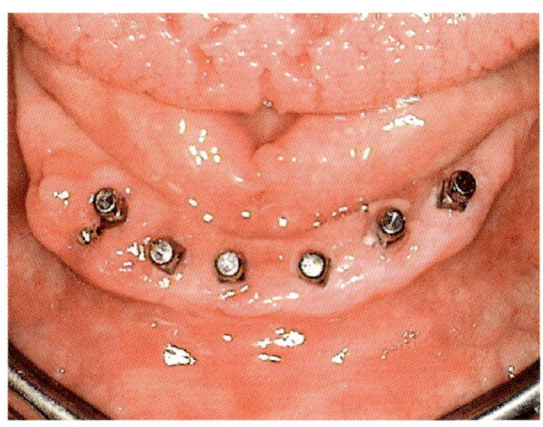

1st postoperative day

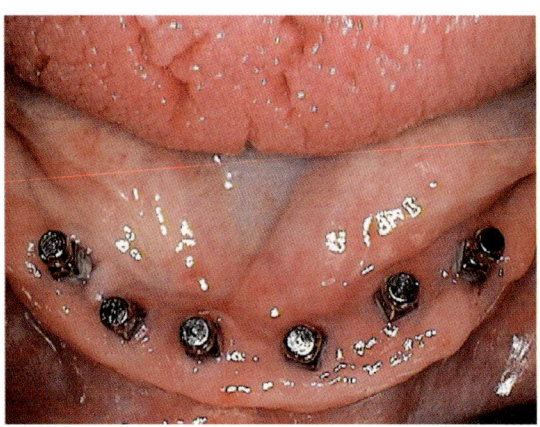

Clinical situation after more than 6 months, occlusal view

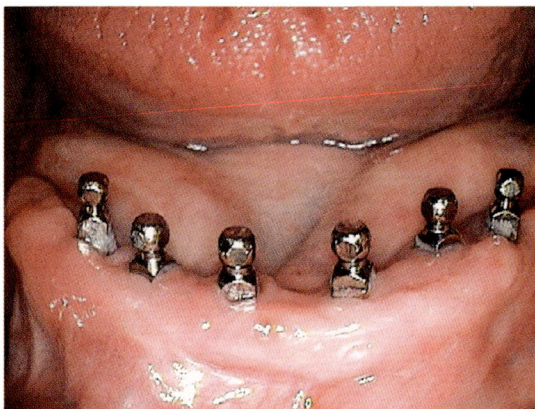

Clinical situation after more than 6 months, anterior view

7.5.6/Case 44

Patient: female, 56 years old

8 upper jaw implants, direct matrix integration

07/02/2011	Upper jaw	Restoration: Reworking to an overdenture Space (tooth 14-24) for implants and matrices as well as for vestibule thickening in order to reduce wrinkles of the upper jaw lip section
	13	extraction
08/02/2011	14-24	8 inserted Champions® "tulips"-implants 8 cured matrices (metal matrices for tulips)
05/04/2011	21	Periotest +22 explantation, no additional implant placement planned planned rebasing
Treatment period:		**2 hours**
Remarks:	21 13	explantation 21 → no additional implant placement! immediate implant placement Always only 1 surgery! That means: we also insert into critical regions upon the danger that individual implants do not osseointegrate. The goal is one surgical procedure without additional implant placement. The empirical benefit of this method is extremely high!

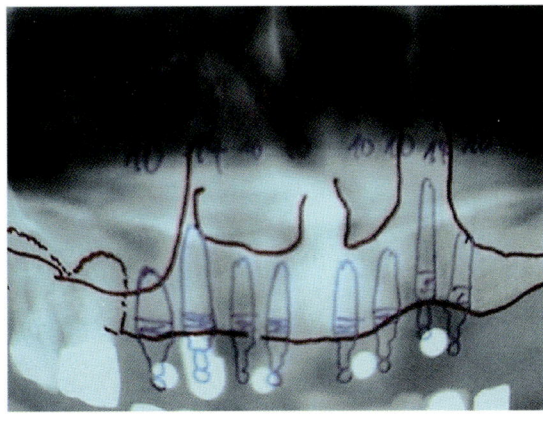

Panoramic radiograph for planned treatment

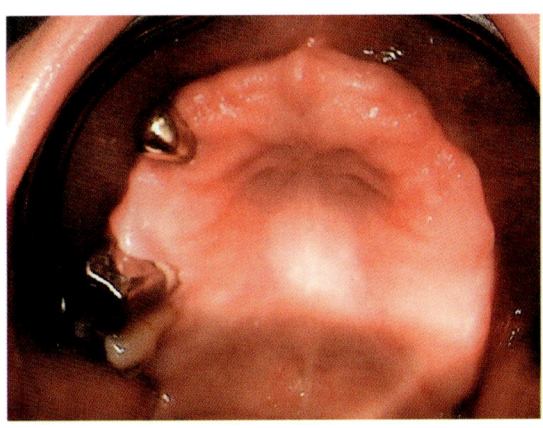

Clinical initial situation

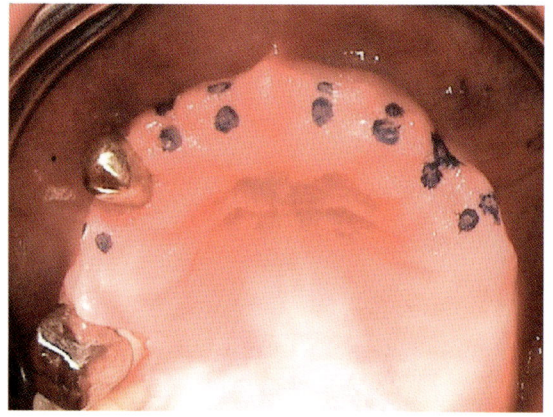

Marked points for planned pilot hole preparation

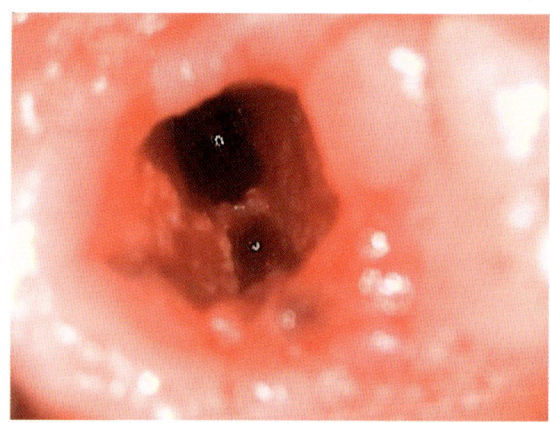

New drilled hole in regio 13

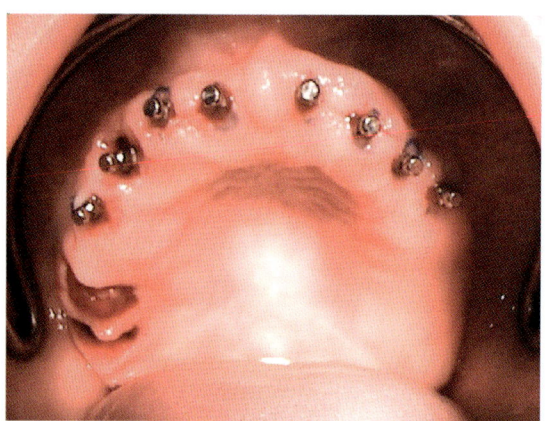

Completed implant placement

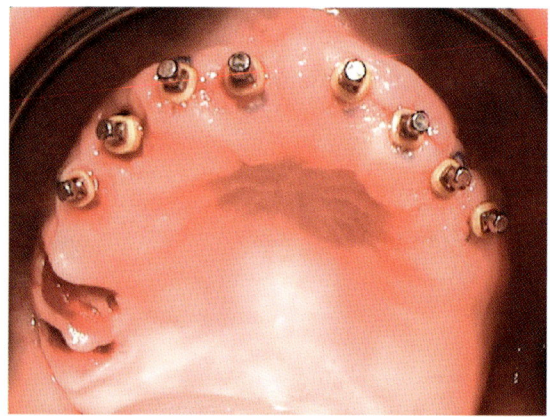

Protection of the implant heads of resin by placed rubber rings

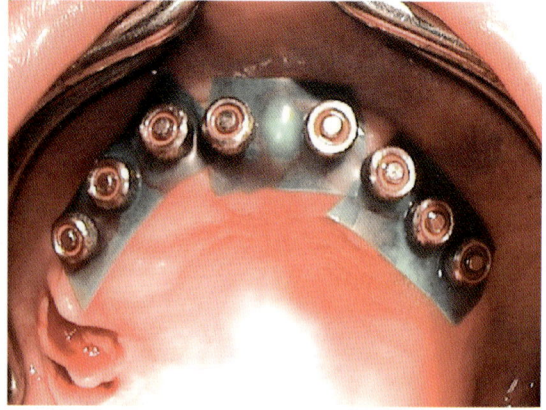

Protection of the gingiva by a rubber dam

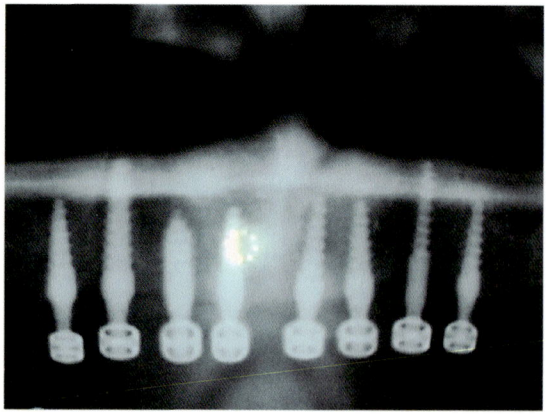

Panoramic radiographic control

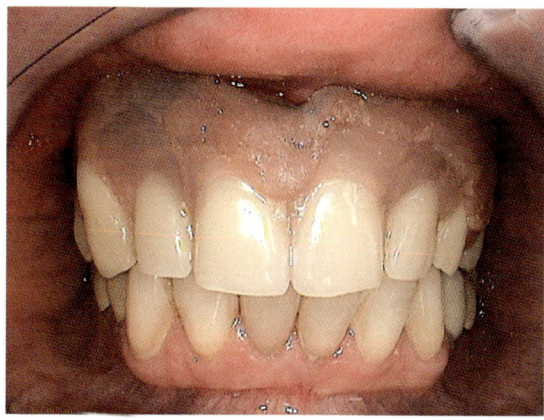

Completed polymerisation process of the matrices, anterior view

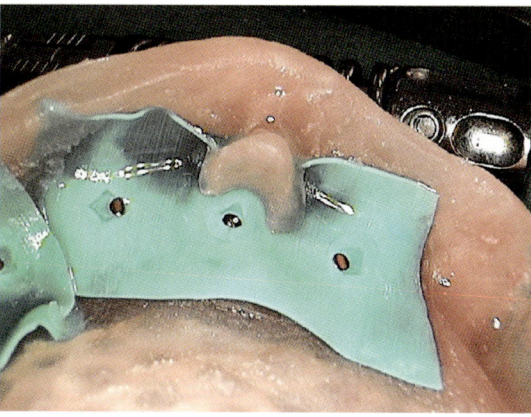

Completed polymerisation process of the matrices, detailed view

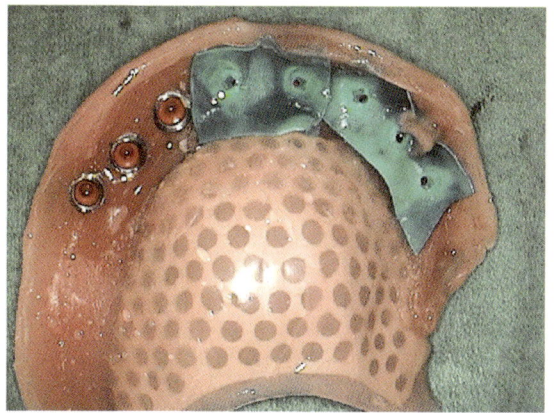

Completed polymerisation process of the matrices, view of the denture base

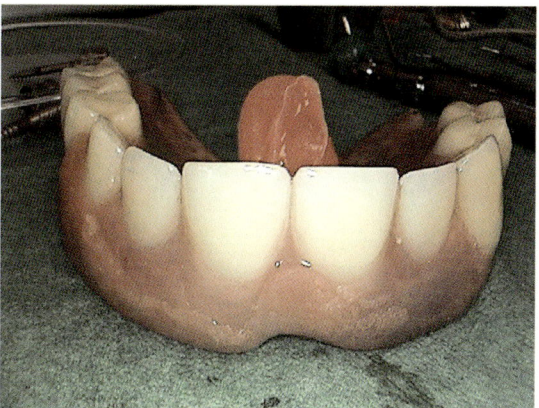

Completed polymerisation process, acrylic-resin surplus

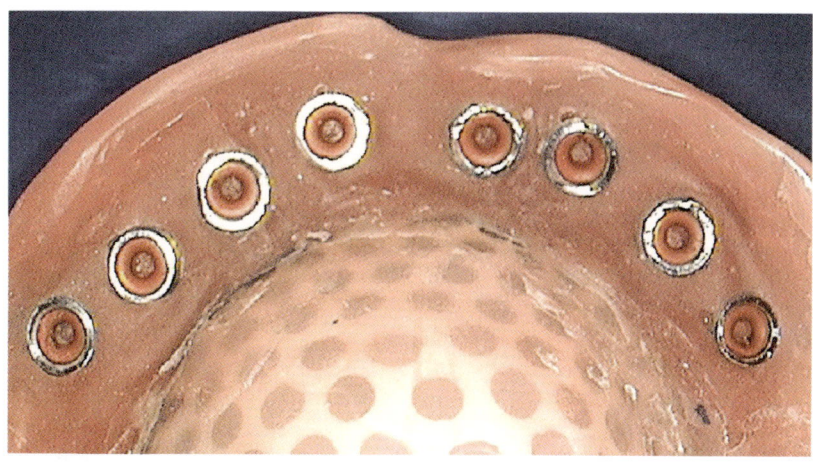

Prepared and polished prosthesis

7.5.7/Case 45

Patient: male, 46 years old

5x extraction, 8 upper jaw implants, augmentation, direct cementing of the matrices into the prosthesis

---

December 2010		Manufactured upper jaw overdenture
03/01/2011	23	osteotomy, autologous bone removed
	15,14,13,21,	extraction
	22	extraction
	15	Champions® implant Ø 4.5 x 10 mm, >30 Ncm
	14	Champions® implant Ø 4.5 x 12 mm, >40 Ncm
	13	Champions® implant Ø 4.0 x 18 mm, 30 Ncm
	12	Champions® implant Ø 4.0 x 12 mm, >50 Ncm
	11	Champions® implant Ø 4.5 x 12 mm, >40 Ncm
	21	Champions® implant Ø 3.5 x 12 mm, >40 Ncm
	22	Champions® implant Ø 4.0 x 14 mm, 30 Ncm
	23	Champions® implant Ø 4.0 x 16 mm, 30 Ncm
	15,14,22,23	bone augmentation, suture
		8 incorporated matrices
04/01/2011		Wound control
Treatment period:		**2.5 hours**
Remarks:		Immediate implant placement
		Immediate loading
		Augmentation with autologous bone
		Due to financial reasons the patient opted for a removable denture solution.

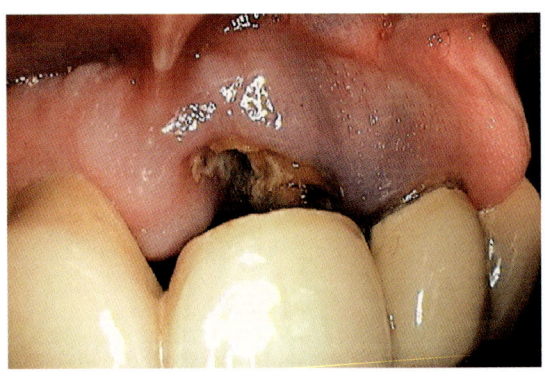

Detailed image of tooth 21

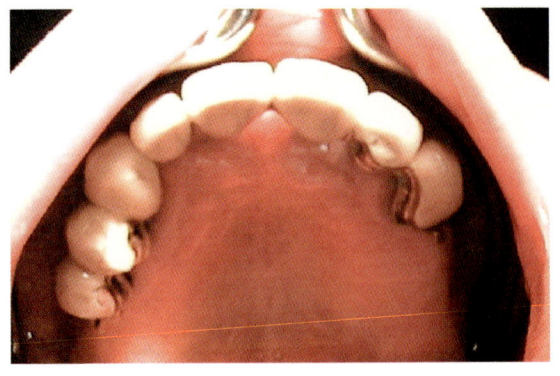

Clinical initial situation

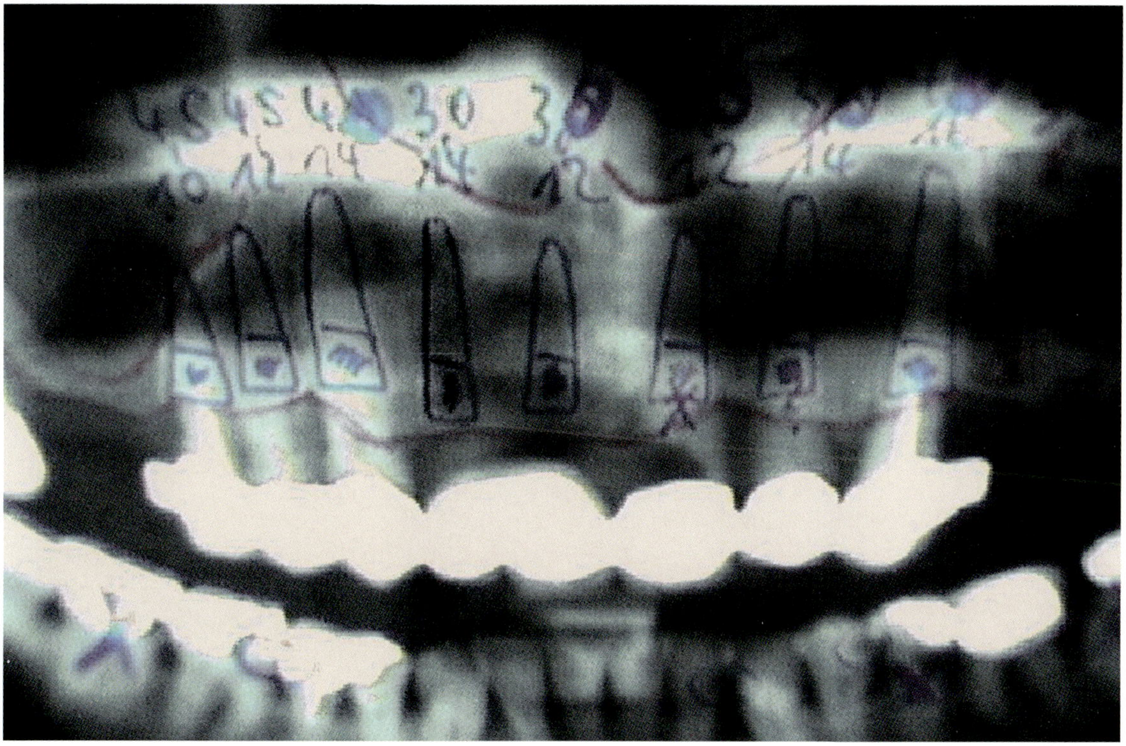

Panoramic radiograph for planned treatment

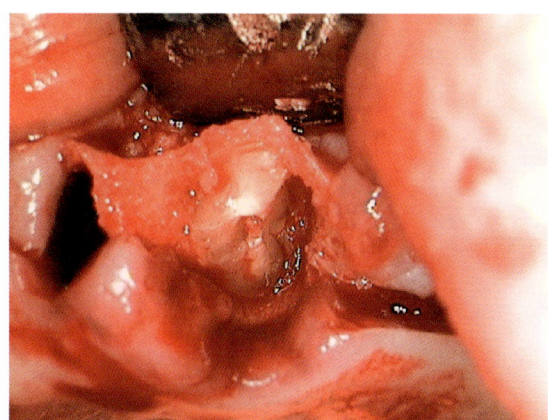

Osteotomy 23

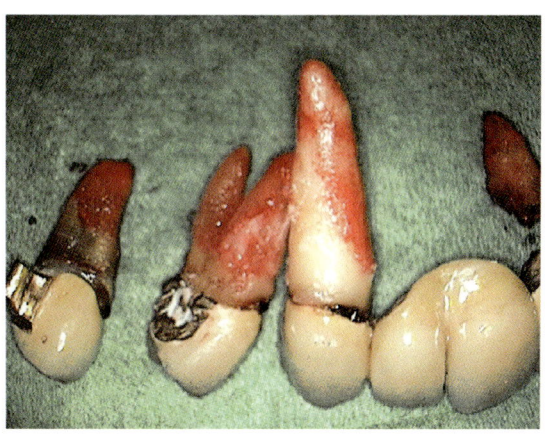

Extracted teeth

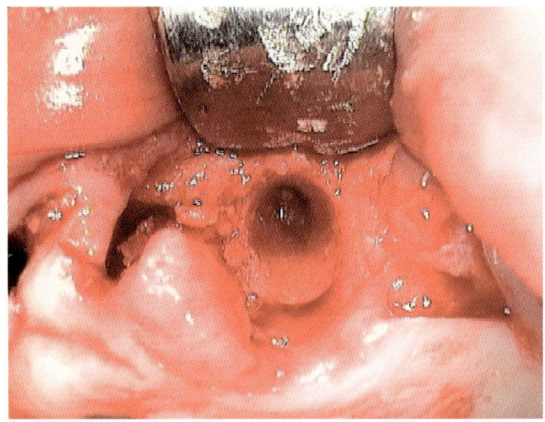

Alveolus 23 after extraction

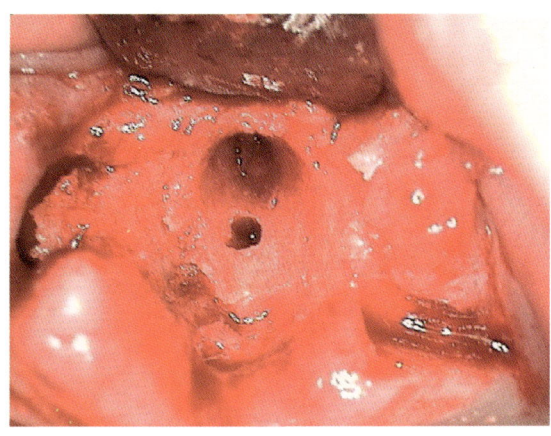

Palatal initial pilot hole preparation in regio 23...

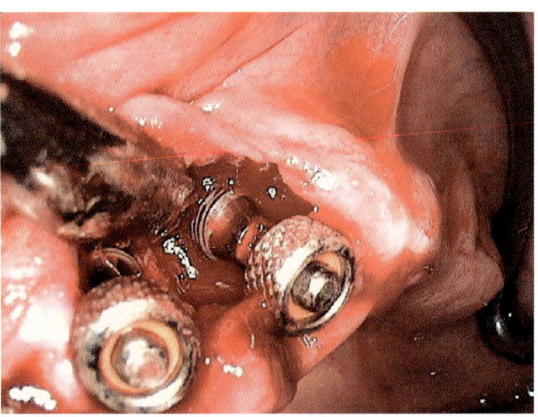

...and implant placement

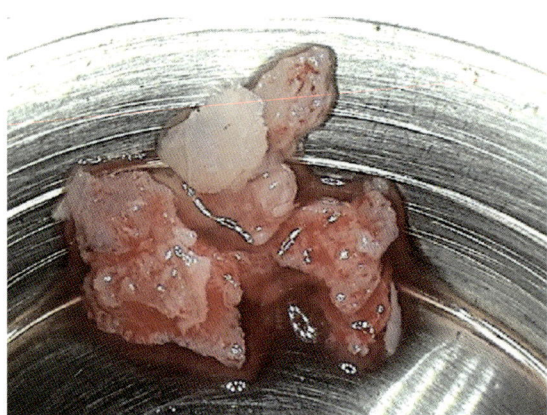

Autologous bone

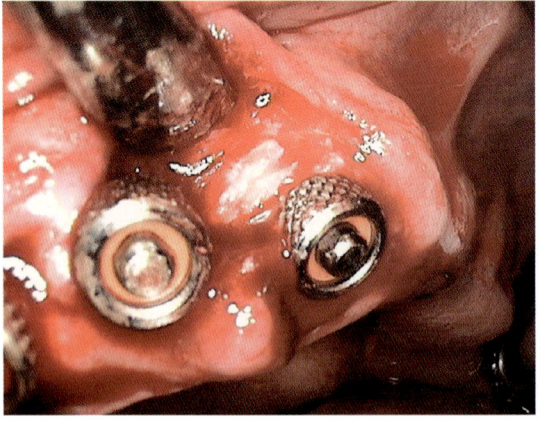

Augmentation in regio 23

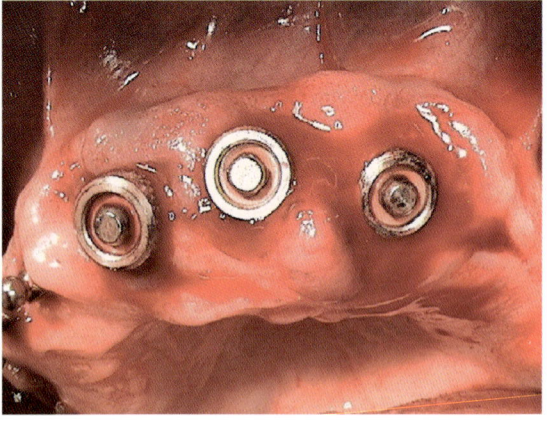

Situation after augmentation in regio 23

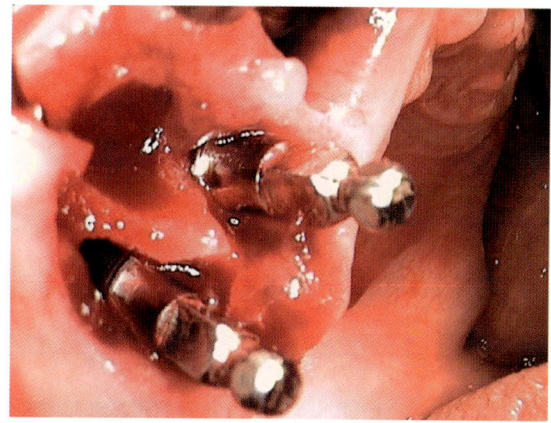

Implant placement in regio 14, 15

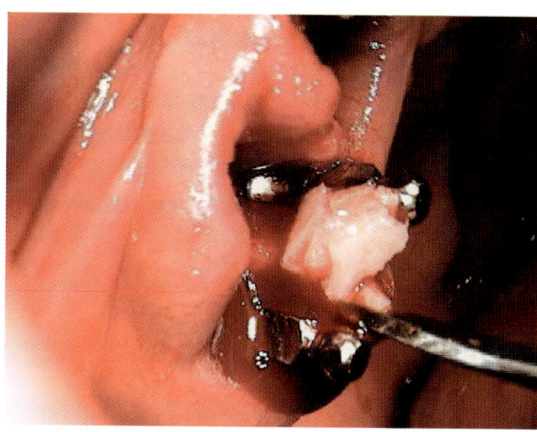

Augmentation in regio 14, 15

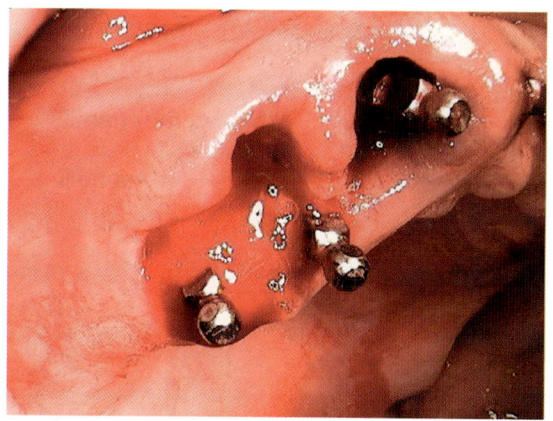

After augmentations in regio 14, 15

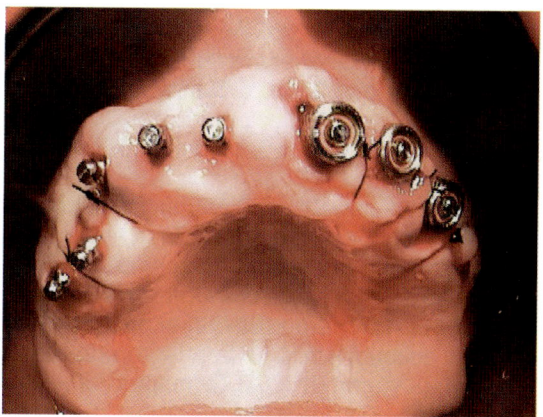

Completed implant placement

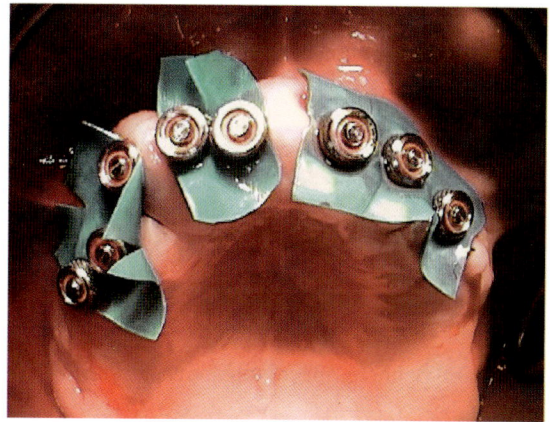

The rubber dam is placed in order to protect the gingiva

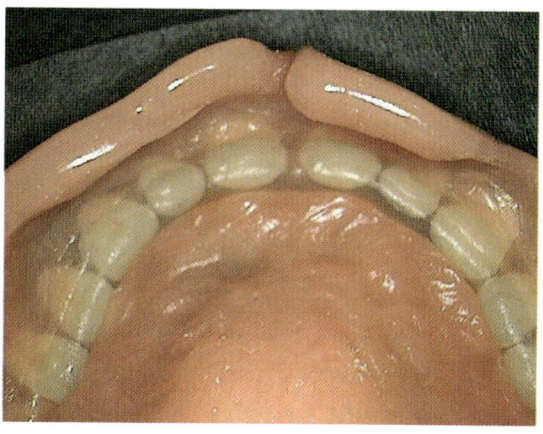

Prepared prosthesis

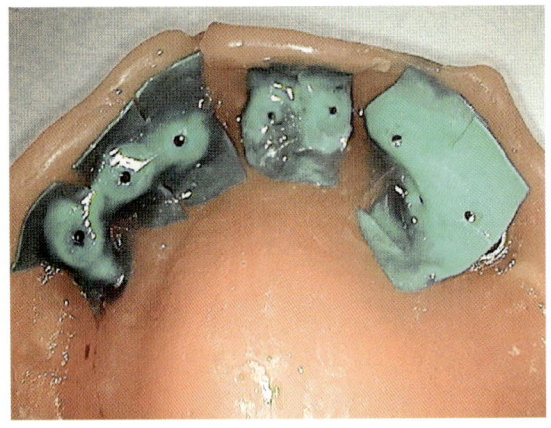

Directly after polymerisation process, basal view

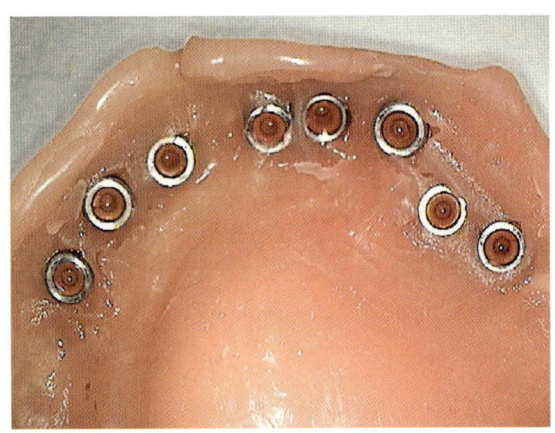

Before prosthesis preparation

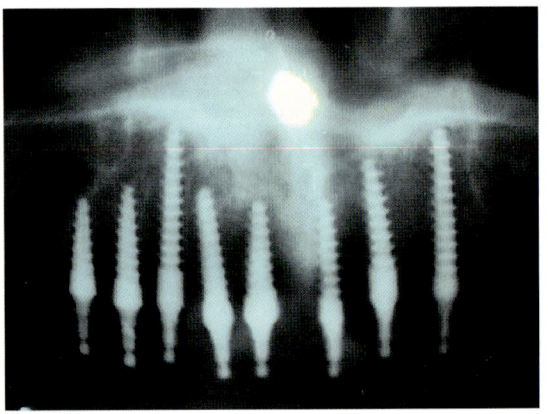

Panoramic radiographic control

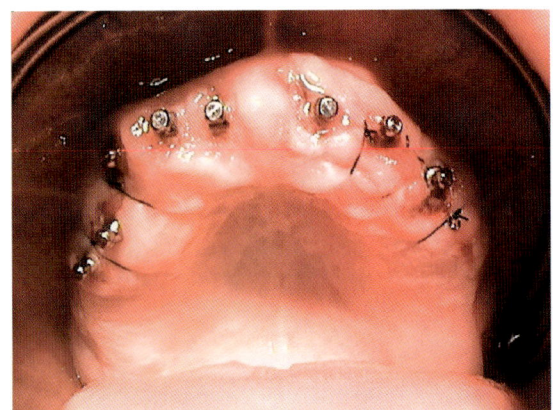

1st postoperative day

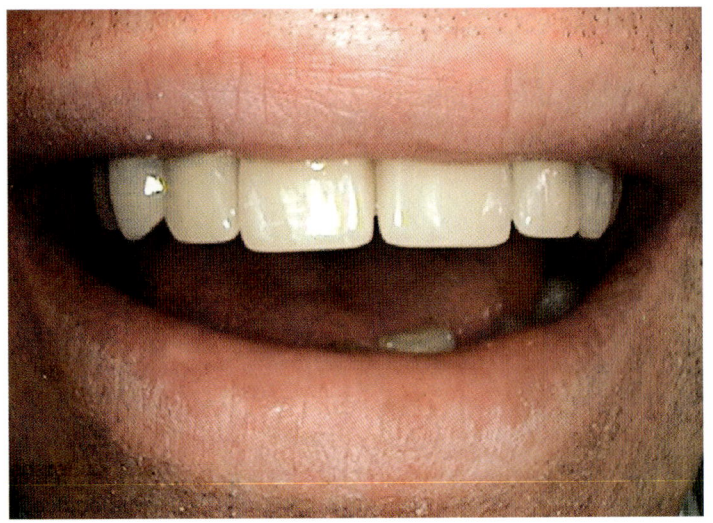

1st postoperative day, lip

7.5.8/Case 46

Patient: female, 50 years old

10 implants in the upper jaw, augmentation, integration of matrices, ball head shortening

---

10/02/2011	13,23	extraction
	15	Champions® implant Ø 3.5 x 10 mm, 30 Ncm
	14	Champions® implant Ø 3.0 x 14 mm, 20 Ncm, open procedure, bone augmentation
	13	Champions® implant Ø 4.0 x 18 mm, 30 Ncm, open procedure, bone augmentation, bone chips
	12	Champions® implant Ø 3.0 x 14 mm, >30 Ncm
	11	Champions® implant Ø 3.0 x 14 mm, >40 Ncm
	21	Champions® implant Ø 3.0 x 14 mm, >30 Ncm
	22	Champions® implant Ø 3.0 x 14 mm, 40 Ncm
	23	Champions® implant Ø 4.0 x 16 mm, 50 Ncm, open procedure, bone augmentation
	24	Champions® implant Ø 4.0 x 14 mm, >30 Ncm, open procedure, bone augmentation
	25	Champions® implant Ø 3.5 x 10 mm, 25 Ncm, open procedure, bone augmentation
11/02/2011	12	wound control vestibular ball head reduction
21/02/2011		Suture removal
04/04/2011	15-25	control after osseointegration images
Treatment period:		**2 hours**
Remarks:		Cysts!
	13,23	immediate implant placement immediate loading augmentation with bone chips ball head implant in regio 12, prepared from vestibular in order to optimise the insertion of the prosthesis

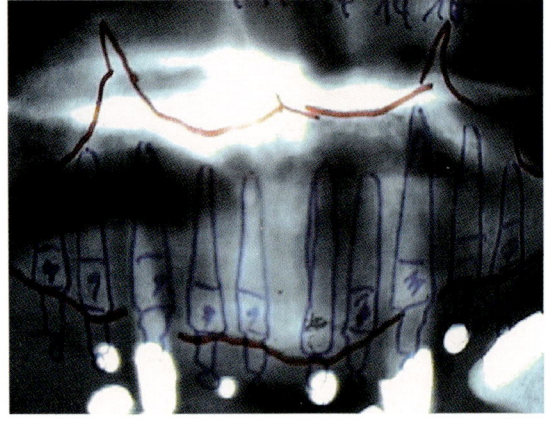

Panoramic radiograph for planned treatment

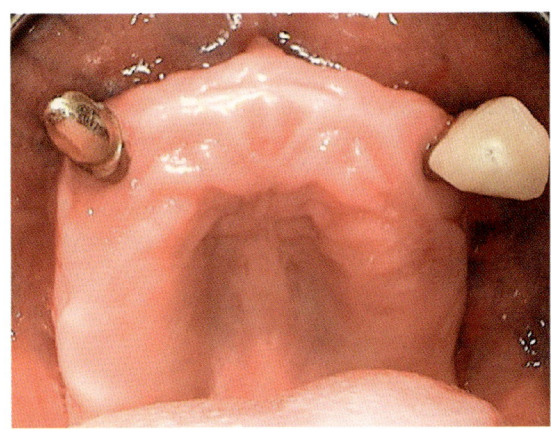

Clinical situation,

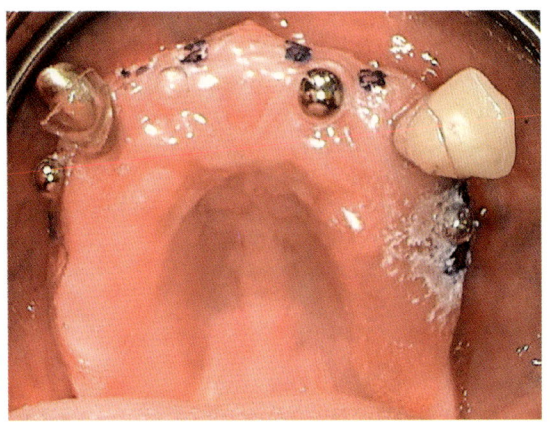

Overlay template in situ

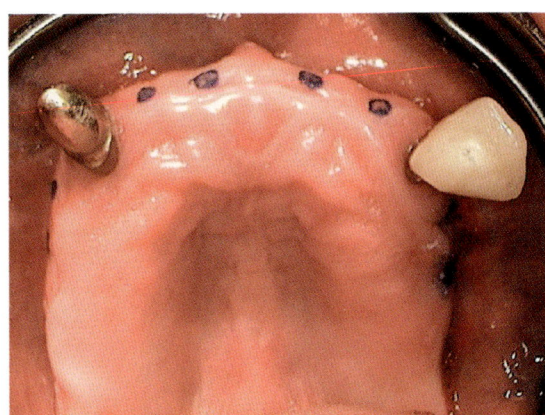

Vestibular markings

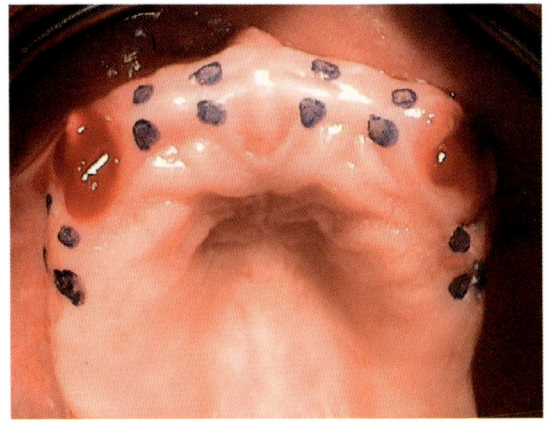

Transfer of the markings to the insertion points

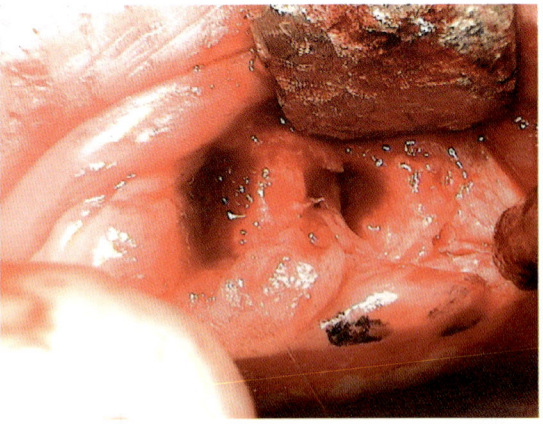

Open procedure in regio 23-25

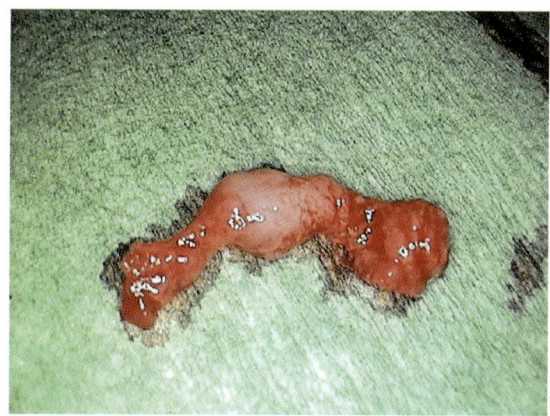

Granulation tissue in regio 23-25

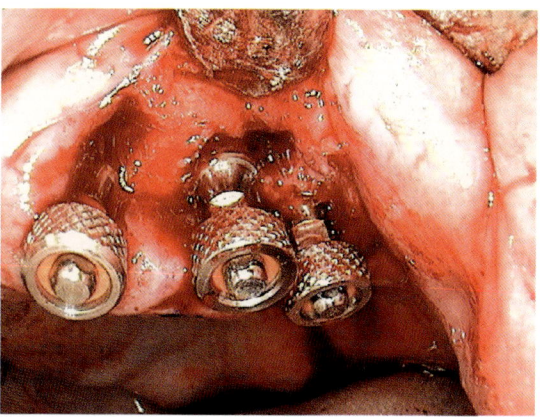

Implant placement in region 23-25 with attached metal matrices for tulips

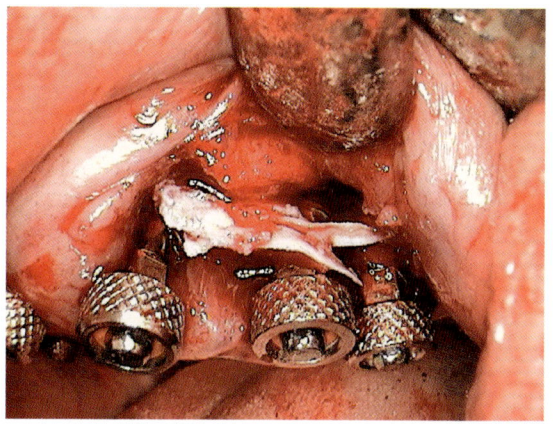

Augmentation in regio 23-25 with bone chips

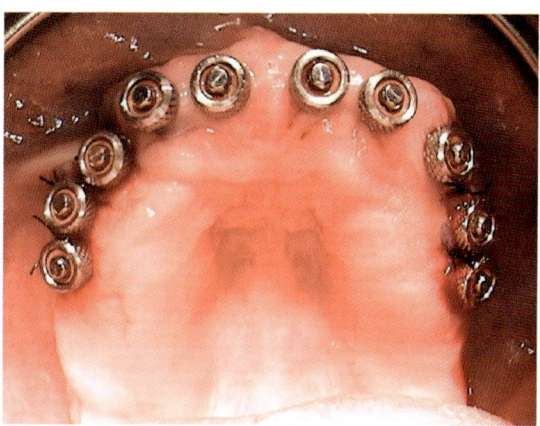

Completed implant placement

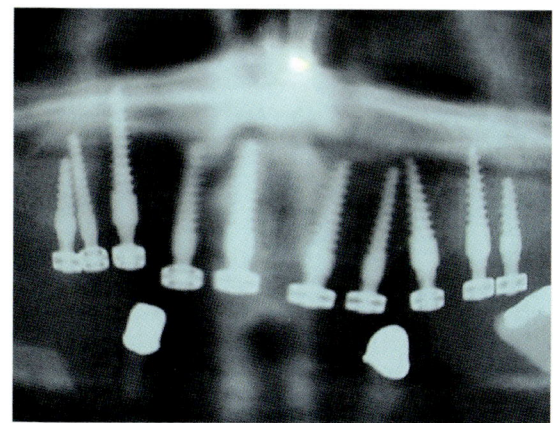

Panoramic radiographic control

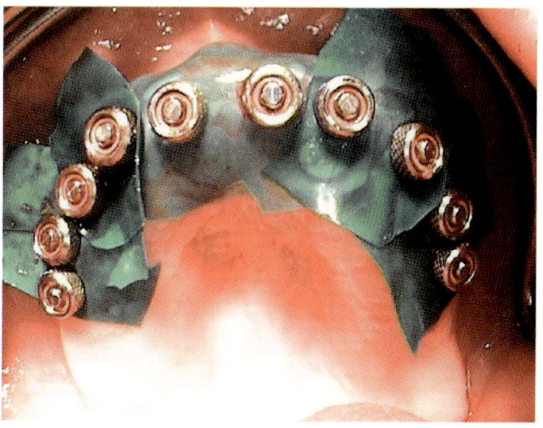

Rubber dam protects the gingiva and the implants from the flowing in of cold -cured polymer

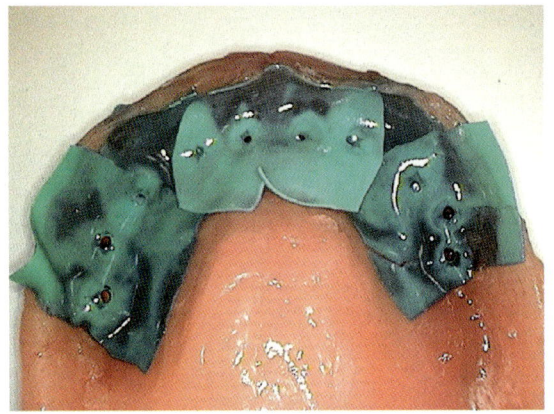

Prosthesis after matrix polymerisation process...

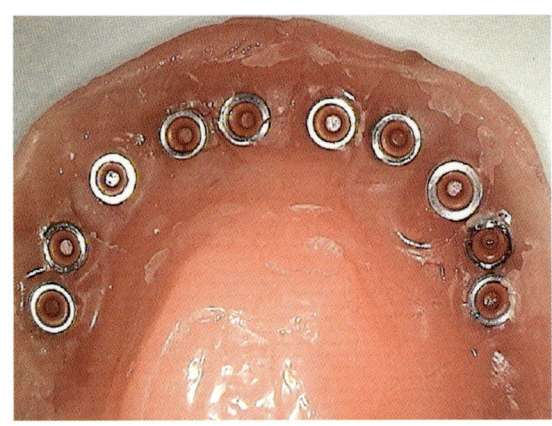

...and removal of the rubber dam...

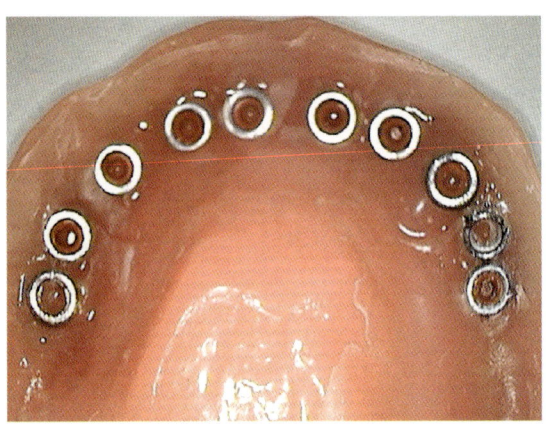

...and dense contouring

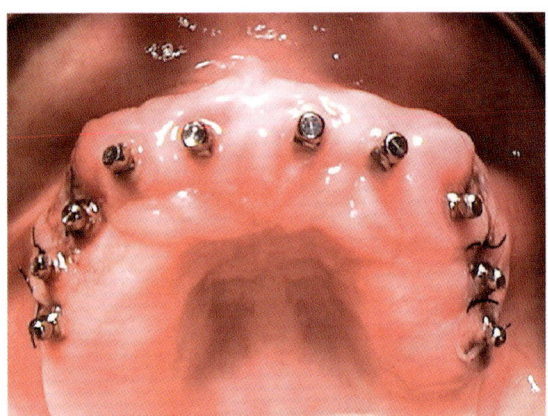

1st postoperative day

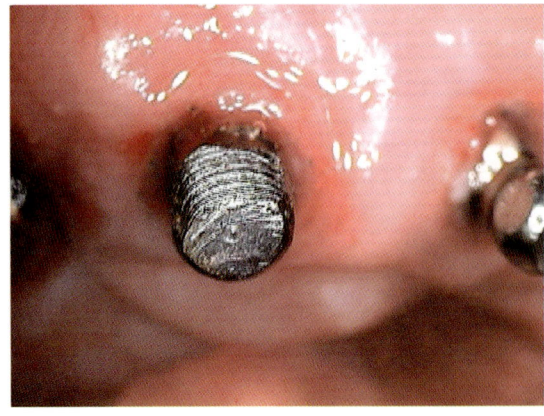

Ball head implant in regio 12, from vestibular reduced...

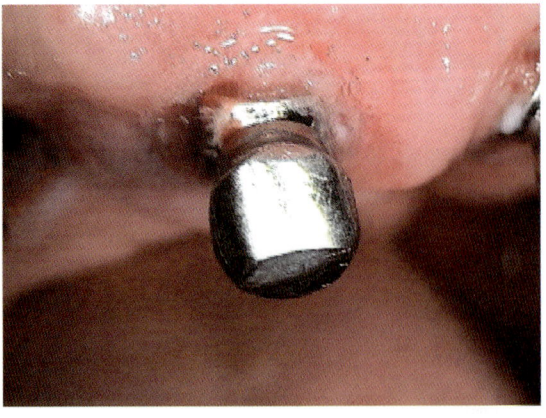

...and polished

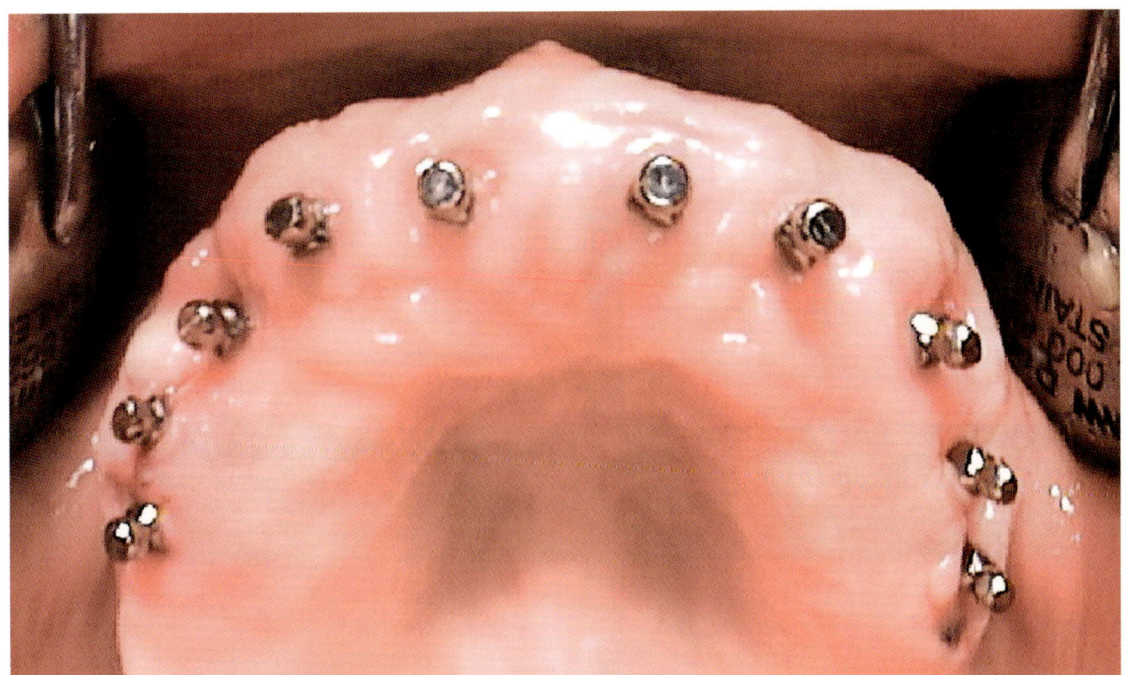

After osseointegration

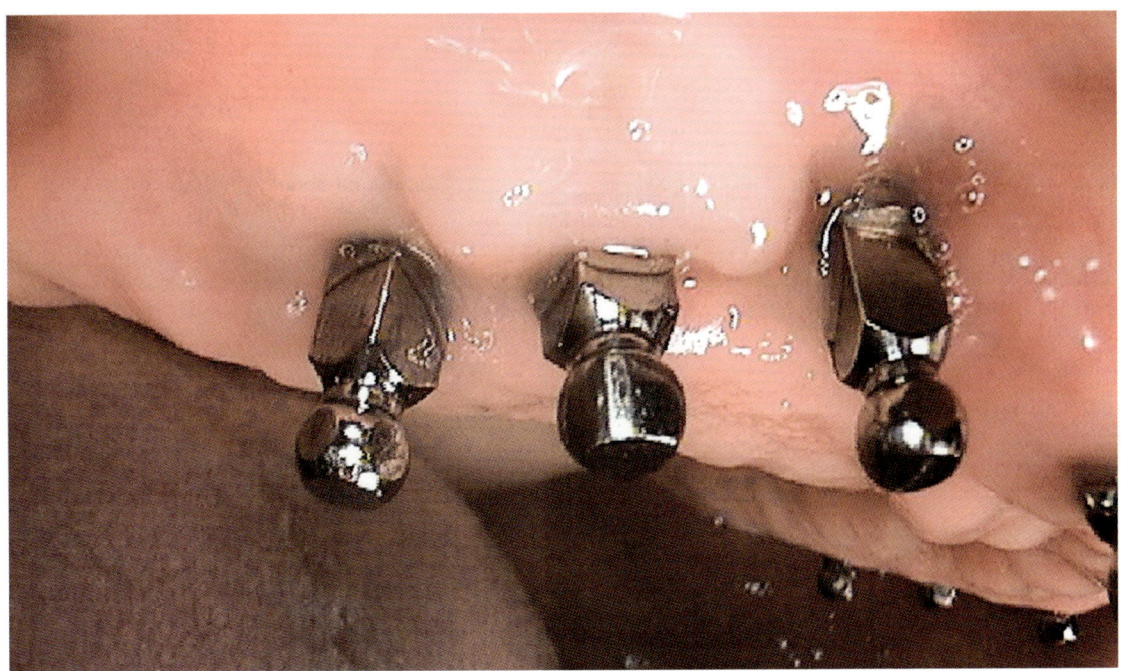

Detailed view

7.5.9/Case 47

Patient: female, 54 years old

6 x upper jaw extraction, 15-25 implants, 15 explanted, palatal free upper jaw prosthesis after osseointegration

---

16/12/2010	17, 16,11	Crown and bridge isolation
	21, 23,26	extraction
	15	extraction
	14	Champions® implant Ø 4.5 x 10 mm, 20 Ncm
	13	Champions® implant Ø 3.5 x 10 mm, 30 Ncm
	12	Champions® implant Ø 3.5 x 12 mm, 40 Ncm
	11	Champions® implant Ø 3.5 x 12 mm, 40 Ncm,
	21	Champions® implant Ø 4.5 x 10 mm, >40 Ncm
	22	Champions® implant Ø 4.5 x 10 mm, >40 Ncm
	23	Champions® implant Ø 3.5 x 12 mm, >40 Ncm
	24	Champions® implant Ø 3.0 x 14 mm, >40 Ncm
	25	Champions® implant Ø 3.5 x 10 mm, >20 Ncm
	24, 25	Champions® implant Ø 4.5 x 10 mm, >20 Ncm
		open maxillary sinus, suture
		Matrices (metal matrices for tulips and Preci-Clix) cured into denture resin
20/12/2010		
		Wound control, panoramic radiograph
23/12/2010	15	
		Wound control
	Upper jaw	explanted
March 2011		
		new palatal free prosthesis
11/10/2011		
		taking of control radiographs due to a planned lower jaw new restoration, images
Treatment period:		
		2.5 hours
Remarks:		
		Endotracheal anaesthesia
		No taking of panoramic radiographs during endotracheal anaesthesia possible.
		No additional implant placement required since 8 implants are sufficient for a palatal free restoration!
		Immediate implant placement
		Immediate loading

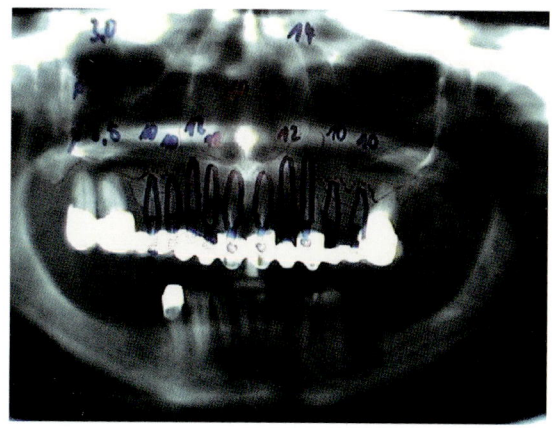

Panoramic radiograph for planned treatment

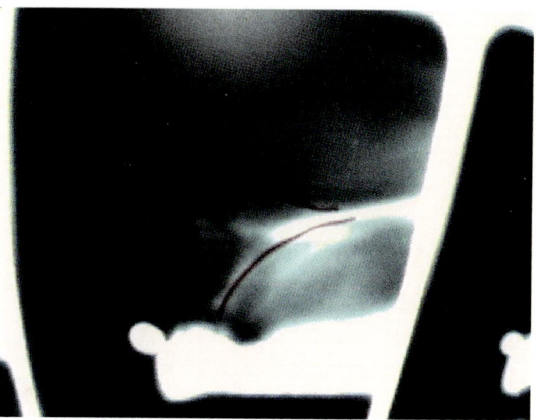

Cross-sectional radiography

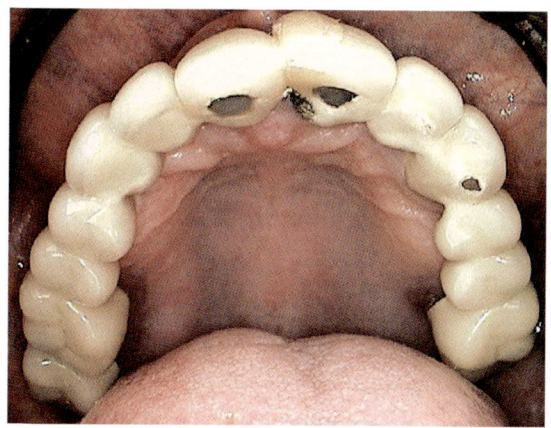

Clinical initial findings, occlusal view

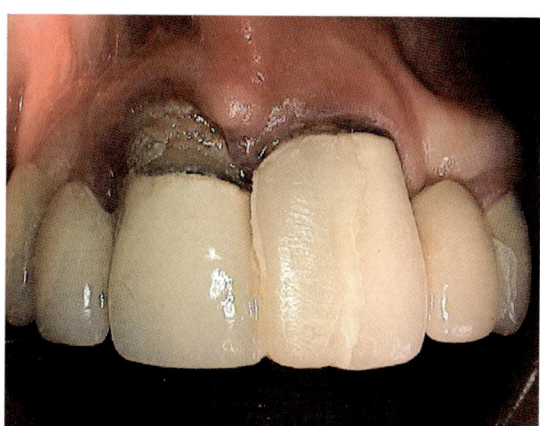

Clinical initial findings,
anterior detailed image

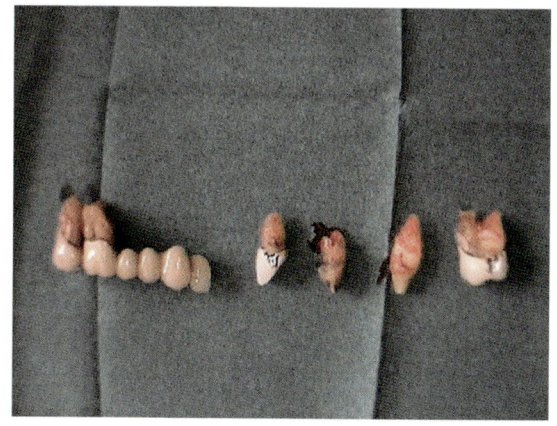

Extracted teeth

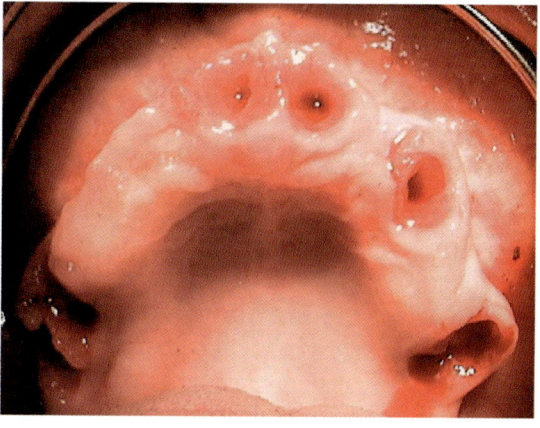

Situation after extraction

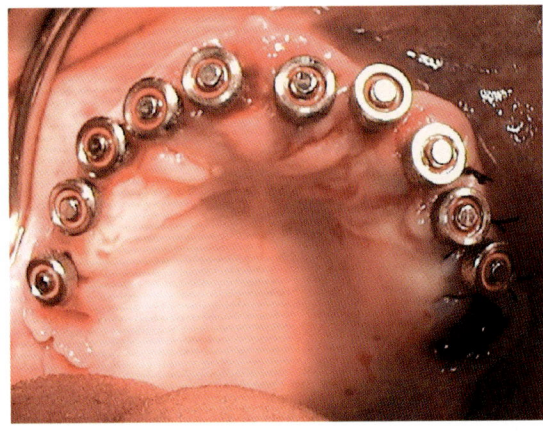

Completed implant placement, attached matrices

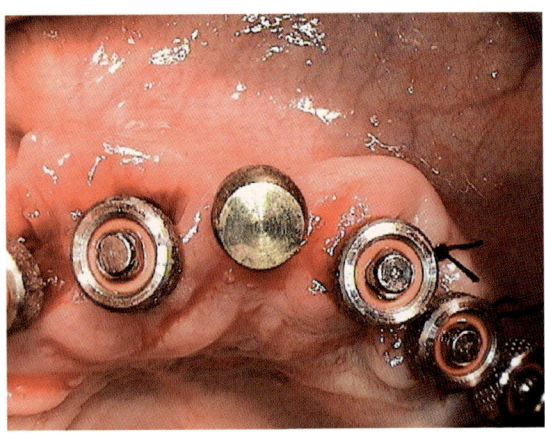

Selection of a Preci-Clix matrix for compensating differences in regio 22

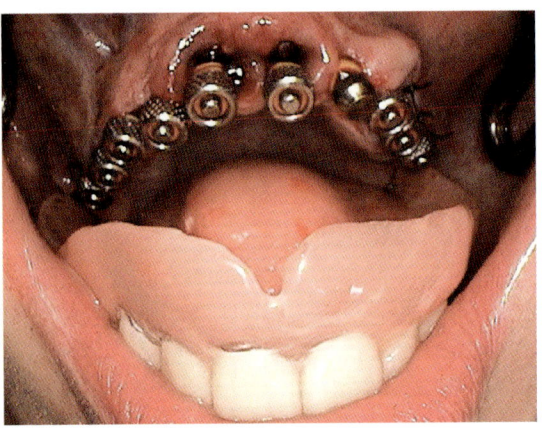

Control of the ground cavity for matrices

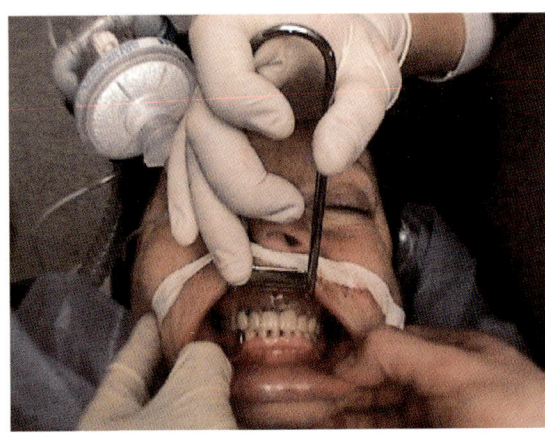

Control of proper occlusion

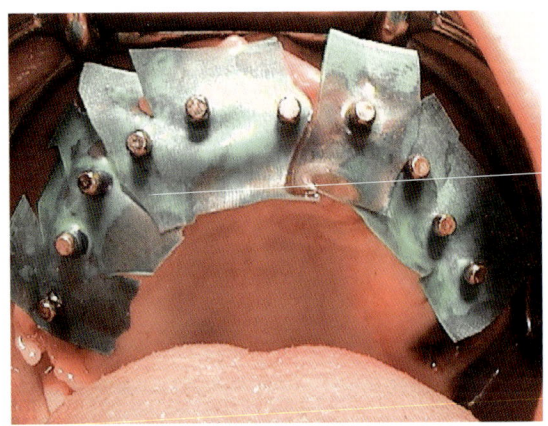

Rubber dam to protect the gingiva

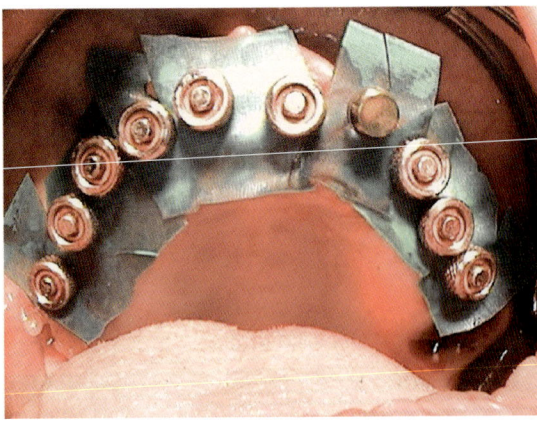

Attached and isolated matrices before the polymerisation process

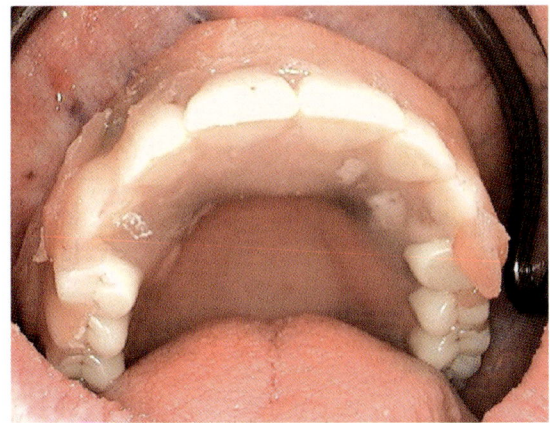

Completed polymerisation process of the matrices, occlusal view

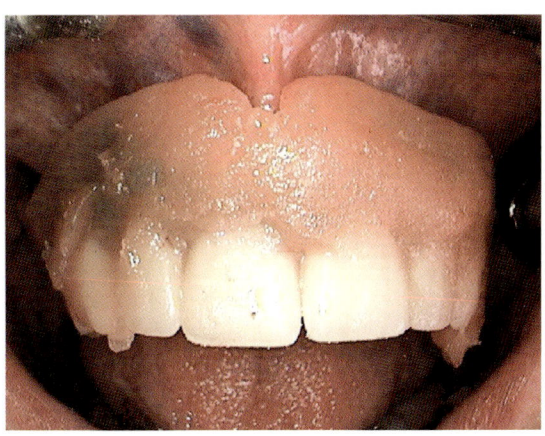

Completed polymerisation process of the matrices, anterior view

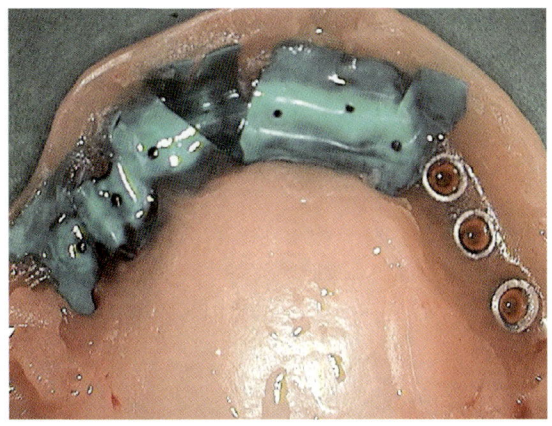

Completed polymerisation process of the matrices, basal view

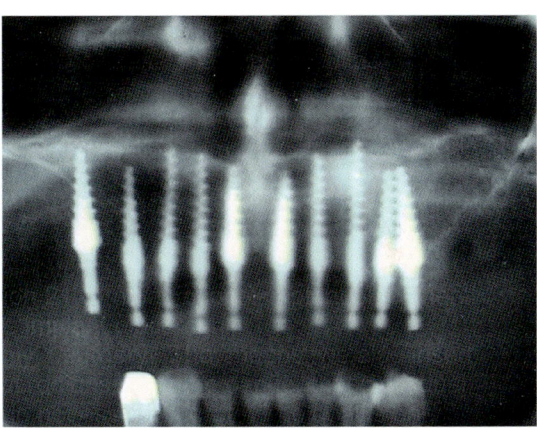

Final radiographic control

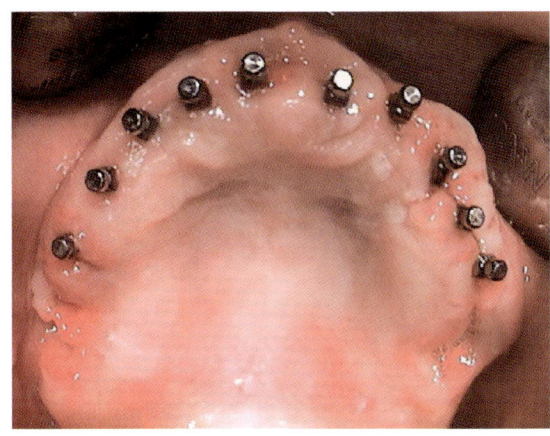

Wound control, before explantation in regio 15

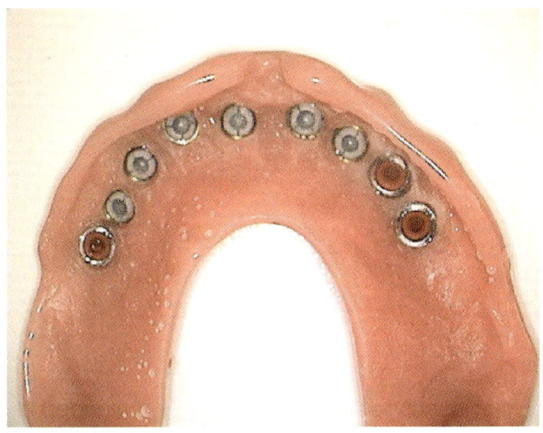

New palatal free prosthesis

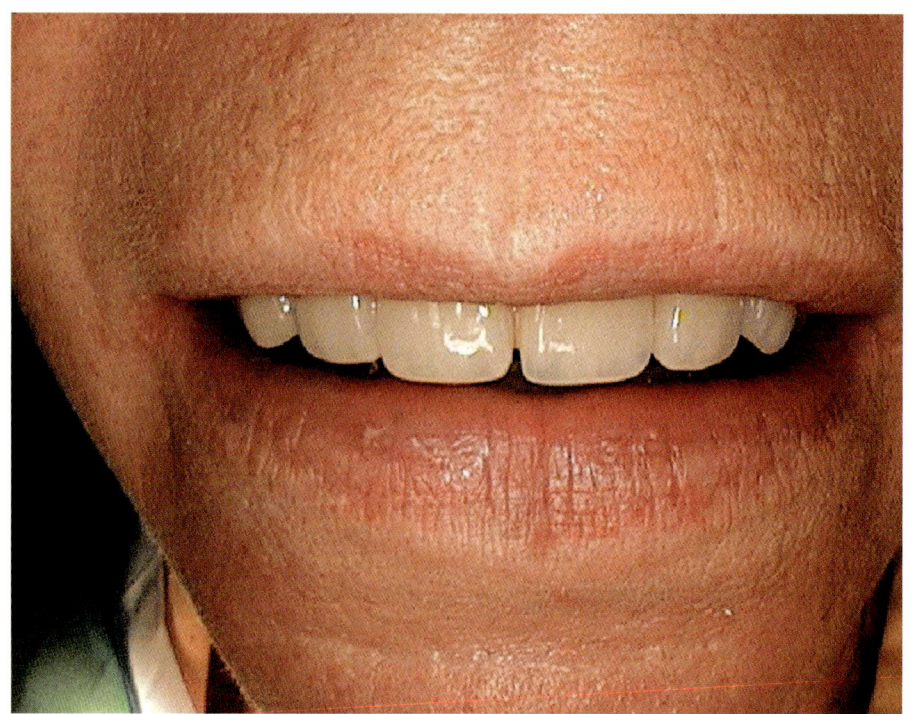

New palatal free prosthesis in situ

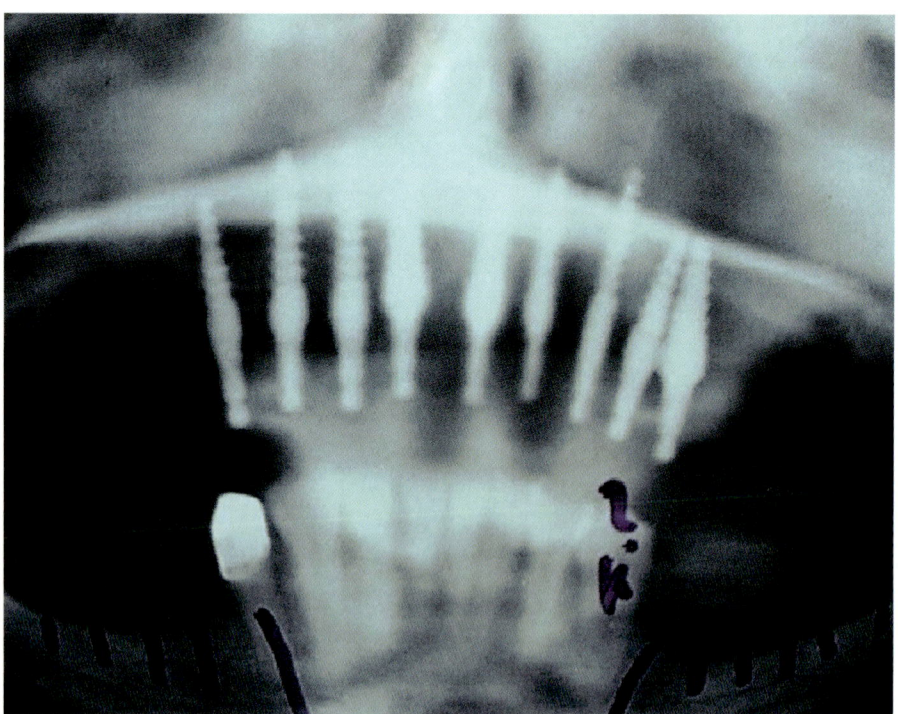

Panoramic radiographic control, situation after 10 months

7.5.10/Case 48

Patient: male, 52 years old

10 upper jaw implants, 10 matrices directly cured into denture resin

---

01/08/2011	15	Champions® implant Ø 3.0 x 8 mm, 40 Ncm, Periotest +2
	14	Champions® implant Ø 3.0 x 12 mm, 40 Ncm, Periotest +1
	13	Champions® implant Ø 3.0 x 12 mm, 40 Ncm, Periotest +2
	12	Champions® implant Ø 3.0 x 12 mm, 40 Ncm, Periotest +2
	11	Champions® implant Ø 3.0 x 12 mm, >50 Ncm, Periotest +2
	21	Champions® implant Ø 3.0 x 12 mm, 60 Ncm, Periotest +2
	22	Champions® implant Ø 3.5 x 10 mm, 60 Ncm, Periotest 0
	23	Champions® implant Ø 3.5 x 10 mm, >40 Ncm, Periotest 0
	24	Champions® implant Ø 3.0 x 8 mm, 40 Ncm, Periotest +4
	25	Champions® implant Ø 4.0 x 8 mm, 30 Ncm, Periotest +3
		Metal matrices for tulips and Preci-Clix matrices cured into denture resin
02/08/2011		Wound control, images
07/07/2011		Periotest: 15 -1, 14 -1, 13 +2, 12 +2, 11 +2 21 +1, 22 +3, 23 -2, 24 +5, 25 +2
Treatment period:		**2 hours**
Remarks:		Different matrices due to limited space. After implant restoration in the lower jaw a new upper jaw an overdenture is planned. Immediate loading

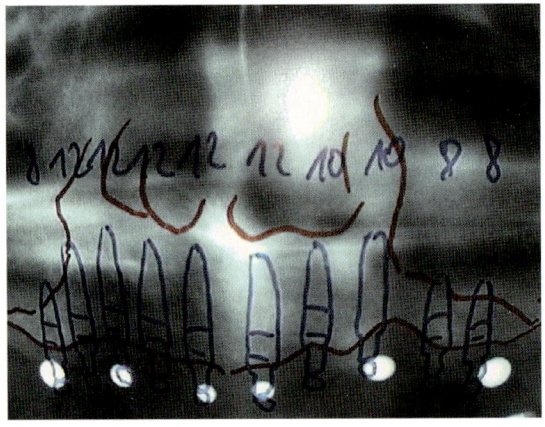

Panoramic radiograph for planned treatment

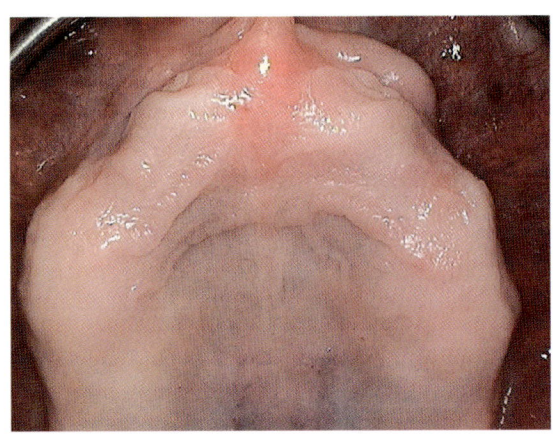

Clinical initial situation

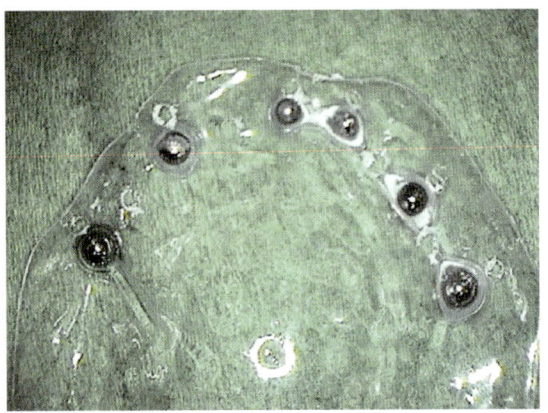

Overlay template

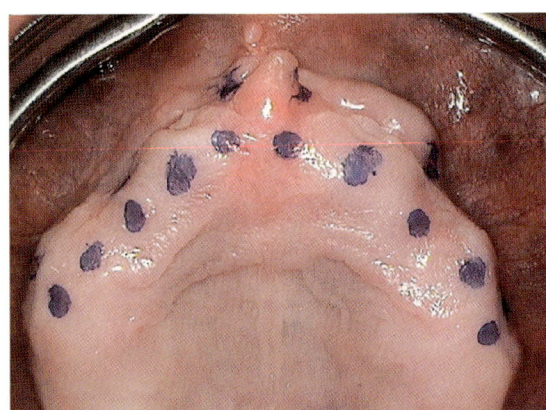

Marked points for initial pilot hole preparation

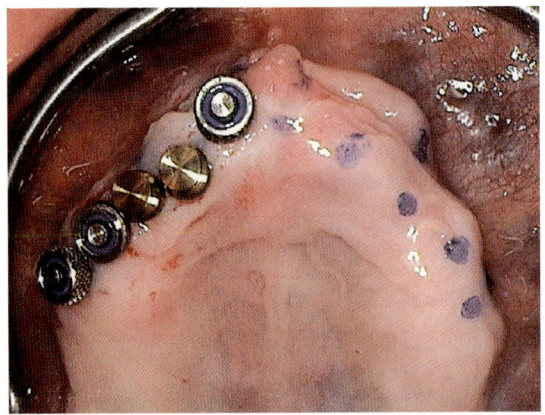

Completed implant placement, right side

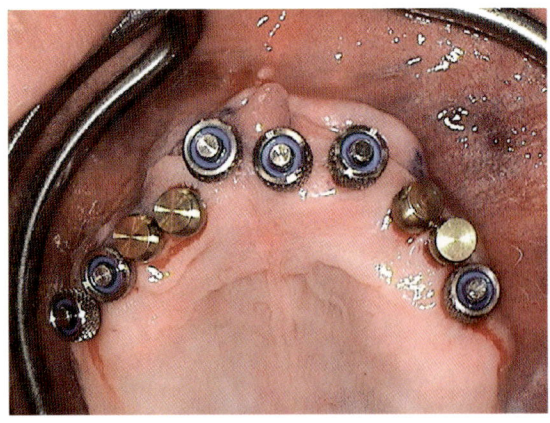

Completed implant placement, left side

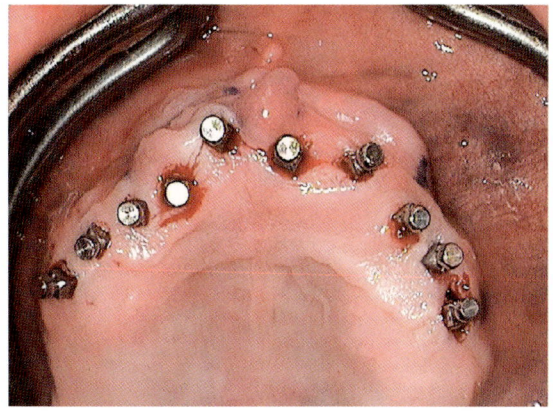

...without matrices

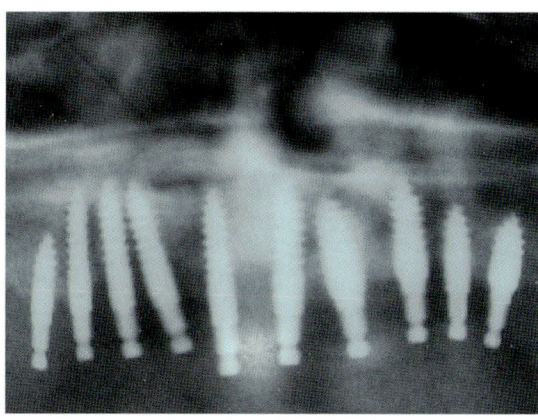

Panoramic radiographic control

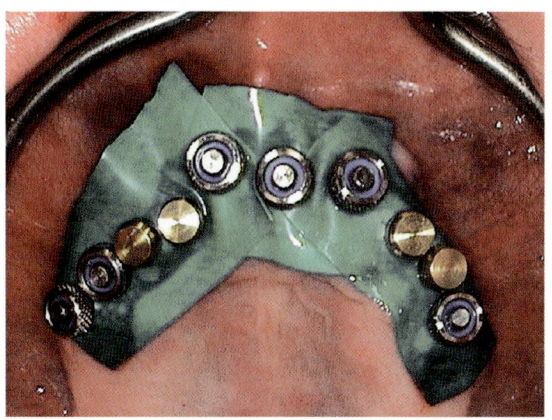

With a rubber dam protected gingiva before polymerisation process

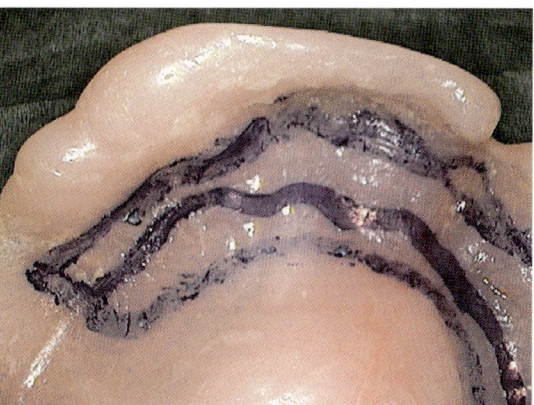

Former prosthesis with marking of the section which has to be ground

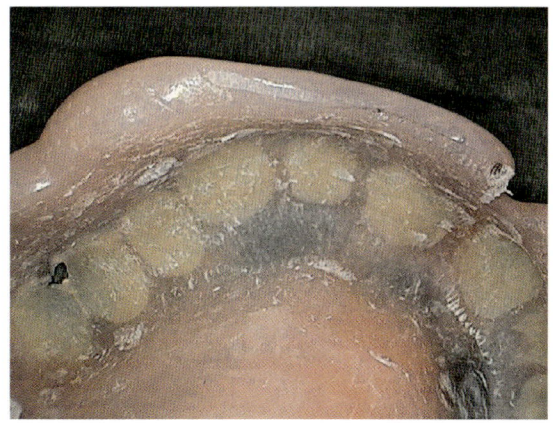

Former prosthesis with ground section

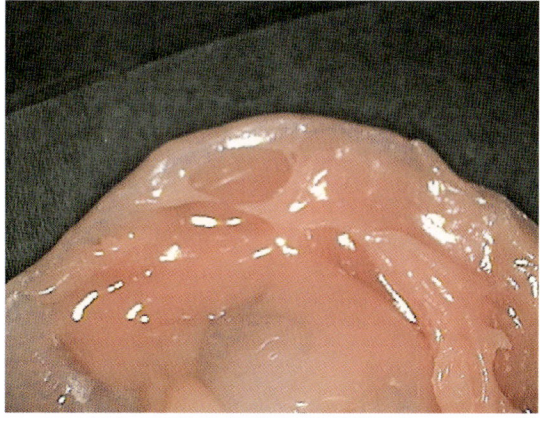

Injected cold-cured polymer

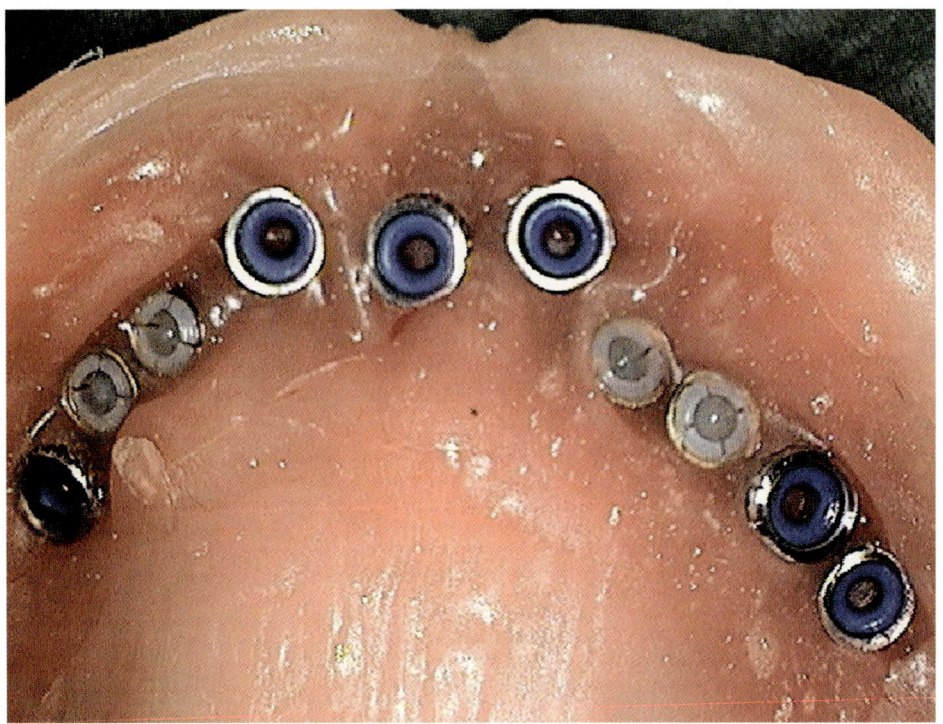

Cured matrices immediately after removal

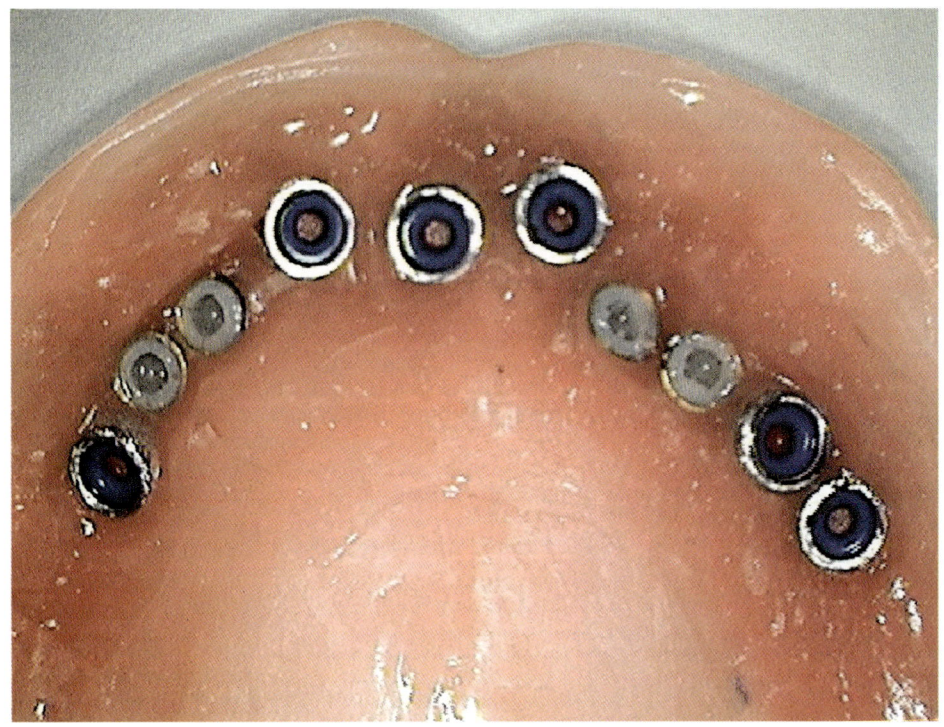

...and after preparation of the prosthesis with final high-gloss polishing

7.5.11/Case 49

Patient: female, 70 years old

15-25 10 tulip head implants with early loading

28/09/2011	Upper jaw	Extension to a metal-free overdenture with gaps in regio 16-26 for matrices
29/09/2011	15	Champions® implant Ø 3.0 x 8 mm, 20 Ncm, Periotest 0
	14	Champions® implant Ø 3.0 x 8 mm, 30 Ncm, Periotest +6
	13	Champions® implant Ø 4.0 x 10 mm, 40 Ncm, Periotest +1
	12	Champions® implant Ø 3.0 x 12 mm, 40 Ncm, Periotest +1
	11	Champions® implant Ø 3.0 x 12 mm, >40 Ncm, Periotest +4
	21	Champions® implant Ø 3.0 x 12 mm, >40 Ncm, Periotest +3
	22	Champions® implant Ø 3.0 x 10 mm, >20 Ncm, Periotest +6
	23	Champions® implant Ø 4.0 x 10 mm, >40 Ncm, Periotest -3
	24	Champions® implant Ø 3.0 x 10 mm, > 30 Ncm, Periotest +3
	25	Champions® implant Ø 3.0 x 8 mm, 20 Ncm, Periotest -3
		10 matrices (blue) cured into the denture resin
04/10/2011		Post-control, images
Treatment period:		**2 hours**
Remarks:		After osseointegration followed the palatal free creation of the prosthesis. Due to financial reasons the patient refused a fixed restoration. Immediate implant placement Immediate loading

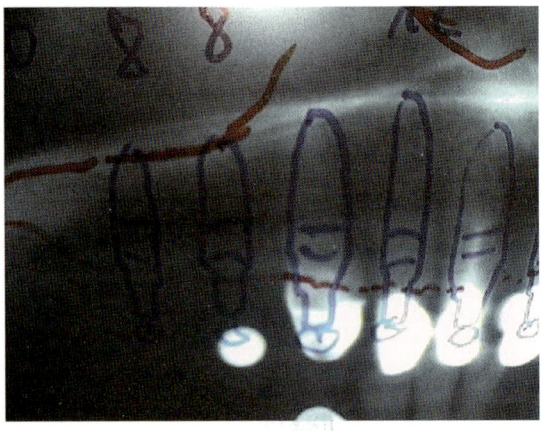

Panoramic radiograph for planned treatment, right side

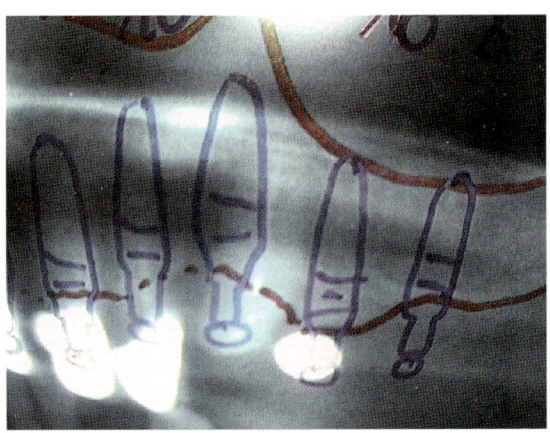

Panoramic radiograph for planned treatment, left side

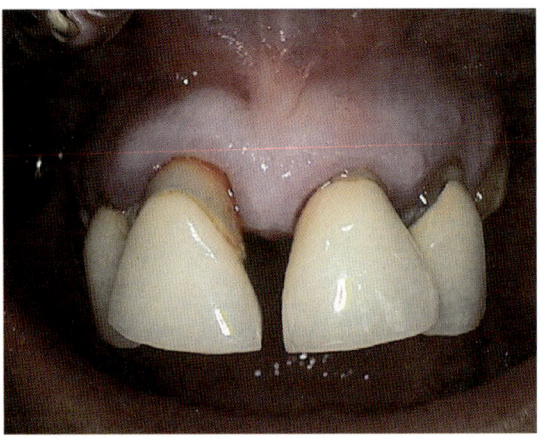

Clinical initial situation, anterior view

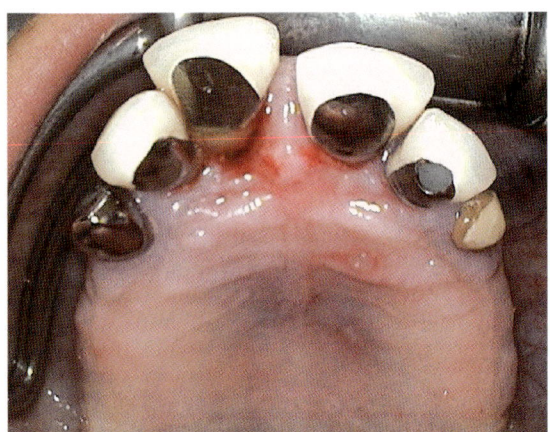

Clinical initial situation, palatal view

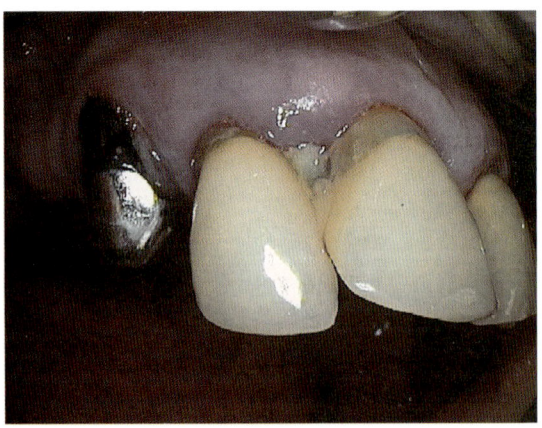

Clinical initial situation, right side

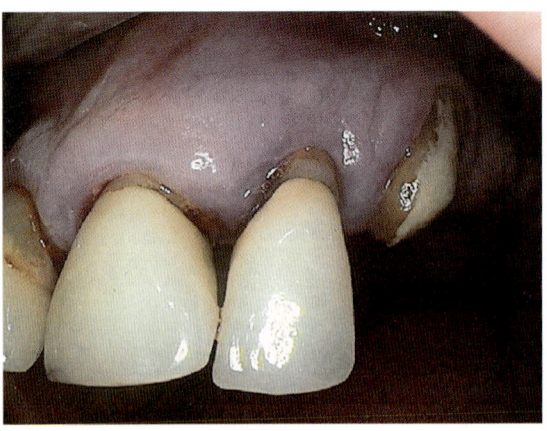

Clinical initial situation, left side

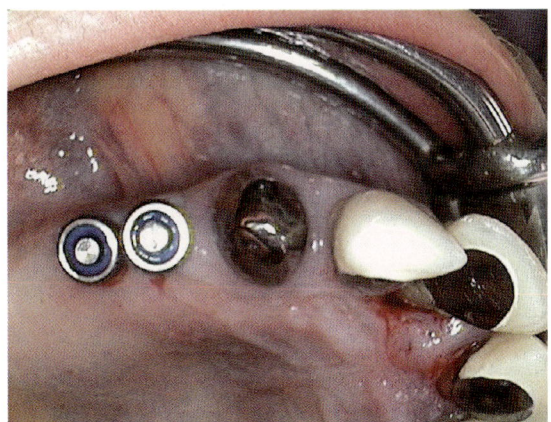

Implant placement, right side

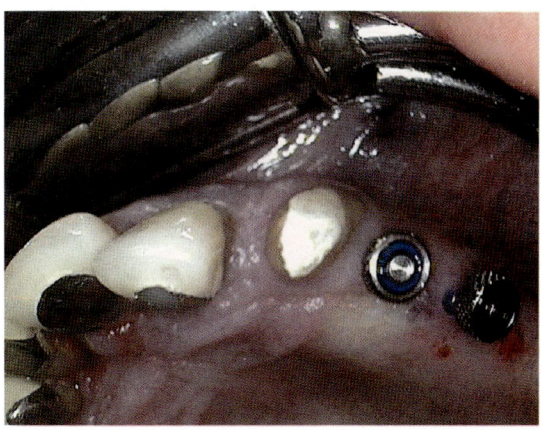

Implant placement, left side

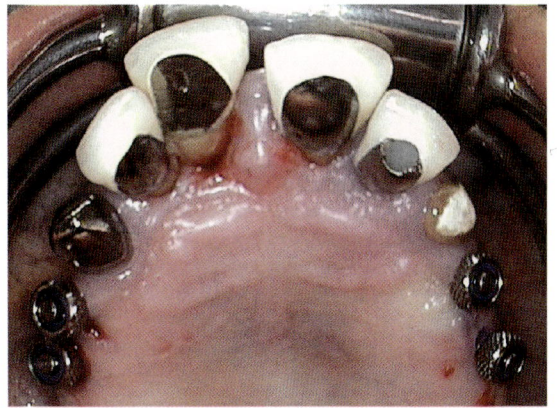

Occlusal view

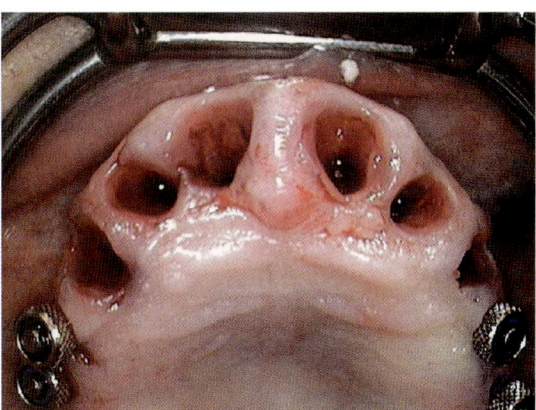

Extraction in regio 13- 23

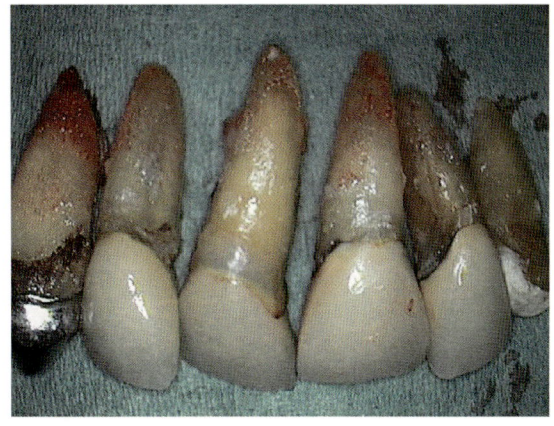

Extracted teeth 13-23

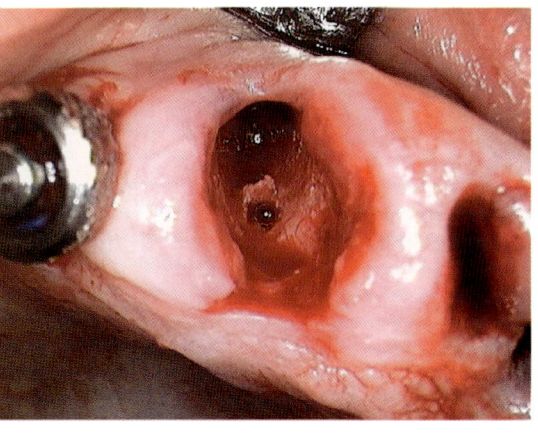

Palatal drilled hole in regio 13

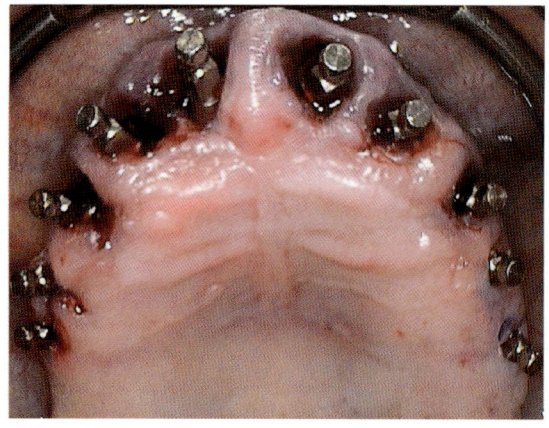

Overview image after implant placement, occlusal view

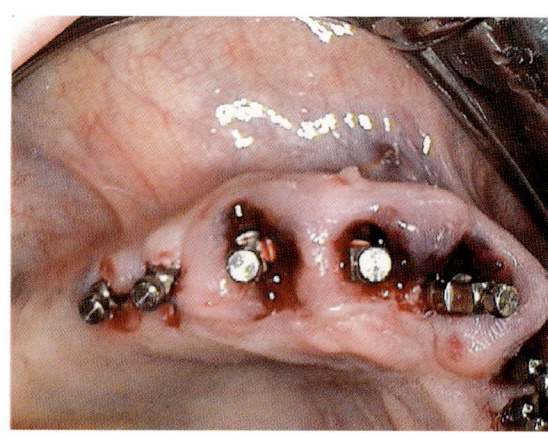

Detailed image, right side

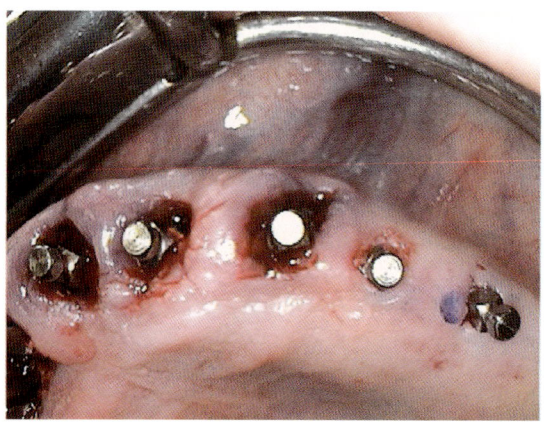

Detailed image, left side

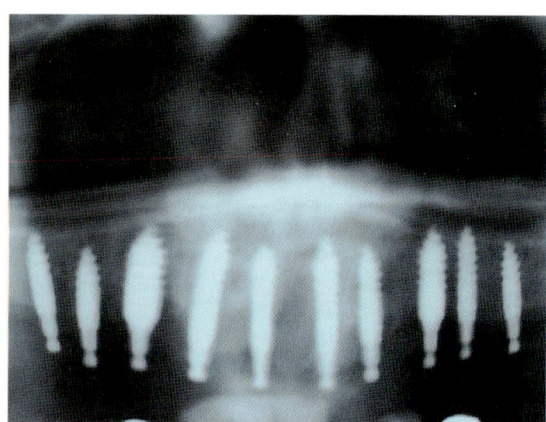

Panoramic radiographic control

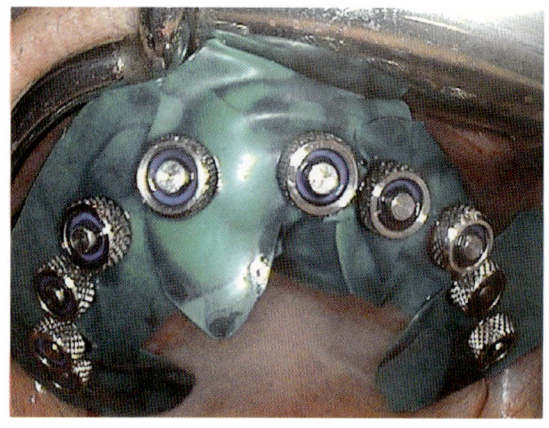

Preparation of the implanted region with rubber dam for the polymerisation process of the matrices

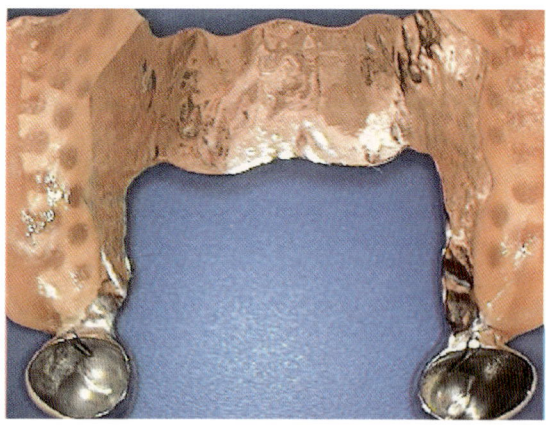

Former prosthesis from the previous day

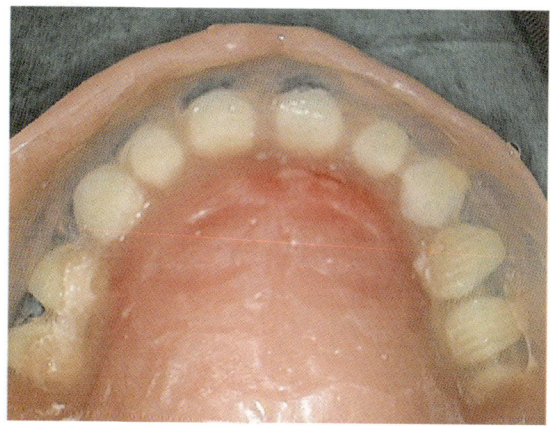

Reworked prosthesis on the day of the surgery session

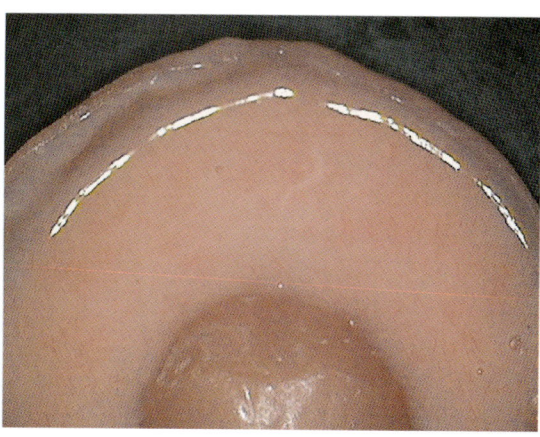

Injected cold-cured polymer

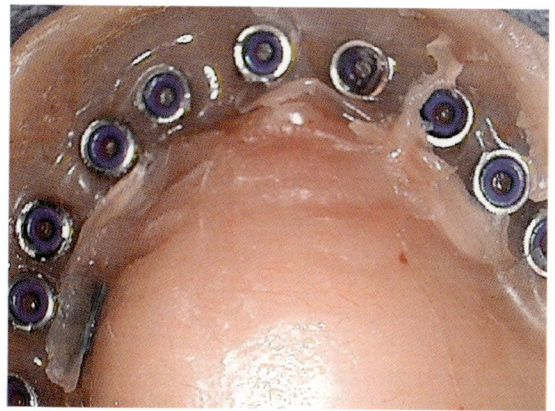

Cured cold-cured polymer

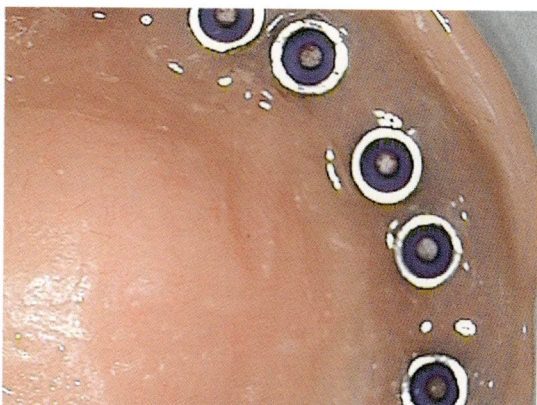

Prepared and polished prosthesis

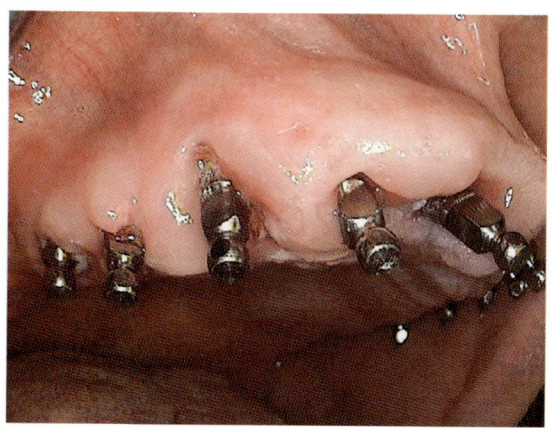

5 days after surgical procedure, right side

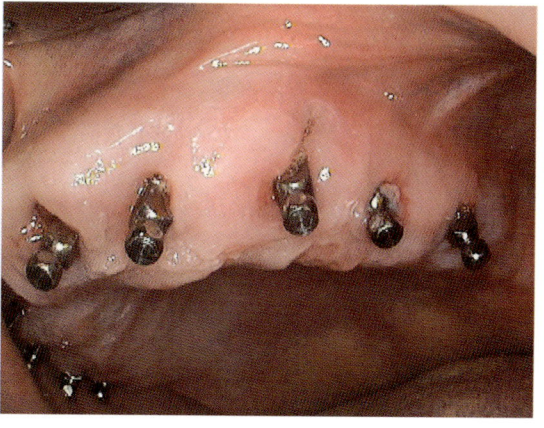

5 days after surgical procedure, left side

7.5.12/Case 50

Patient: male, 68 years old

10 upper jaw implants for a palatal free prosthesis

09/05/2011	Upper jaw	Restoration, metal removal, reworking to an overdenture with gaps for matrices (15-25)
10/05/2011	15-25	Champions® implant Ø 3.0 x 8 mm, >20 Ncm, Periotest 0
		Champions® implant Ø 3.0 x 8 mm, >30 Ncm, Periotest +6
		Champions® implant Ø 4.0 x 10 mm, >40 Ncm, Periotest +1
		Champions® implant Ø 3.0 x 12 mm, >40 Ncm, Periotest +1
		Champions® implant Ø 3.0 x 12 mm, >40 Ncm, Periotest +4
		Champions® implant Ø 3.0 x 12 mm, >40 Ncm, Periotest +3
		Champions® implant Ø 3.0 x 10 mm, >20 Ncm, Periotest +6
		Champions® implant Ø 4.0 x 10 mm, >40 Ncm, Periotest -3
		Champions® implant Ø 3.0 x 10 mm, >30 Ncm, Periotest +3
		Champions® implant Ø 3.0 x 8 mm, >20 Ncm, Periotest -3
		regio 12 fracture of an implant, explantation, additional implant placement.
		10 matrices directly cured into denture resin (metal matrices for tulips, blue - light pulling force)
11/07/2011		Final control, palatal freedom
Treatment period:		**2 hours**
Remarks:		Late implant placement, immediate loading Creation of palatal freedom at the existing prosthesis after osseointegration. A new upper jaw overdenture is planned.

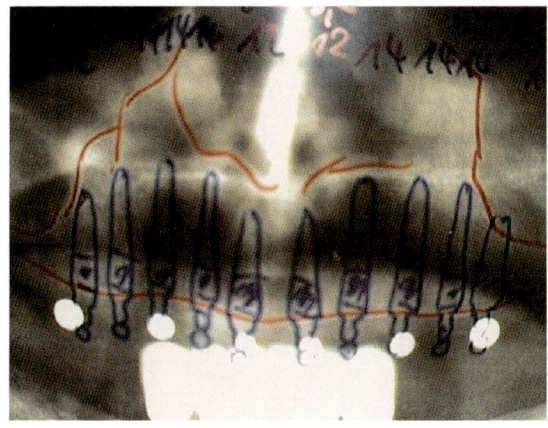

Panoramic radiograph for planned treatment

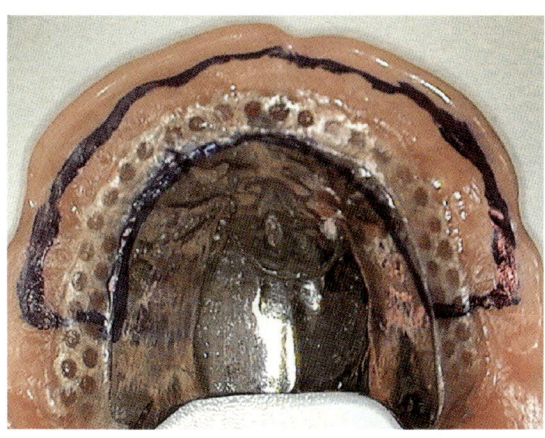

Initial prosthesis

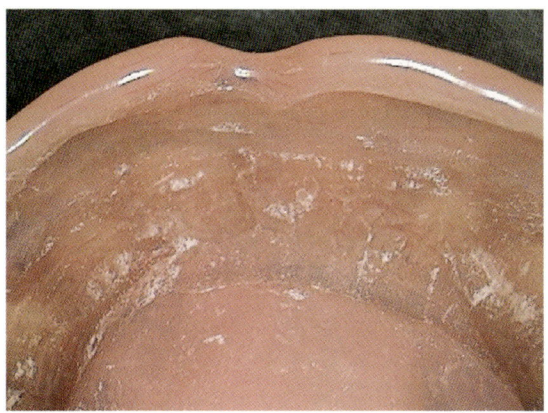

Modified prosthesis

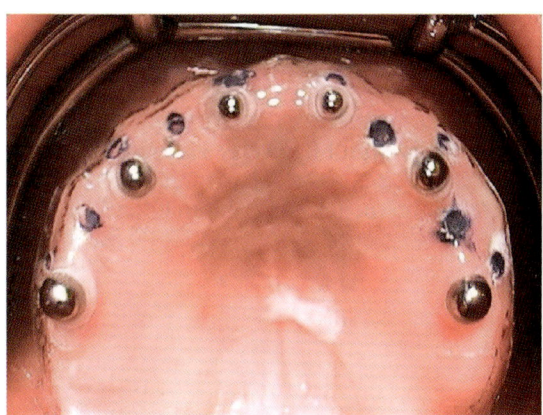

Overlay template in situ

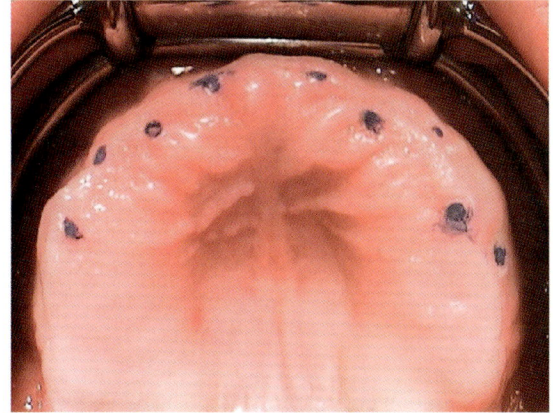

Marked points...

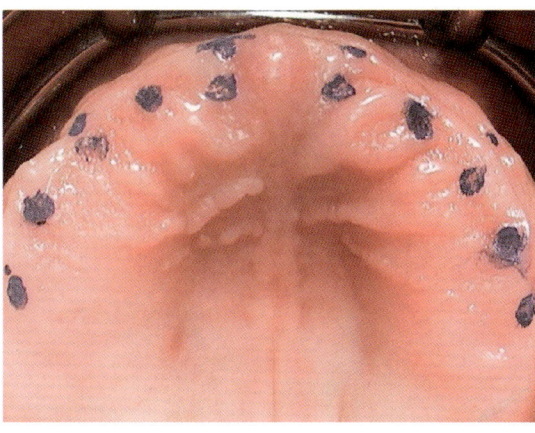

... Transfer for the planned "beginning"

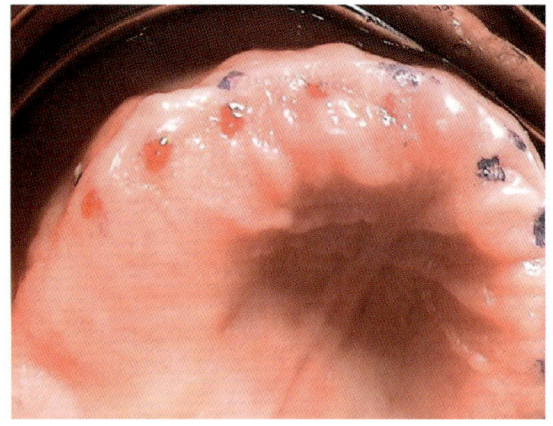

Upper jaw right side, pilot hole preparation

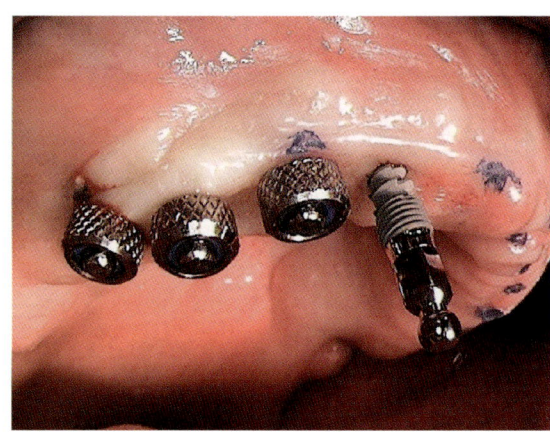

Implant placements

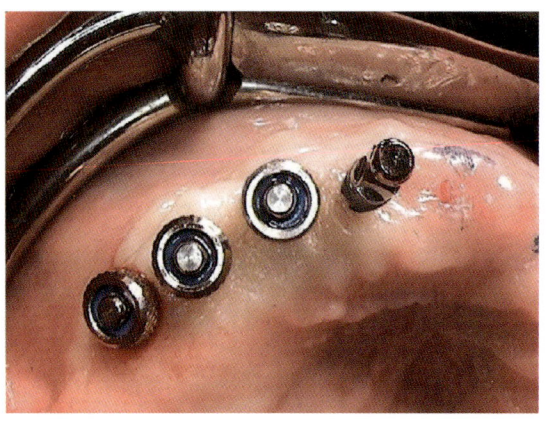

12- Insertion at the beginning...

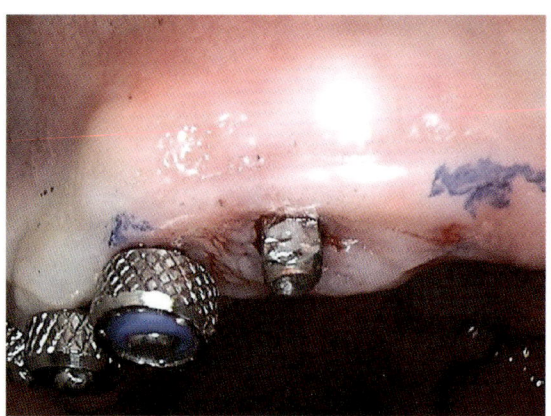

...implant fracture...

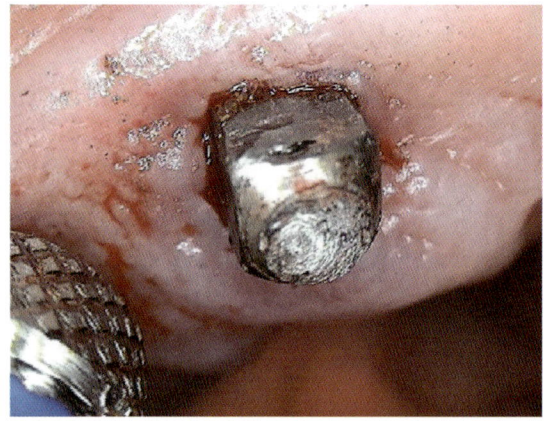

...in macro view...

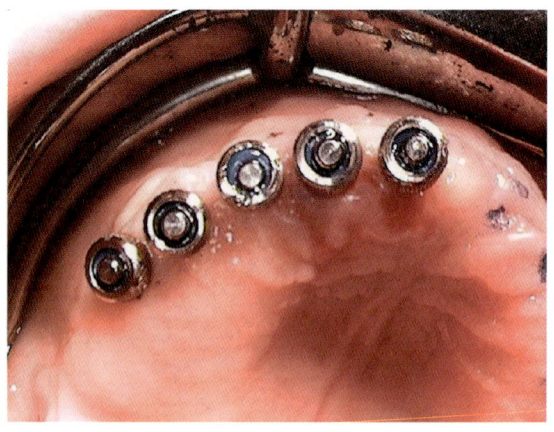

explantation, additional implant placement

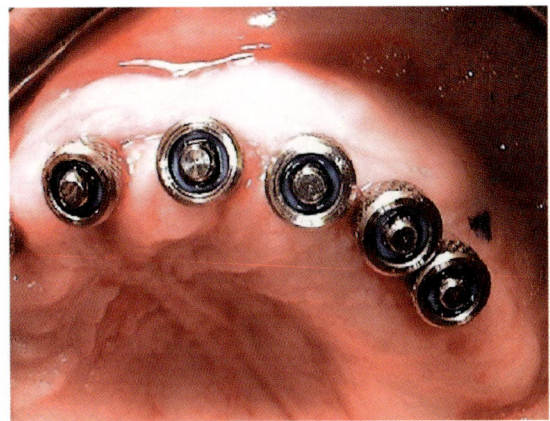

Implant placement, upper jaw and left side

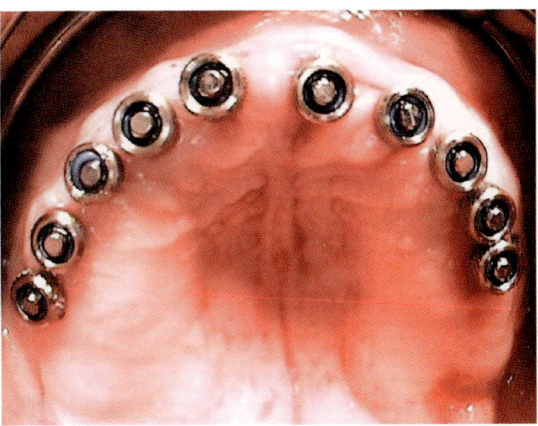

Completed implant placement, with attached metal matrices

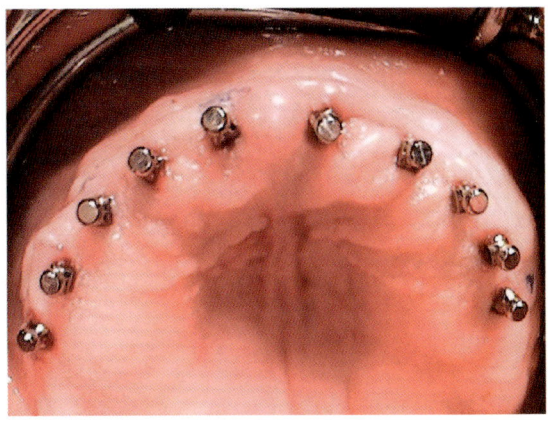

Completed implant placement, without matrices

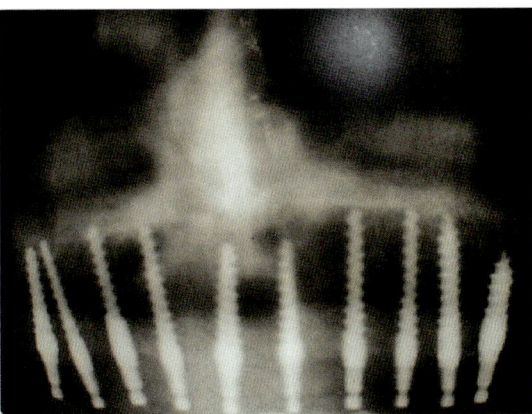

Panoramic radiographic control

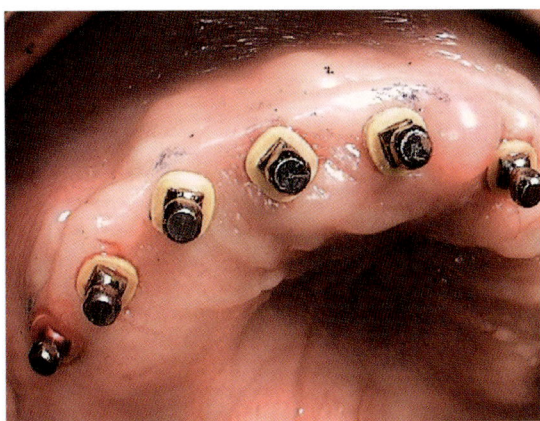

Rubber rings to prevent non-removal of the prosthesis after the cementing of the matrices into the prosthesis

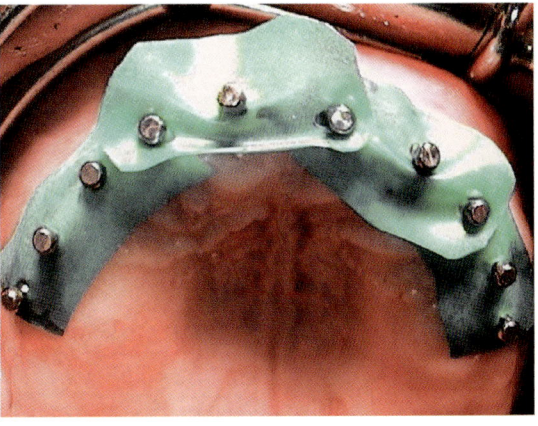

Rubber dam to protect the gingiva and the implants

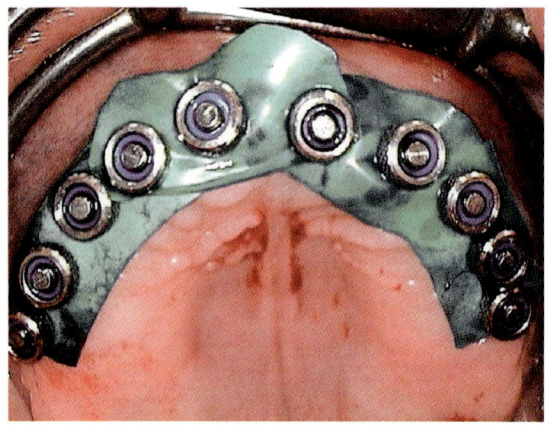

Metal matrices with underlaid rubber dam

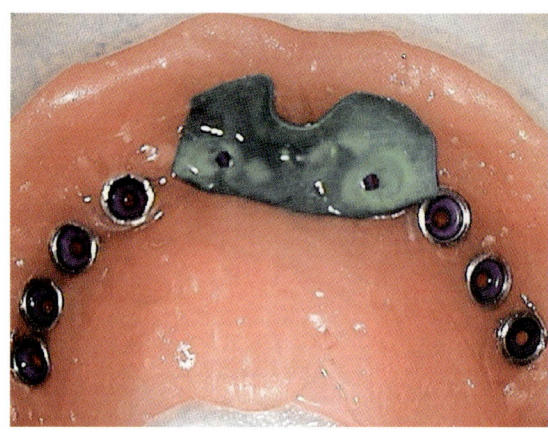

Matrices cemented into the prosthesis after curing

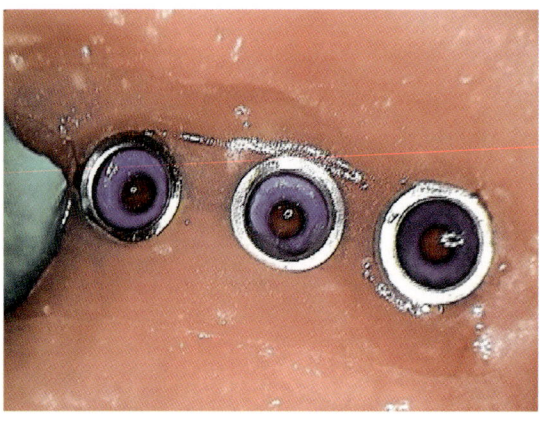

Matrices cemented into the prosthesis after curing, detailed view

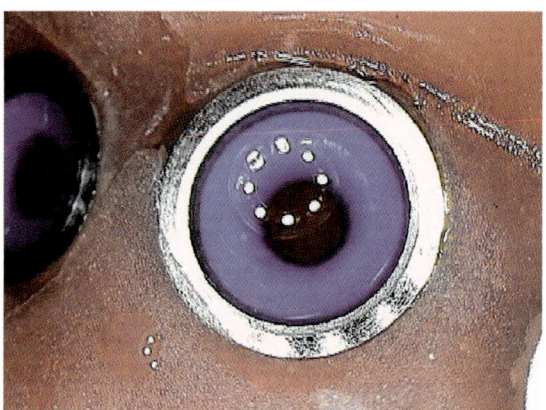

Matrices cemented into the prosthesis after curing, macro view

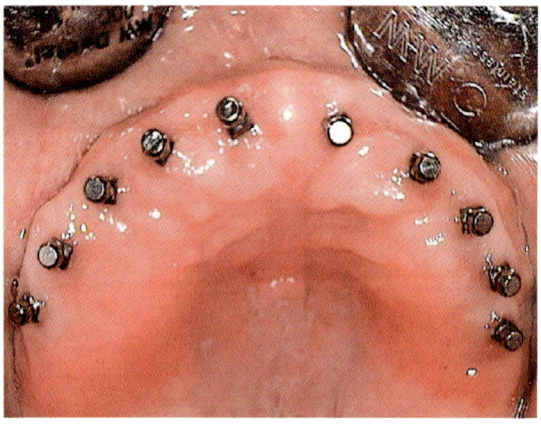

Situation after osseointegration

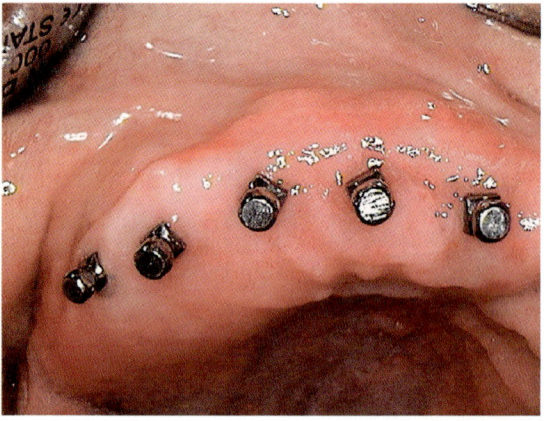

Situation after osseointegration, right side

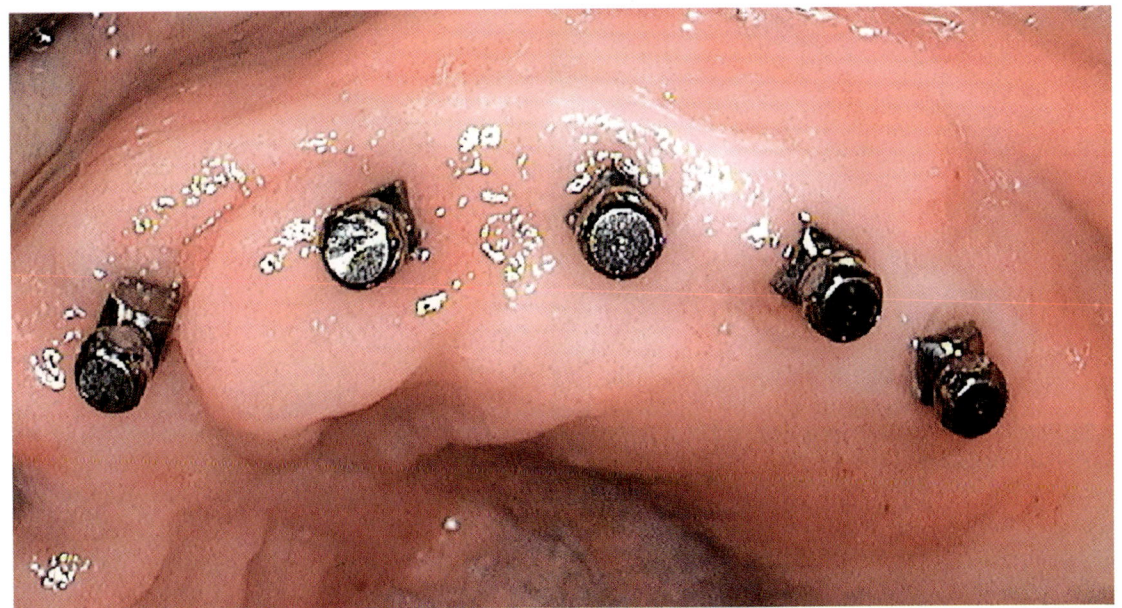

Situation after osseointegration, left side

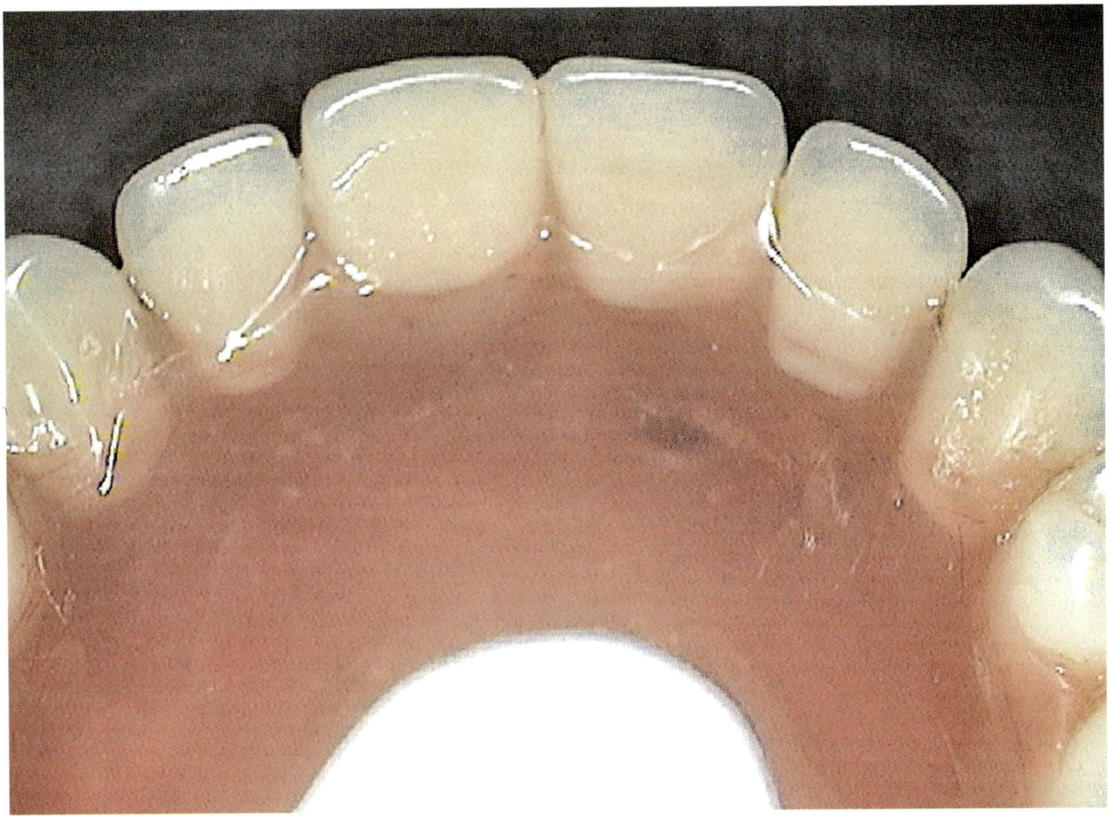

Palatal free prosthesis

Acknowledgement

Oh my dear,

So many people helped me.

My first thanks go to my team who had and still has to handle the daily stress with me. Even though if the journey is the reward - you had to struggle through "our perfectionism".
Permanently in weekly half-our lasting team meetings you were challenged to implement the constantly changing parameters and working procedures.
Thank you so much!

I wish to thank my long-term mate Bert Siegemund, who has not only produced DVDs on traditional implant placements with me, but who also has brought this book forward to you. Thanks for burning the midnight oil, so it looks like you like me, really like me.

I thank Dr. Armin Nedjat the "Champions inventor" who has the substance of a genius in the Champions implantology for providing me with his illustrations.

I thank Dr. Ulrich Brause for his meticulous proofreading and his advice.
For all the time you sacrificed.
Seriously: Thanks a lot for doing a great job.

I also thank all the other many "Champions" who ensured suggestions and improvements.

I thank both my dental laboratories (Dentaltec Michael Schmidt and Dentallabor Thomas Reckrühm) for their professional denture works and in particular you, Thomas for your efforts to fulfil my ambitious expectations.

I thank my parents who raised me to be the person that I am today.

I thank my sweetheart for her patience to do without me in the small hours..
For her affectionate willingness to endure my impatience and for her calmness to tolerate without complaints my daily shoptalk as a dental layman.

Most of all I wish to thank you, who read my first book. For the fact that you hopefully let me know what I have forgotten or what I have done wrong in order to maybe quench your thirst for knowledge in "Implantology 2 - immediate implant placement forever."

Yours,
Frank Schrader

Additional literature

Nikellis I, Levi A, Nicolopoulus C.Immediate loading of 190 endosseous dental implants:a prospective oberservational study of 40 patient treatments with up to 2-year data. Int J Oral Maxillofac Implants.19 (1):116-23.

Henry PJ, van Steenberghe D, Blombäck U, Polizzi G, Rosenberg R, Urgell JP, Wendelhag I. Prospective multicenter study on immediate rehabilitation of edentulous lower jaws according to the Branemark Novum protocol. Vlin Implant Dent Relat Res.2003; 5(3):137-42.

Degidi M, Nardi D, Piatelli A. Immediate versus one-stage restoration of small-diameter implants for a single missing maxillary lateral incisor:a 3-year randomizied clinical trial. J Periodontol.2009 Sep;80 (9):1393-8.

DegidiM, Piattelli A, Shibli JA, Perrotti V, Iezzi G.Early bone formation around immediately restored implants with and without occlusal contact: a juman histolgic and histomorphometiric evaluation. Case report: Int J Oral Maxillofax Implants. 24(4): 734-9.

Cannizzaro G, Torchio C, Leone M, Esposito M. Immediate versus early loading of flapless-planced implants supporting maxillary full-arch prostheses: a randomised controlled clinical trial. Eur J Oral Implantol.2008; 1 (2):127-39.

Chiapasco M. Early and immediate restoration and loading of implants in completely edentulous patients.Int J Oral Maxillofax Implants.2004;19 Suppl:76-91.

Ioannidou E, Doufexi A. Does loading time affect implant survival? A metaanalysis of 1.266 implants. J Periodontol.2005 Aug; 76(8):1252-8.

Misch CE, Wang HL, Misch CM, Sharawy M, Lemons J, Judy KW. Rationale for the application of immediate load in implnat dentistry: Part I. Implant Dent.2004 Sep; 13(3): 207-17.

Misch CE, Wang HL, Misch CM, Sharawy M, Lemons J, Judy KW. Rationale for the application of immediate load in implnat dentistry: Part II. Vlin Implant Dent Relat Res.2004; 13(4):310-21.

Romanos GE, Toh CG, Siar CH, Swaminathan D. Histologix and histomorphometric evaluation of peri-implant bone subjected to immediate loading: an experimental study with Macaca fascicularis. Int J Oral Maxillofac Implants.17 (1):44-51.

Testori T, Del Fabbro M, Galli F, Francetti L, Taschieri S, Weinstein R. Immediate occlusal loading the same day or the after implant placement: comparison of 2 different time frames in total edentulous lower jaws. J Oral Implantol.2004;30(5):307-13.

Urive R, Penarrocha M, Balaguer J, Fulfueiras N. Immediate loading in oral implants. Present situation. Med Oral Patol Oral Cir Bucal. 2005.

Ryser MR, Block MS, Mercante DE. Correlation of papilla to crestal bone levels around single tooth implants in immediate or delayed crown protocols. J Oral Maxillofac Surg.2005 Aug;63(8): 1184-95.

Tarnow DP; Emtiaz S, Classi A. Immediate loading of threaded implanta at stage 1 surgery in edentulous arches: ten consectuive case reports with1-to 5-year data. Int J Oral Maxillofac Implants.12(3): 319-24.

Neugebauer J, Weinländer M, Lekovic V, von Berg KH, Zoeller JE. Mechanical stability of immediately loaded implants with various surfaxes and designs:a pilot study in dogs. Int J Oral Maxillofax Implants. 24(6): 1083-92.

Cordaro L, Torsello F, Roccuzzo M. Implant loading protocols for the partially edentulous posterior mandible. Int J Oral Maxillofac Implants.2009;24Suppl:158-68.

Degidi M, Piattelli A, Shibli JA, Perrotti V, Iezzi G. Bone formation around immediately loaded and submerged dental implants with a modified sandblasted and acid-etched surface after 4 and 8 weeks: a human histologic and histomorphometric analysis. Int J Oral Maxillofac Implants.24(5): 896,-901

Dos Santos MV, Elias CN; Cavalcanti Lima JH. The Effects of Superficial Roughness and Design on the Primary Stability of Dental Implants. Clin Implant Dent Relat Res. 2009 Sep 9; (Epub ahead of print)

Dierens M, Collaert B, Deschepper E, Browaeys H, Klinge B, De Druyn H. Patient-centrered outcome of immediately loaded implants in the rehabilitation of fully edentulous jaws. Cin Oral Implants Res. 2009 Oct; 20(10): 1070-7.

Neugebauer J, Iezzi G, Perrotti V, Fischer JH, Khoury F, Piattelli A, Zoeller JE. Experimental immediate loading of dental implants in conjunction with grafting procedures. J Biomed Mater Res B Appl Biomater.2009 Nov; 91(2): 604-12.

Alsabeeha N, Atieh M, Payne AG. Loading protocols for mandibular implant overdentures: A systematic review with meta-analysis. Clin Implant Dent Relat Res. 2009 Sep 23; (Epub ahead of print)

Fabbri G, Ban G, Mancini R. Immediate loading and flapless, postextraction, single-tooth implant restoration: advantages and indications. Pract Proced Aesthet Dent. 20(10): 633-9.

Danza M, Fanali S, Quaranta A, Vozza I. The importance of immediately loaded immediate post-extractive implants in esthetical rehabilitation: case series. Minerva Stomatol.2010 Apr;59(4): 215-22.

Esposito M, Grusovin MG, Coulthard P, Worthington HV. Different loading strategies of dental implants: a Cochrane systematic review of randomised controlled clinical trials. Eur J Oral Implantol.2008,1(4): 259-76.

Schrader F, Sofortimplantation von 6 Kugelkopfimplantaten und Sofortversorgung. Dentalbarometer 1_2011:46-47.

Schrader F, Prothesenstabilisierung: Minimalinvasiv implantieren und sofort belasten. ZMK 2010 Mai Jg. 26 Ausgabe 5: 294-297.

Schrader F, Zahnärztliche Kooperation bei Implantation und prothetischer Versorgung. ZMK 2011 Jan./Feb. Jg. 27 Ausgabe 1-2: 62-64.

Schrader F, Sofortbelastung eines Champions-Implantates – ein Fallbeispiel. ZMK 2009 Nov. Jg. 25 Ausgabe: 782-786.

Schrader F, Einfach und schonend. Deutscher Ärzte Verlag, Dental Magazin 2010; 28(3): 150-153.

Schrader F, Einfachste Zusammenarbeit zwischen Hauszahnarzt und Implantologen. Dentalbarometer 2_2011: 66-67.

Schrader F, Komplette Oberkieferrehabilitation durch eine Hybridbrücke. Dentalbarometer 6_2011: 38-39.

Schrader F, Sofortbelastung von sechs Kugelkopfimplantaten mit einer Totalprothese. ZAHN PRAX 13,3, 168-171 (2010).

Schrader F, Einfache Zusammenarbeit zwischen Hauszahnarzt und Implantologen. Dentalbarometer 5_2011: 40-41.

Schrader F, Region 41 Implantation mit Sofortversorgung und gleichzeitiger Wurzelspitzenresektion bei 31. Dentalspiegel 5/2010: 34-37.

Schrader F, Sofortimplantation und Sofortversorgung. Dentalbarometer 7_2011: 40-43.

Schrader F, Extraktion 12 mit dem Benex-System. Dentalbarometer 4_2009. 22,-23

Schrader F, Sofortbelastung von sechs Kugelkopfimplantaten mit einer UK-Totalprothese. ZMK 2009 Sept. Jg. 27 Sonderausgabe 32-34.

The author

DS Frank Schrader, Albertstr. 33, D-39261 Zerbst/Anhalt

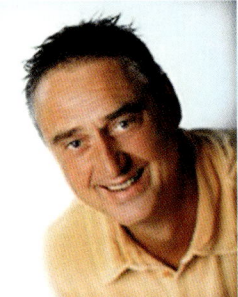

1981–86

- Studies of dental medicine at the Martin-Luther-Universität in Halle-Wittenberg in Germany

1986

- State examination
- Diploma thesis with a Master's degree in Stomatology

1991

- own dental office in Zerbst

1998

- Member of the German Association for Dental, Oral and Orthodontic Medicine (Deutsche Gesellschaft für Zahn-, Mund-, und Kieferheilkunde, DGZMK)

1999

- Member of the Implant Association for Dentists (IGfZ eG, Implantologische Genossenschaft für Zahnärzte)
- Member of implant associations: German Association of Dental Implantology (Deutsche Gesellschaft für Implantologie, DGI), Middle German State Association for Dental Implantology (Mitteldeutsche Landesverband für Zahnärztliche Implantologie, MVZI)
- Presentations for patients
- Presentations and training for dentists
- National and International publications in the field of implantology

2007

- Foundation of an Implantology continuing education centre
- Live- surgical procedures
- Hands-on courses
- Live-broadcast from the operating room into the conference room
- Dental training for dentists
- More than 700 implants per year
- Reference and training practice for the German company CHAMPIONS®-IMPLANTS-GMBH

2012

- Publishing of the implant book „Teeth in a day" part I

2013

- Publishing of the implant book „Teeth in day" part II

Fon +49(0)3923/2097
Fax +49(0)3923/612521
info@zahnarzt-zerbst.de

www.zahnarzt-zerbst.de
www.teethinaday.de
www.implantologisches-zentrum-zerbst.de